Gastroenterology: A Case-Based Approach

Gastroenterology: A Case-Based Approach

Editor: Marissa Brown

AMERICAN
MEDICAL PUBLISHERS
www.americanmedicalpublishers.com

AMERICAN
MEDICAL PUBLISHERS
www.americanmedicalpublishers.com

Cataloging-in-Publication Data

Gastroenterology: a case-based approach / edited by Marissa Brown.
p. cm.
Includes bibliographical references and index.
ISBN 979-8-88740-638-1
1. Gastroenterology. 2. Digestive organs--Diseases.
3. Digestive organs--Diseases--Treatment. I. Brown, Marissa.
RC801 .G37 2023
616.33--dc23

American Medical Publishers,
41 Flatbush Avenue,
1st Floor, New York,
NY 11217, USA

ISBN 979-8-88740-638-1 (Hardback)

Contents

Preface

I am honored to present to you this unique book which encompasses the most up-to-date data in the field. I was extremely pleased to get this opportunity of editing the work of experts from across the globe. I have also written papers in this field and researched the various aspects revolving around the progress of the discipline. I have tried to unify my knowledge along with that of stalwarts from every corner of the world, to produce a text which not only benefits the readers but also facilitates the growth of the field.

The organs involved in digestion, such as the esophagus, stomach, small intestine, large intestine, liver, gallbladder and pancreas together make up the gastrointestinal tract. The diagnosis and treatment of disorders related to the gastrointestinal tract are conducted within a medical specialty known as gastroenterology. Some of the diseases and disorders which are treated within this field are peptic ulcer disease, irritable bowel syndrome and gastrointestinal bleeding. The open sores which may form on the upper portion of the small intestine or the inside lining of the stomach are known as peptic ulcers. Irritable bowel syndrome refers to a functional disorder which is characterized by abdominal pain, bloating, and changes in bowel habits without any evidence of structural abnormalities. Gastroenterology also deals with the management of medical conditions that cause bleeding in the digestive tract. These conditions may include diverticulosis, gastrointestinal tumors and varices. This book unravels the recent studies in the field of gastroenterology. It will provide comprehensive knowledge to the readers.

Finally, I would like to thank all the contributing authors for their valuable time and contributions. This book would not have been possible without their efforts. I would also like to thank my friends and family for their constant support.

Editor

1

Extraintestinal Amoebiasis in Women after 6th Day of Delivery

Awoke Minwuyelet,[1] Yibeltal Aschale,[2] and Solomon Ayenew[1]

[1]*Bichena Primary Hospital, Amhara Region, Ethiopia*
[2]*Department of Medical Laboratory Science, College of Health Science, Debre Markos University, Debre Markos, Ethiopia*

Correspondence should be addressed to Yibeltal Aschale; yibea33@gmail.com

Academic Editor: Hirotada Akiho

Background. Extraintestinal amoebiasis is more common in countries with lower socioeconomic status. Complication related to amoebiasis is common in pregnant patients with malnutrition and others. Severe cases can be associated with high fatality rates. We would like to report a patient with a presumptive diagnosis of extraintestinal amoebiasis who was on the 6th postpartum day after intrauterine fetal death (IUFD). *Case Presentation.* The patient was a 31 year-old female who was on 6th postpartum day after IUFD after the 9th month of amenorrhea. She presented with severe epigastric pain, hiccups, and bloody vomiting of ingested matter for 5 days. She also had right upper quadrat pain and fatigue. In addition, she had generalized body weakness and yellowish discoloration of the eyes for one week. Moreover, she had pruritus, fever, and a history of watery diarrhea 6 days ago which got subsided during the presentation. Laboratory investigation indicated leukocytosis and increased level of alkaline phosphatase and direct and total bilirubin. Trophozoite of *E. histolytica* was seen on stool microscope, negative for viral marker and *Helicobacter pylori*. Abdominal ultrasonography showed normal liver parenchyma and biliary system. She was treated onsite with 500 mg metronidazole and 500 mg ceftriaxone for five days and discharged with metronidazole 500 mg PO three times a day and cloxacillin 500 mg PO four times a day for 7 days. *Conclusions.* Extraintesinal amoebiasis can be resolved if it is diagnosed early and treated with metronidazole. Clinicians should not neglect amoebiasis in patients presenting with jaundice and right upper quadrant pain.

1. Background

Entamoeba histolytica is a protozoan that causes intestinal and extraintestinal amoebiasis. In an endemic area, 90% of *E. histolytica* infections are limited to the lumen of the intestine and are asymptomatic. However, gastroenterology reports showed that nearly 50 million people become symptomatic with about 100,000 deaths yearly in the world [1]. Amoebic infections are more prevalent in countries with lower socioeconomic status and poor public health due to ingestion of amoebic cysts through fecal-oral contact, usually through contaminated food or water resources. Trophozoites can invade the intestinal mucosa or blood vessels, reaching extraintestinal sites such as the liver, brain, and lungs [2–4].

Even though the majority of infections restricted to the lumen of the intestine ("luminal amoebiasis") are asymptomatic, amoebic colitis, or invasive intestinal amoebiasis, occurs when the mucosa is invaded. Trophozoites of *E. histolytica* kill epithelial cells and invade colonic epithelium, progressing to the submucosa. Necrosis progresses laterally and downwards forming "flask-shaped" necrotic tissue which leads to different organ damage and causes secondary bacterial infections. The report indicated that extraintestinal amoebiasis is 3 times more likely to affect middle-aged men between the ages of 18 and 50 [4].

Symptoms include severe dysentery and associated complications. Severe prolonged infections may lead to complications such as perforations, peritonitis, and the formation of amoebic granulomas (amoeboma). Amoebic liver abscesses are the most common form of extraintestinal amoebiasis [5]. We report a patient who initially delivered with intrauterine fetal death (IUFD) after the 9th month of amenorrhea and treated for intestinal amoebiasis with tinidazole but was later found to have extraintestinal amoebiasis related to pregnancy.

2. Case presentation

Our client was a 31-year-old female who was on the 6th postpartum day after intrauterine fetal death (IUFD). She claimed to be amenorrheic for nine months, and delivery was at the hospital by spontaneous vaginal delivery. There was a nuchal cord on the freshly dead fetus. On February 28, 2021, she was admitted to Bichena Primary Hospital with severe epigastric pain, hiccups, and bloody vomiting of ingested matter of 5 days. She had also right upper quadrat abdominal pain and fatigue. In addition, she had yellowish discoloration of the eyes for one week. Moreover, she had pruritus, fever, and had a history of watery diarrhea six days ago which got subsided during the presentation.

On physical examination, the patient was acutely sick seeming with pain. Vital signs: blood pressure was 150/100 mmHg, pulse rate was 92 bpm, respiration rate was 32 breaths/min, temperature was 36.6°C, and oxygen saturation was 96% with atmospheric air. On head and neck evaluation, she had icteric sclera and pink conjunctiva. On abdominal examination, she had tenderness at the right upper quadrant of the abdomen. Otherwise, there was no finding in the remaining systems.

Her laboratory investigations revealed serum total bilirubin of 9.4 mg/dL, direct bilirubin of 3.55 mg/dL, alkaline phosphatase of 213 μ/L, aspartate transaminase of 42 μ/L, alanine transaminase of 40 μ/L, creatinine of 0.6 mg/dl, and blood urea nitrogen of 16 mg/dl. She had also bloody urine (blood 3+), no protein and ketone on urine analysis, and trophozoites of *E. histolotica/dispar* were seen in stool microscopically. Her total white blood count was 13000 cell/mm^3 (neutrophils cover 53.1%; lymphocytes, 10.4%; eosinophils, 2.8%; basophils, 19.6%; and monocytes, 14.1%); red blood cells, 3,700,000 cells/μ; Hgb, 12 mg/dl; Hct, 32%; and platelets, 79,000cell/mm^3. She was negative for hepatitis viral markers and *Helicobacter pylori* in stools.

A diagnosis of obstructive jaundice secondary to choledocholithiasis with ascending cholangitis and intestinal amoebiasis was made, and the patient kept nothing per mouth (NPO). She was admitted and started management with diclofenac 75 mg intramuscularly as needed, cimetidine 400 mg loading intravenous, then 200 twice a day, ceftriaxone 1 gm intravenous twice a day, metrindazone 500 mg intravenous three times a day, nifedipine 20 mg PO twice a day and maintenance fluid with normal saline, ringers lactate, and 5% dextrose as required. On the second day of admission, abdominal ultrasound was done and showed a normal biliary system and no stone at the common bile duct. But, there were multiple lesions on the right lobe of liver parenchyma which were most likely small multiple amebic live abscesses. She was treated onsite with metronidazole 500 mg TID and ceftriaxone 500 mg QID for five days considering extraintestinal amoebiasis that is amoebic liver abscess. Then, she was discharged with metronidazole 500 mg PO three times a day and cloxacillin 500 mg PO four times a day for seven days and appointed for two weeks later.

After two weeks of discharge, a patient come back to the hospital with normal vital signs and tested for hematological profile, liver function, stool sample, and abdominal ultrasound. Her total white blood cell count was 11,000 cell/mm^3 (neutrophils (56%), lymphocytes (24%), eosinophils (2.3%), basophils (8%), and monocytes (9%)). Red blood cell count was 4.3 million cells/mm^3; Hgb, 13 mg/dl; Hct, 38%; and platelets, 156,000 cells/mm^3. Total bilirubin was 3.6 mg/dL; direct bilirubin, 1.2 mg/dL; alkaline phosphatase, 135 μ/L; aspartate transaminase, 52 μ/L; alanine transaminase 45 μ/L; creatinine, 0.5 mg/dl; and blood urea nitrogen, 14 mg/dL. From her stool sample, no ova or parasite is seen and few pus cells were observed. Abdominal ultrasound confirmed absence of lesions on the right lobe of liver parenchyma. We were unable to show the endoscopic images of this patient because of absence of endoscopy access.

3. Discussion

Extraintestinal amoebiasis is more likely to occur in the developing world. It especially affects pregnant women on corticosteroid treatment, malignancy, malnutrition, and alcoholic individual. However, we can easily manage this disease if we have appropriate anticipation and correct diagnosis. The reasons for misdiagnosis and late presentation of the disease are not only limited to illiteracy, poverty, lack of awareness, and lack of social support but also because we have limited diagnostic methods and poor exposure of clinicians for the extraintestinal amoebiasis. In developing countries, infection with *E. histolytica* is usually neglected and marginalized [6].

Our patient presented after the 6th day of IUFD delivery and was diagnosed to have amoebic liver abscess. She was admitted for 5 days and treated with metronidazole three times per day intravenous together with antibiotics. A study done in England reported that extraintestinal amoebiasis has a strong association with pregnancy [4]. Trophozoites of *E. histolotica* adhere to colonic epithelial cells through a specific parasite protein: galactose-N-acetyl galactosamine lectin, amebapore, and proteases. Invasion is mediated by the killing of epithelial cells, neutrophils, and lymphocytes by trophozoites, and the colonic epithelial cells were killed through cytolysis and apoptosis, as consequences of interleukin-1α and precursor interleukin-1 release. Those cells also produce cytokines and other inflammatory mediators such as COX-2, interleukin-1, interleukin-8, INF α, and others. These cytokines and inflammatory mediators subsequently attract neutrophils and macrophages, and this state aggravates mucosal inflammation, thickening, ulcers, and necrosis which can subsequently lead to perforation [4].

In addition, Gal/GalNAc-specific lectin has antigenic cross-reactivity to CD59, a human leukocyte antigen that prevents the assembly of the complement C5b–C9 membrane attack complex. Amoebic cysteine proteinases rapidly degrade the complement anaphylatoxins C3a and C5a [7]. The cysteine proteinases also degrade secretory IgA and serum IgG, possibly protecting amoebae from opsonization

[8]. Finally, amoebae appear to suppress both the macrophage respiratory burst and antigen presentation by class II major-histocompatibility complex (MHC) molecules that probably result in fetal distress and cause fetal death.

Our patient had antenatal care follow-up (ANC), and there was no danger sign, there was no history of abortion, and she has an O blood group and RH is positive. She was also dewormed by mebendazole and took iron foliate for two months. She had seen by ultrasound during ANC follow-up, the fetus was actively mobile, and the fetal heartbeat was normal. The amniotic fluid and placenta were good at 6 months of gestational age. Generally, she did not have any known illness. Probably, extraintestinal amoebiasis infection might have triggered toxic substance release (probably vesicles) and inflammatory cells to pass to the fetus through the placenta that caused the IUFD.

Our patient presented with yellowish discoloration of eyes with severe epigastric pain, hiccups, and bloody vomiting of ingested matter of 5 days. She had also right upper quadrant abdominal pain and fatigue. She also presented with yellowish discoloration of eyes. Reports indicated that gastrointestinal symptoms occur in 10 to 35 percent of patients, which include nausea, vomiting, abdominal cramps, abdominal distention, diarrhea, and constipation. Hepatomegaly with point tenderness over the liver, below the ribs, or in the intercostal spaces is a typical finding [9, 10]. Our patient had right upper quadrant abdominal tenderness and icteric sclera. The study showed that less than 10 percent of patients have jaundice [11]. After the patient has discharged, the yellowish discoloration of the eyes decreased, and there was no body swelling.

Laboratory investigation of our patient showed leukocytosis and an increased level of alkaline phosphatase and direct and total bilirubin. Common laboratory findings include leukocytosis without eosinophilia, elevated alkaline phosphatase, transaminitis, and elevated erythrocyte sedimentation rate [10]. In addition, actively motile trophozoites were visualized with an Olympus microscope from a stool sample.

Finally, our patient was treated with diclofenac 75 mg intramuscularly as needed, cimetidine 400 mg intravenous state, then 200 two times a day, ceftriaxone 1 gm intravenous two times a day, and metronidazole 500 mg intravenous three times a day. The study indicated that patients with fulminant amebic colitis will additionally require fluid resuscitation, broad-spectrum antimicrobial therapy for peritonitis, intensive supportive care, and surgical intervention for bowel perforation and bowel necrosis. However, our patient did not have a sign of peritonitis. Metronidazole is highly effective in eliminating invading trophozoites and remains the recommended therapy for amebic colitis and amoebic liver disease. Tinidazole has a longer half-life and is better tolerated, but metronidazole is as effective at clearing parasites [12].

4. Conclusions

Amoebiasis is a common parasitic infection, especially in developing countries. Immunocompromised individuals are at a risk of extraintestinal amoebiasis and its complication. Health workers could give attention and open communication especially in obtaining a good history will be critical in early diagnosis and treatment.

Abbreviations

ANC: Antenatal care
C: Complement
CD: Cluster of differentiation
E. histolytica: *Entamoeba histolytica*
Gal/GalNAc: Galactose-N-acetyl galactosamine
IL: Interleukin
Im: Intramuscle
IUFD: Intrauterine fetal death
Iv: Intravenous.

Authors' Contributions

AM conceived the study, performed laboratory tests, and prepared the first draft of the manuscript. SA diagnosed and followed up the patient strictly. YA critically reviewed the manuscript. All authors read and approved the final manuscript.

Acknowledgments

The authors would like to thank the clinical staff of Bichena Primary Hospital who participated in case diagnosis and strict follow-up of the case.

References

[1] T. E. Bercu, W. A. Petri, and B. W. Behm, "Amebic colitis: new insights into pathogenesis and treatment," *Current Gastroenterology Reports*, vol. 9, no. 5, pp. 429–433, 2007.

[2] I. E. Salit, K. Khairnar, K. Gough, and D. R. Pillai, "A possible cluster of sexually transmitted Entamoeba histolytica: genetic analysis of a highly virulent strain," *Clinical Infectious Diseases*, vol. 49, no. 3, pp. 346–353, 2009.

[3] A. C. Billet, A. Salmon Rousseau, L. Piroth, and C. Martins, "An underestimated sexually transmitted infection: amoebiasis," *BMJ Case Reports*, vol. 12, no. 5, Article ID e228942, 2019.

[4] S. L. Stanley, "Amoebiasis," *Lancet (London, England)*, vol. 361, 2003.

[5] R. Haque, C. D. Huston, M. Hughes, E. Houpt, and W. A. Petri, "Amebiasis," *New England Journal of Medicine*, vol. 348, no. 16, pp. 1565–1573, 2003.

[6] D. A. Shirley, L. Farr, K. Watanabe, and S. Moonah, "A review of the global burden, new diagnostics, and current therapeutics for amebiasis," *Open Forum Infectious Diseases*, vol. 5, no. 7, Article ID ofy161, 2018.

[7] L. L. Braga, H. Ninomiya, J. J. McCoy et al., "Inhibition of the complement membrane attack complex by the galactose-specific adhesion of Entamoeba histolytica," *Journal of Clinical Investigation*, vol. 90, no. 3, pp. 1131–1137, 1992.

[8] S. L. Reed, J. A. Ember, D. S. Herdman, R. G. DiScipio, T. E. Hugli, and I. Gigli, "The extracellular neutral cysteine proteinase of Entamoeba histolytica degrades anaphylatoxins C3a and C5a," *The Journal of Immunology*, vol. 155, no. 1, pp. 266–274, 1995.

[9] E. B. Adams and I. N. MacLeod, "Invasive amebiasis. II. Amebic live abscess and its complications," *Medicine*, vol. 56, no. 4, pp. 325–334, 1977.

[10] D. Katzenstein, V. Rickerson, and A. Braude, "New concepts of amebic liver abscess derived from hepatic imaging, serodiagnosis, and hepatic enzymes in 67 consecutive cases in San Diego," *Medicine*, vol. 61, no. 4, pp. 237–246, 1982.

[11] S. Anil Kumar, A. Mishra, N. Malhotra, and M. Alpana, "Hyperbilirubinemia in patients with amoebic liver abscess: a study of 75 cases," *Journal of Gastrointestinal & Digestive System*, vol. 3, no. 138, 2013.

[12] D.-A. Shirley and S. Moonah, "Fulminant amebic colitis after corticosteroid therapy: a systematic review," *PLoS Neglected Tropical Diseases*, vol. 10, no. 7, Article ID e0004879, 2016.

2

Gallstone Dislodgement in the Airway during ERCP: A Case Report and Review of the Literature

Hisham Hurreiz,[1] **Amira Babikir**,[2] **and Edward Black**[2]

[1]*Al Ain Hospital, Al Ain, UAE*
[2]*Tawam Hospital, Al Ain, UAE*

Correspondence should be addressed to Hisham Hurreiz; hishamhurreiz@yahoo.co.uk

Academic Editor: Antonio Macrì

Endoscopic retrograde cholangiopancreatography (ERCP) is a diagnostic and therapeutic procedure with many studied complications. We are presenting a rare complication of ERCP in choledocholithiasis: gallstone dislodging into the airway upon retrieval. The patient is a 37-year-old female admitted with obstructive jaundice. She was evaluated, and her management plan included a referral for an ERCP to extract the impacted common bile duct stones. Upon retrieval of the gallstone, it fell out the basket and lodged into the airway which was confirmed on bronchoscopy and successfully retrieved. This report describes successful management of a rare but potentially dangerous complication of ERCP to remove impacted CBD stones. The possible complications of delayed removal or inability to remove gallstones from the airway have yet to be studied and reported but are likely to include recurrent chest infections, bronchiectasis, and empyema of the lung.

1. Introduction

Endoscopic retrograde cholangiopancreatography (ERCP) is a diagnostic and therapeutic procedure with many studied complications. Some of which include pancreatitis, bleeding, perforation, and cholangitis. It is commonly used to evaluate the biliary system for dilatation as well as locate tumors and impacted gallstones in obstructive jaundice patients. It is also used to obtain biopsies for tissue diagnosis as well as administer therapeutic measures such as placement of biliary stents and extraction of impacted common bile duct stones. We are presenting a rare complication of ERCP in choledocholithiasis: gallstone dislodging into the airway upon retrieval.

2. Case History

A 37-year-old female, known to have cholelithiasis, presented to our emergency department with recurrent attacks of upper abdominal pain associated with nausea. On examination, her abdomen was soft with localised tenderness in the right upper quadrant. Her blood investigations showed hyperbilirubineamia. She underwent ultrasound (US) examination and magnetic resonance cholangiopancreatography (MRCP) (Figure 1) which revealed dilatation of the biliary tree with stones seen within the common bile duct (CBD). She was therefore referred for an ERCP to remove the stone impacted in the distal CBD. She underwent ERCP (Figure 2) 4 days after admission. The initial cholangiogram confirmed the presence of a stone in the distal CBD. A papillotomy was carried out with balloon sweeping and extraction of the CBD stone via endoscopic dormia basket under monitored anaesthesia using propofol for sedation. During extraction, the stone dislodged from the basket and was aspirated into the upper airway. A rigid bronchoscopy was performed, and this demonstrated the presence of the stone in the trachea which was successfully extracted. The patient recovered well after the procedure and underwent laparoscopic cholecystectomy within the same admission. She was discharged home 2 days later, and on subsequent review at the surgical clinic 2 weeks after the surgery, she demonstrated an uneventful recovery.

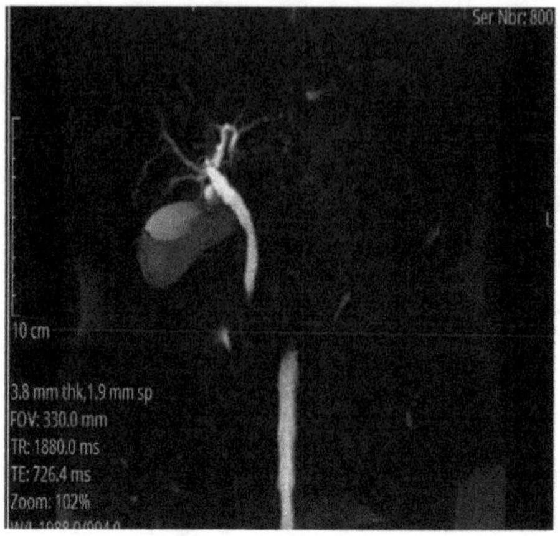

FIGURE 1: MRCP, coronal view, showing the dilated CBD with a distal filling defect.

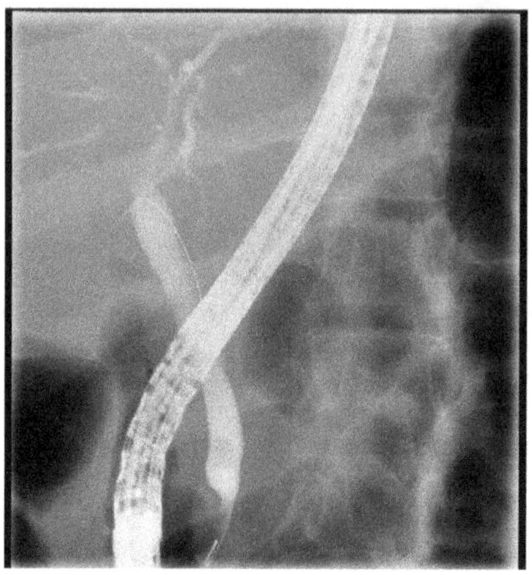

FIGURE 2: Fluoroscopy during ERCP showing the dilated CBD and contrast reaching the hepatic ducts.

3. Discussion

The most frequent complications of endoscopic retrograde cholangiopancreatography (ERCP) and endoscopic biliary sphincterotomy are pancreatitis (3.5%), cholangitis (1%), haemorrhage (1.3%), and duodenal perforation (0.6%) [1–4]. A number of less common adverse events have also been described including cardiopulmonary complications, contrast allergy, impaction of a retrieval basket, and numerous other events reported in only small numbers of patients or individual case reports. These unusual adverse events, which may be difficult to manage, can be associated with significant morbidity and mortality [5, 6]. Factors affecting morbidity and mortality during ERCP include operator experience and patient comorbidity [7].

No previous reports exist of gallstone dislodgement into the airway during ERCP. There were, however, reports of possible sequelae after the presence of gallstone in chest cavity rather than within the bronchopulmonary tree, namely, biliothoraces and cholecystothoracic fistulas [8].

Another report documented complications of basket malfunction or disruption in which metallic fragments of the basket were left in situ and removed at a later date using endoscopy [9]. The risk of leaving gallstones within the bronchial tree are theoretically similar to presence of other foreign bodies, which includes pneumonia, atelectasis, bronchiectasis, respiratory distress if the stone is big enough to obstruct the upper airway, as well as bleeding or erosion into nearby structures, but to our knowledge, there are no reports in the literature describing the sequelae of the presence of gallstones in the airway and demonstrating if any difference exists between the different types of stones.

4. Conclusion

This report describes successful management of a rare but potentially dangerous complication of ERCP to remove impacted CBD stones. In the presence of experienced endoscopy and bronchoscopy teams, such stones can be safely removed endoscopically, avoiding the risk of major surgery. The possible complications of delayed removal or inability to remove gallstones from the airway have yet to be studied and reported but are likely to include recurrent chest infections, bronchiectasis, and empyema of the lung.

References

[1] A. Andriulli, S. Loperfido, G. Napolitano et al., "Incidence rates of post-ERCP complications: a systematic survey of prospective studies," *The American Journal of Gastroenterology*, vol. 102, no. 8, pp. 1781–1788, 2007.

[2] M. L. Freeman, D. B. Nelson, S. Sherman et al., "Complications of endoscopic biliary sphincterotomy," *New England Journal of Medicine*, vol. 335, no. 13, pp. 909–919, 1996.

[3] E. Masci, G. Toti, A. Mariani et al., "Complications of diagnostic and therapeutic ERCP: a prospective multicenter study," *The American Journal of Gastroenterology*, vol. 96, no. 2, pp. 417–423, 2001.

[4] S. Loperfido, G. Angelini, G. Benedetti et al., "Major early complications from diagnostic and therapeutic ERCP: a prospective multicenter study," *Gastrointestinal Endoscopy*, vol. 48, no. 1, pp. 1–10, 1998.

[5] C.-I. Kwon, S. H. Song, K. B. Hahm, and K. H. Ko, "Unusual complications related to endoscopic retrograde cholangiopancreatography and its endoscopic treatment," *Clinical Endoscopy*, vol. 46, no. 3, p. 251, 2013.

[6] D. Chavalitdhamrong, S. Donepudi, L. Pu, and P. V. Draganov, "Uncommon and rarely reported adverse events of endoscopic retrograde cholangiopancreatography," *Digestive Endoscopy*, vol. 26, no. 1, pp. 15–22, 2014.

[7] D. Kingsley, C. Schermer, and M. Jamal, "Rare complications of endoscopic retrograde cholangiopancreatography: two case reports," *JSLS Journal of the Society of Laparoscopic & Robotic Surgeons*, vol. 5, no. 2, pp. 171–173, 2001.

[8] F. Delcò, G. Domenighetti, D. Kauzlaric, D. Donati, and G. Mombelli, "Spontaneous biliothorax (thoracobilia) following cholecystopleural fistula presenting as an acute respiratory insufficiency," *Chest*, vol. 106, no. 3, pp. 961–963, 1994.

[9] N. M. Kelly and G. R. Caddy, "Successful endoscopic management of fractured dormia basket during endoscopic retrograde cholangiopancreatography for choledocholithiasis," *The Ulster Medical Journal*, vol. 77, no. 1, pp. 56–58, 2008.

3

Esophageal Plasmacytoma Revealed by Persistent Hiccups: A Case Report and Literature Review

Khaoula Khalil, Fatima Ezzahra Lahlimi, and Illias Tazi

Department of Hematology and Bone Marrow Transplantation, Mohammed VI University Hospital, Cadi Ayyad University, Marrakesh 40080, Morocco

Correspondence should be addressed to Khaoula Khalil; khaoulakhalil90@gmail.com

Academic Editor: Yoshihiro Moriwaki

Introduction. Solitary extramedullary plasmacytoma (SEP) is a rare neoplasm that is derived from monoclonal proliferation of plasma cells in the soft tissues or organs arising outside the bone marrow. It is present in about 3% of all plasma cell tumors and originates mainly from the upper respiratory tract and nasopharynx. Involvement of the esophagus is exceptionally seen in cases of SEP. *Case Presentation.* We report a novel case of a 74-year-old male patient attended with a 6-month history of hiccupping further associated with dysphasia and weight loss all caused by esophageal plasmacytoma. Histological and immunohistochemical examination of the tumor confirmed the diagnosis of plasmacytoma. Workup for the multiple myeloma came out to be negative, thus confirming the diagnosis of SEP. The patient was treated with radiotherapy alone, leading to complete remission (at 30 months of follow-up). *Conclusion.* Esophageal plasmacytoma, an exceptional presentation of extramedullary plasmacytoma, should be kept in mind while dealing with patients presenting with intractable hiccups.

1. Introduction

Solitary extramedullary plasmacytoma (SEP) is a rare form of plasma cell dyscrasia derived from monoclonal proliferation of plasma cells and located in the soft tissues or organs arising outside the bone marrow [1]. The gastrointestinal tract accounts for less than 5% of SEP [2]. The esophagus appears to be the least common location for the SEP to originate. We report a novel case of esophageal plasmacytoma in a 74-year-old male patient disclosed by refractory hiccupping and treated with radiation monotherapy alone. A brief overview of the relevant literature is given focusing on the presentation, the diagnosis, and the treatment of an exceptional site and presentation of SEP.

2. Case Presentation

A 74-year-old man presented, in October 2018, with a 6-month history of persistent hiccupping. Since 3 months before the visit, his hiccups had worsened disturbing his sleep and daily life and were associated with intermittent dysphagia and recurrent postprandial vomiting. There was no history of alcohol consumption or cigarette smoking. He did not present with fever, night sweats, hiatus hernia symptoms, abdominal pain, a recent change in diet, bone pain, or any pathological fracture in the recent past. Physical examination revealed an old man in no apparent distress except for hiccups. At presentation, his temperature was 37.3°, pulse rate was 82/min, respiratory rate was 18/min, and blood pressure was 120/70 mmHg. He did not present any significant alterations beyond weight loss. There was no pallor, icterus, lymphadenopathy, bone pains, or any bleeding manifestations such as ecchymosis or petechiae. Esophagoscopy identified a 4-centimetre circumferential ulcerated mass of the distal third of the esophagus. The biopsy results of the esophagus showed abundant sheets of small lymphoid mononuclear cells (plasma cells) (Figure 1). Immunohistochemistry analysis showed positive expression for CD138, CD79a, and EMA and negative expression for CD20, CD3, and pan-cytokeratin. Ki-67 index value was 20% (Figure 2). These pathological features were consistent with extramedullary plasmacytoma diagnosis.

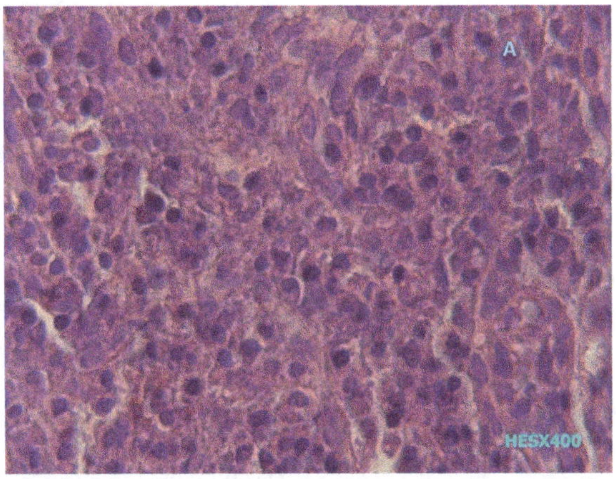

FIGURE 1: Histological examination of esophagus biopsy showing the presence of sheets of plasma cells.

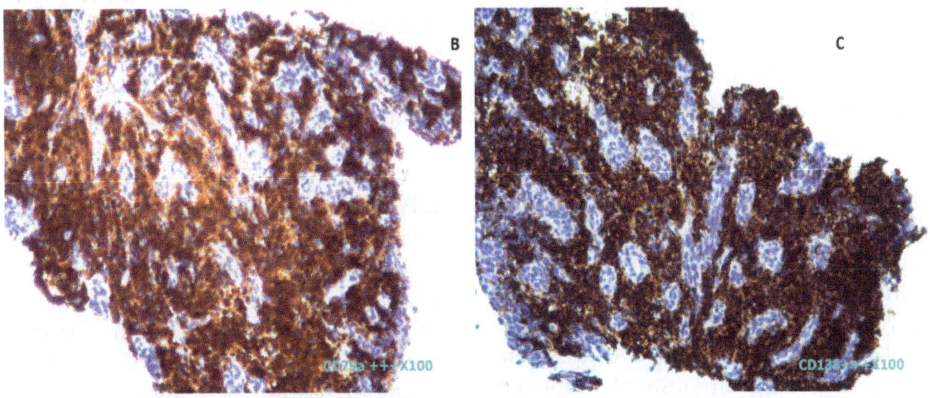

FIGURE 2: (a) Immunohistochemical examination of biopsy sample showing positivity in majority of tumor cells for CD79a and (b) CD138.

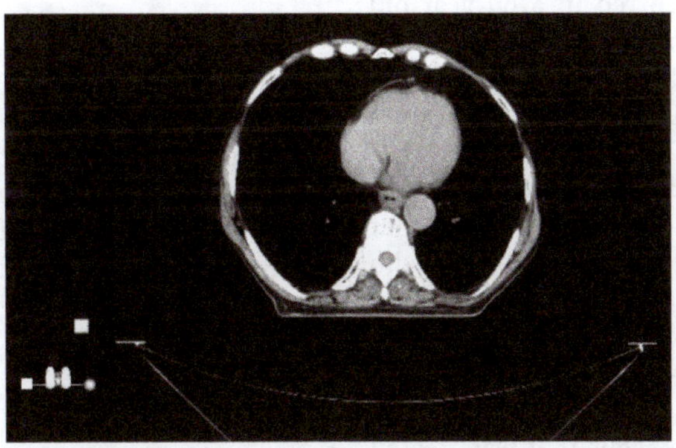

FIGURE 3: Pretreatment computed tomography showing circumferential esophageal wall thickening located at the distal third of the esophagus.

Computed tomography of the chest and abdomen revealed a circumferential esophageal wall thickening of 9 mm that was located at the distal third of the esophagus measuring 38.3 mm (Figure 3). No enlarged lymph nodes, other organ involvement, or osteolytic lesions were found. Complete blood count (CBC) showed hemoglobin of 13.5 g/dl, total leucocyte count of 6400/mm^3, normal platelet count of 211,000/mm^3, and erythrocyte sedimentation rate (ESR) of 12 mm/1st hour and B2 microglobulin of 3.13 mg/L. Serum creatinine and calcium levels were within the normal range.

Bone marrow tests (aspiration and biopsy) did not show the presence of myeloma cells. Serum protein electrophoresis and immunofixation were also negative for any monoclonal gammopathy.

Urine examination was negative for Bence-Jones proteins. All the investigations listed above confirmed the diagnosis of solitary extramedullary plasmacytoma of the esophagus. The patient was referred to the radiotherapy department where three-dimensional conformal radiotherapy (3DCRT) was applied to the involved site (oesophagus) with curative intent. The prescribed dose of 40 Gy was delivered in 20 fractions over a period of 4 weeks. Radiotherapy was well-tolerated, and the patient's hiccupping resolved progressively during treatment with only a few episodes noted while eating or drinking that have persisted after the end of treatment. During the last thirty months of follow-up, no recurrence or progression to myeloma were noted.

3. Discussion

Solitary extramedullary plasmacytoma (SEP) is a proliferation of neoplastic monoclonal plasma cells in soft tissues outside the bone marrow. It accounts for 3% of plasma cell tumors and involves males in 75% of cases [1, 2]. The diagnosis of SEP is based on the exclusion of systemic involvement and an absence of end-organ damage attributable to plasmacytoma [3]. It arises mainly from the upper respiratory tract (nasal cavity, paranasal sinuses, and nasopharynx). The stomach and small bowel are the most usual primary sites when the gastrointestinal system is involved. The esophagus is an extremely rare primary location for the SEP to originate, and only 6 cases of esophageal extramedullary plasmacytoma have been reported in the literature to date. Morris and Pead described a case of a 59-year-old woman who presented with weight loss and progressively worsening intermittent dysphagia [4]. The SEP was a protuberant mass that occurred in the lower esophagus. Ahmed et al. reported a case of a 67-year-old man who had dysphagia, weakness, and weight loss [5]. The case of Davies and Boxer occurred in a 69-year-old man who only had a 2-week history of dysphagia with no other significant alterations [6]. The tumor was polypoid, measured 4 cm in diameter, and involved the distal one-third of the esophagus. Chetty et al. reported a case of a 58-year-old man who presented with dysphagia for solids over a period of 2 months [7]. The fifth case belongs to Rimmer et al. describing a 62-year-old man, with no dysphagia, who presented with cardiac chest pain and was worked up for possible acute myocardial injury [8]. Zhou et al. reported in 2012 the sixth case of an 80-year-old-woman with a primary isolated extramedullary plasmacytoma on the left posterior wall of the proximal esophagus that was treated with endoscopic submucosal dissection [9].

Plasmacytomas commonly show a protuberant mass on endoscopy. The most common clinical presenting features of esophageal plasmacytoma are similar to those of carcinomas such as worsening dysphagia due to mass effect, anorexia, and weight loss [5]. Hiccupping, the primary and main ongoing symptom in our case, has never been reported in the literature. It may be due to a direct effect of the tumor itself or to a secondary dilatation of the esophagus above a stenotic lesion leading to raised pressure that stimulates a reflex action or perhaps to the disruption to esophageal motility that occurs in esophageal cancer [10].

Despite the consideration of local radiotherapy as the preferred treatment modality for solitary plasmacytoma, there are no treatment guidelines for esophageal plasmacytoma. Many authors reported achieving complete remission with radiotherapy followed by esophagectomy: the gold standard treatment for esophageal cancer [11]. We opted for radiotherapy alone using 3-dimensional conformal radiotherapy (3DCRT) with curative intent in a daily fraction of 2 Gy, 5 days a week. The dose used for our patient was 40 Gy as recommended by the International Lymphoma Radiation Oncology Group. Interestingly, Elsayad et al. have shown in their international multicenter analysis that using radiotherapy dose-escalation (above 40 Gy) and modern irradiation techniques as intensity-modulated radiotherapy (IMRT) and proton therapy seem to improve the local control and reduce the rate of relapse in patients with solitary bone or solitary extramedullary plasmacytoma, without a significant effect on survival rates [12]. Imaging examinations, such as positron emission tomography (PET) computed tomography (CT), are required for the management of suspected SEP, as well as to monitor the therapeutic response to radiotherapy and the possibility of recurrence and progression of into multiple myeloma [13].

A follow-up CT scan 6 months after 3DCRT showed a normal structure of the esophagus. Endoscopic examination with multiple biopsies of the plasmacytoma site and surrounding tissues attested to the good radiotherapy results showing normal esophageal mucosa without plasma cell infiltration of the scars and the surrounding tissue. Also, neither recurrence nor progression to myeloma was noted during the last thirty months of follow-up.

4. Conclusion

We have presented a novel case of an extramedullary plasmacytoma revealed by intractable hiccupping and effectively treated with local radiotherapy. Hiccups are common and often idiopathic, but persistent hiccups could be an unrecognized symptom of many esophageal cancers not only common ones like carcinoma but also the rare ones like extramedullary plasmacytoma.

Authors' Contributions

All authors contributed to this work and commented on the manuscript at all stages, and finally, the final version was approved for publication.

References

[1] P. Galieni, M. Cavo, A. Pulsoni et al., "Clinical outcome of extramedullary plasmacytoma," *Haematologica*, vol. 85, no. 1, 2000.

[2] M. A. Dimopoulos and G. Hamilos, "Solitary bone plasmacytoma and extramedullary plasmacytoma," *Current Treatment Options in Oncology*, vol. 3, no. 3, pp. 255–259, 2002.

[3] S. V. Rajkumar, M. A. Dimopoulos, A. Palumbo et al., "International Myeloma Working Group updated criteria for the diagnosis of multiple myeloma," *The Lancet Oncology*, vol. 15, no. 12, pp. e538–e548, 2014.

[4] W. T. Morris and J. L. Pead, "Myeloma of the oesophagus," *Journal of Clinical Pathology*, vol. 25, no. 6, pp. 537-538, 1972.

[5] N. Ahmed, S. Ramos, J. Sika, H. H. LeVeen, and V. A. Piccone, "Primary extramedullary esophageal plasmacytoma.First case report," *Cancer*, vol. 38, no. 2, pp. 943–947, 1976.

[6] R. A. Davies and D. I. Boxer, "Primary plasmacytoma of the oesophagus," *British Journal of Radiology*, vol. 61, no. 732, pp. 1180-1181, 1988.

[7] R. Chetty, A. Bramdev, and A. D. Reddy, "Primary extramedullary plasmacytoma of the esophagus," *Annals of Diagnostic Pathology*, vol. 7, no. 3, pp. 174–179, 2003.

[8] C. Rimmer, A. Hazra, V. M. Gulli, R. Siderits, M. Castaldi, and Z. Zamir, "Esophageal plasmacytoma diagnosed in a patient presenting with cardiac symptoms: a novel case," *Case Reports in Gastrointestinal Medicine*, vol. 2013, Article ID 121670, 2013.

[9] Y. Zhou, X. Xu, L. Xu et al., "Treatment of primary isolated extramedullary plasmacytoma of esophagus with endoscopic submucosal dissection," *Clinical Gastroenterology and Hepatology*, vol. 10, no. 3, pp. e21–e22, 2012.

[10] T. Khorakiwala, R. Arain, J. Mulsow, and T. N. Walsh, "Hiccups: an unrecognized symptom of esophageal cancer?" *American Journal of Gastroenterology*, vol. 103, no. 3, p. 801, 2008.

[11] D. Gerry and E. J. Lentsch, "Epidemiologic evidence of superior outcomes for extramedullary plasmacytoma of the head and neck," *Otolaryngology-Head and Neck Surgery*, vol. 148, no. 6, pp. 974–981, 2013.

[12] K. Elsayad, M. Oertel, L. König et al., "Maximizing the clinical benefit of radiotherapy in solitary plasmacytoma: an international multicenter analysis," *Cancers*, vol. 12, no. 3, p. 676, 2020.

[13] S. Rachh, K. Puj, and A. Parikh, "18F-FDG PET/CT in the evaluation of solitary extramedullary plasmacytoma: a case series," *Asia Oceania journal of nuclear medicine & biology*, vol. 9, no. 1, pp. 56–61, 2021.

4

Dramatic Response of Lupus Enteritis, Nephritis and Pancytopenia to Plasmapheresis and Rituximab

Adan Aftab, Nida Saleem, Syed Farhat Abbas, Zafar Ullah, and Muhammad Haneef

Shifa International Hospital, H-8/4, Pitras Bukhari Road, Islamabad, Pakistan

Correspondence should be addressed to Nida Saleem; nidasaa1968@gmail.com

Academic Editor: Hirotada Akiho

Background. Although lupus enteritis is a rare manifestation of systemic lupus erythematosus yet results in significant distress. This disorder contributes to diagnostic and therapeutic dilemma leading to enhanced mortality. *Case Description.* We report a case history of a 29-year-old female who presented with severe abdominal pain, watery stools, and vomiting, and later on, she developed pancytopenia and renal impairment. On intensive workup, diagnosis of lupus-associated enteritis, nephritis, and pancytopenia was discovered. She improved drastically on initiation of plasmapheresis followed by low-dose intravenous rituximab. One year posttreatment, she remained in complete remission. *Conclusion.* From this case, it can be suggested that in a young female with intractable abdominal pain, the remote possibility of lupus enteritis must be kept in mind. Besides this, plasmapheresis can have a potential role in refractory lupus enteritis. Furthermore, low-dose intravenous rituximab can be a safe and cost-effective treatment option in achieving sustained remission of clinical and laboratory parameters in lupus enteritis.

1. Introduction

Systemic lupus erythematosus (SLE) is a multisystem autoimmune disorder affecting predominantly young females. Many gastrointestinal manifestations can occur in SLE, which can be related to disease itself, superimposed infections, and gastrointestinal side effects of immunosuppressant given for its management. The reported incidence of these manifestations is between 1.3 and 27.5% [1]. Lupus enteritis is a rare manifestation of SLE with a reported prevalence of around 3.5–5.8% in Asian population [2], caused by formation of immune complexes against small vessels of the gut, predominantly the jejunum and ileum [3], leading to necrotizing vasculitis. The classical manifestation of this disorder is severe acute abdominal pain. Abdominal pain in SLE can be secondary to peritonitis, pancreatitis, acalculous cholecystitis, gastroenteritis, mesenteric ischemia, intestinal pseudoobstruction, and peptic ulcer disease [1, 3, 4], thus making diagnosis of this rare debilitating condition even more difficult. Lupus enteritis, if remained undiagnosed, can lead to gastrointestinal ischemia, infarction leading to bleeding, and perforation requiring emergent surgical intervention [1] and is associated with a high mortality rate. Therefore, deeper understanding of this disease entity is necessary. Several studies have mentioned the therapeutic role of several immunosuppressive medications in improving clinical and laboratory parameters. However, no study has described about the potential role of plasmapheresis and low-dose intravenous rituximab in achieving sustained remission. We report the first case of severe acute onset lupus enteritis with nephritis and pancytopenia responded immediately upon initiation of plasmapheresis with no recurrence after low-dose intravenous rituximab therapy.

2. Case Report

The patient, a 29-year-old female resident of Gujrat, Pakistan, married, with no known comorbidities, admitted to our hospital through emergency department with severe abdominal pain, loose stools, and vomiting for one week. These symptoms had not responded to the intravenous antibiotics and analgesics, which she received at some local hospital. Her symptoms worsened three days before admission. At that time, there was an increase in the severity of pain, and loose stools became more watery in consistency with mucus in them. However, there was no blood in stools. Besides this, she had unintentional weight loss of around seven kilograms with generalized weakness and joint pains for the last three months. Her family history was insignificant for any bowel or autoimmune disorder.

On examination, she was pale. Her blood pressure was 100/60 mmHg, pulse was 92/min, and she was afebrile. Her abdominal examination was significant for severe abdominal tenderness with hypoactive bowel sounds. Rest of the systemic examination was unremarkable. Postadmission, her workup was performed, as given in Table 1.

As given in Table 1, there is evidence of pancytopenia, raised serum creatinine, proteinuria, folic acid deficiency, hypokalemia, and presence of mucus with white blood cells on stool routine examination.

She was kept nil per oral due to ongoing diarrhea and vomiting. She received intravenous fluids for volume depletion. She also received intravenous meropenem and metronidazole along with syrup vancomycin for suspected infectious diarrhea. Also, intravenous tramadol and nalbuphine on as need basis was prescribed for abdominal pain relief. To control vomiting and dyspeptic symptoms, omeprazole infusion and intravenous ondansetron were administered. Intravenous folinic acid was given for correction of folic acid deficiency.

At this point, diagnosis of inflammatory bowel disease and mesenteric ischemia was suspected. In order to identify the exact cause of her symptoms, CT vascular angiography was performed which showed extensive mucosal enhancement, thickening, and marked submucosal edema in the rectum, sigmoid, and descending colon up to the splenic flexure. However, there was relative sparing of ascending and transverse colon. Moreover, there was mild hepatosplenomegaly and ascites. All the vessels were patent with no evidence of engorgement of mesenteric vasculature. These findings were suggestive of severe acute proctocolitis.

Considering her history and radiological findings, upper GI endoscopy and colonoscopy were done as shown in Figure 1.

Multiple biopsies from different segments including the sigmoid colon, rectum, gastric body, and ileum were taken. Figures 2 and 3 show light microscopic appearance of different GI segments at different power fields.

As shown in above figures, there is no evidence of malignancy and granulomatous disease. Congo red staining was negative for amyloidosis as well.

In addition to this, diagnostic laparoscopy was performed which showed moderate abdominopelvic ascites. Her peritoneal fluid cytology was negative for malignancy. Contrast enhanced CT scan abdomen (CECT) was repeated, which showed worsening of the disease process with panenteritis involving large and small bowel up to the esophagus. Figure 4 shows CECT abdomen images.

As her condition deteriorated further, her autoimmune workup was done to identify any autoimmune pathology.

Results are given in Table 2.

As given in Table 2, there are low serum complement levels (c3, c4) and positive ANA, anti-Ro, and anti-La antibodies, indicating the possible diagnosis of systemic lupus erythematosus.

Keeping in view of the above, diagnosis of lupus enteritis was made. She was then started on intravenous methylprednisolone 250 mg once daily, for 3 days, which was then increased to 500 mg once daily, for 5 days after no symptomatic improvement. In spite of these interventions, no symptomatic relief was obtained and her abdominal pain persisted. In order to relieve her abdominal pain, pain management department was consulted and epidural bupivacaine infusion was started. Despite of opioids administration and even the neuromuscular blocking agent, her pain continued.

Meanwhile, tablet mycophenolate mofetil (MMF) was initiated at a low dose (250 mg twice daily) due to low total leucocyte count. After 3 days, MMF was increased to 500 mg twice daily. However, no symptomatic relief was achieved. Later, after 4 days, plasmapheresis was initiated using albumin as a replacement fluid. She responded dramatically to 5 daily sessions of plasmapheresis with complete resolution of all her symptoms in the next few days, and later on, she was off the analgesics as well. As her serum creatinine was 3 mg/dL with ongoing proteinuria, therefore, her renal biopsy was performed. Figure 5 shows histopathological images obtained after renal biopsy.

The above figure shows marked endocapillary hypercellularity consistent with diffuse proliferative glomerulonephritis (class IV lupus nephritis) and moderate tubular injury. Immunofluorescence showed granular IgG and c3 deposits in glomerular basement membrane and mesangium. Mesangial IgM and C1q containing immune deposits were focally positive as well. There was no evidence of tubulointerstitial fibrosis. She remained stable post-plasmapheresis, her complete blood count normalized, serum creatinine decreased to around 2 mg/dL, and later on, she was discharged on mycophenolate mofetil 1000 mg twice daily, hydroxychloroquine (HCQ) 200 mg twice daily, and tapering doses of steroids.

On follow up, 7 days later, she again developed lupus-associated pancytopenia. As she was young female, in her reproductive age group, therefore, intravenous cyclophosphamide was not considered. She was successfully treated with 100 mg weekly doses of intravenous rituximab. After total 4 doses of rituximab, her total leucocyte count, hemoglobin, and platelet count normalized.

One year following 5 sessions of plasmapheresis and 4 doses of rituximab, steroids, MMF, and HCQ, she is in complete remission from all perspectives, which include settlement of abdominal pain and diarrhea, normalization of complete blood picture, and most importantly, renal parameters. Her current serum creatinine is 0.65 mg/dL and urine albumin to creatinine ratio is 33 mg/g. The flowchart in Figure 6 shows the treatment received by the patient.

3. Discussion

As previously reported [3–5], acute intense abdominal pain and vomiting is the predominant clinical feature of lupus

Table 1: Postadmission laboratory investigations.

Post-Admission Laboratory Investigations (Table 1):			
Total leucocyte count	2500/μL	Serum amylase	57 U/L
Platelet count	112000/μL	Serum protein electrophoresis	No paraproteins
Hemoglobin	10.4 g/dL	Serum creatinine	3 mg/dL
Reticulocyte count	0.9%	BUN[e]	40 mg/dL
Transferrin saturation	37%	Sodium	143 meq/L
Vitamin B12	256 pm/L	Potassium	3.1 meq/L
Folic acid	<3.1 ng/mL	Chloride	112 meq/L
LDH[j]	238 U/L	Bicarbonate	20 meq/L
Coombs direct	Positive	Ionized calcium	4.3 mg/dL
Peripheral film	1% schistocyte	C-reactive protein	9.45 mg/dL
AST[a]	38 U/L	ESR[f]	11 mm/h
ALT[b]	12 U/L	Urine R/E[d]	3+ protein, 1+ blood
Total bilirubin	0.59 mg/dL	Albumin to creatinine ratio	1.343 g/g
GGT[c]	13 U/L	Stool R/E[d]	Mucus ++, 8–10 WBCs[i]
Alkaline phosphatase	37 U/L	Stool for *Clostridium difficile* (PCR[h])	Negative
Serum lipase	17 U/L	Stool and blood C/S[g]	Negative

[a]Aspartate aminotransferase, [b]alanine aminotransferase, [c]gamma glutamyl transferase, [d]routine examination, [e]blood urea nitrogen, [f]erythrocyte sedimentation rate, [g]culture and sensitivity, [h]polymerase chain reaction, [i]white blood cells, [j]lactate dehydrogenase.

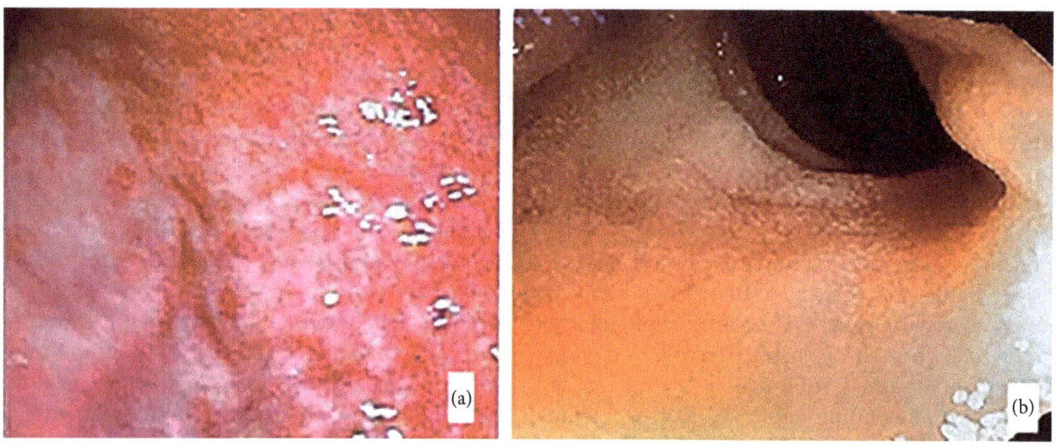

Figure 1: (a) Endoscopic image showing the evidence of hemorrhagic gastritis. (b) Colonoscopic view showing the presence of bowel wall edema.

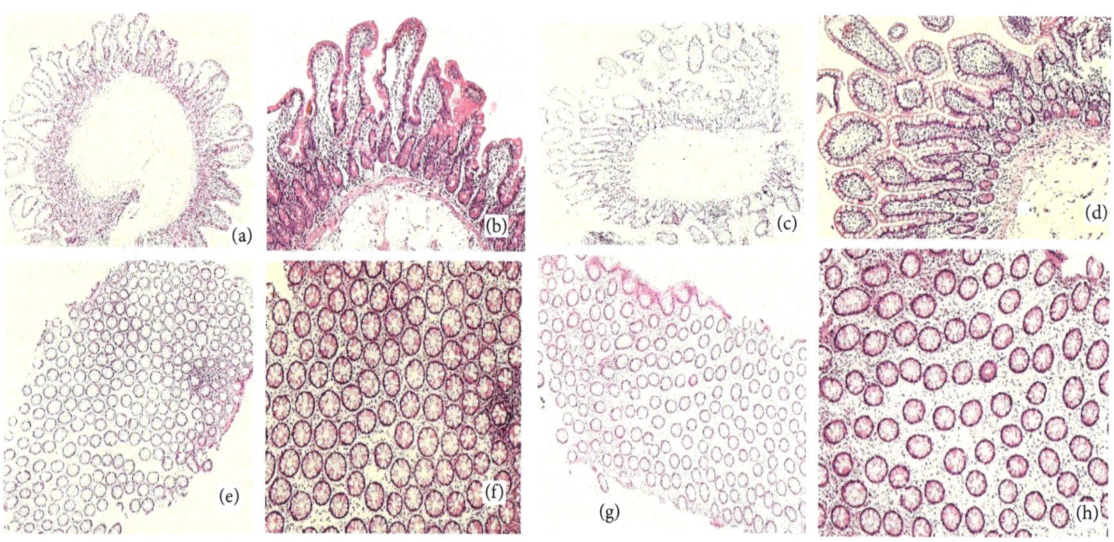

Figure 2: Light microscopic images (H&E staining). Normal duodenal lining: (a) (4X). (b) (10X). Normal ileal lining: (c) (4X). (d) (10X). Normal rectal lining: (e) (4X). (f) (10X). Normal lining of sigmoid colon: (g) (4X). (h) (10X).

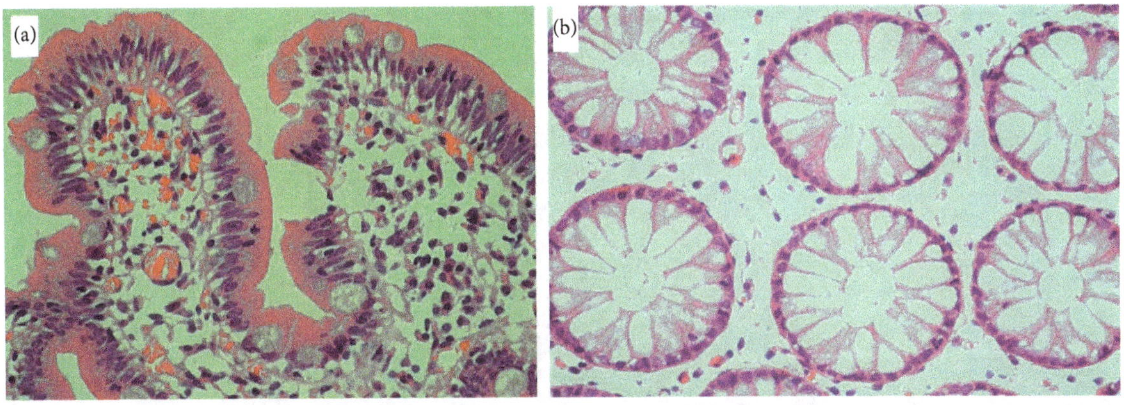

FIGURE 3: Light microscopic images (H&E staining). (a) Normal duodenal lining (40X). (b) Normal colonic lining (40X).

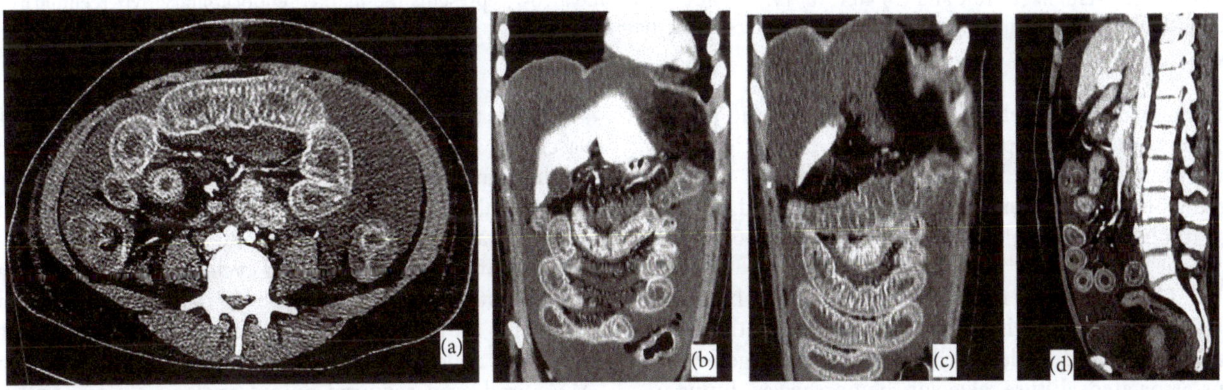

FIGURE 4: Markedly thickened edematous bowel loops at different segments of GI tract with extensive mucosal enlargement. Patent abdominopelvic vessels with no evidence of ischemia. (a) Axial view, (b)-(c) coronal view, and (d) sagittal view.

TABLE 2: Autoimmune workup.

Autoimmune workup (Table 2):			
c3[a]	0.43 G/L ↓	Lupus anticoagulant	Negative
c4	0.15 G/L ↓	Anticardiolipin IgG, IgM	Negative
p-ANCA[b]	Negative	Anti-ds[f]DNA antibody	Negative
c-ANCA[c]	Negative	ANA[d]	2 positive nucleolar patterns
Anti-Ro	87 ↑	Antihistone antibody	Negative
Anti-La	61↑	Anti-TTG[e] IgA antibody	Negative
Fecal calprotectin	Negative	Antiendomysial antibody	Negative

[a]Complement-3, [b]perinuclear antineutrophilic cytoplasmic antibodies, [c]circulating antineutrophilic cytoplasmic antibodies, [d]antinuclear antibody, [e]tissue transglutaminase antibody, [f]double stranded.

enteritis. Our patient had similar clinical manifestations, which were not responding to antimicrobial medications and wide range of analgesics. Therefore, it can be concluded that in a young female with nonresponding abdominal pain and ongoing vomiting and diarrhea, the remote possibility of lupus-induced gastrointestinal (GI) vasculopathy must be kept in mind.

As abdominal pain in SLE can be due to multiple causes and there is no available confirmatory investigation that has high sensitivity and specificity [1], multiple diagnostic clues can aid in accurate diagnosis of lupus enteritis. These include the preexisting history of SLE with hypocomplementemia suggestive of active lupus, nonresponding abdominal pain, extensive bowel wall edema, mesenteric vascular engorgement and enhanced mesenteric fat attenuation on abdominal CT scan, nondiagnostic histopathological evidence, and endoscopic findings.

Few case studies have been published regarding degree of GI involvement in lupus-induced vasculopathy. According to our knowledge, this is the third case report describing about extensive involvement of the gastrointestinal tract from the esophagus to the rectum [5, 6].

There are several reported causes of pancytopenia in SLE patients. These include nutritional deficiency, autoimmune myelofibrosis [7], destruction of cell lines by circulating immune complexes [8], hypersplenism, and haemophagocytic lymphohistiocytosis [9]. Pancytopenia in our patient was likely secondary to immune complex-mediated

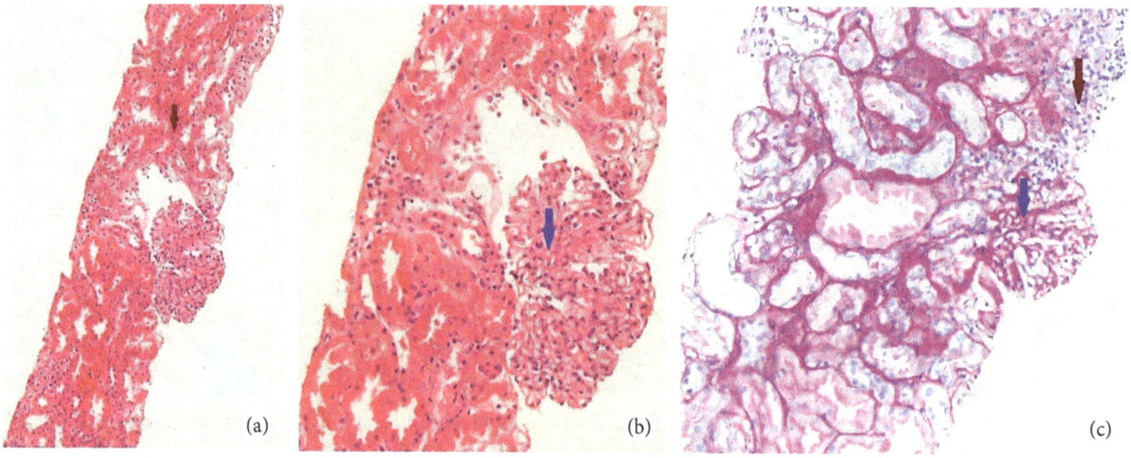

Figure 5: H&E stain at (a) 10X and (b) 40X. (c) PAS stain at 40X. Blue arrow represents the marked endocapillary hypercellularity and proliferation. Maroon arrow represents the tubulointerstitial inflammation.

destruction of blood cell lines as indicated by the positive Coombs test and superimposed folic acid deficiency. However, this cannot be said conclusively, as no bone marrow biopsy was done. Our patient responded immediately upon initiation of four weekly doses of 100 mg intravenous rituximab.

In SLE, several potential therapeutic roles of high-dose intravenous rituximab have been mentioned in the literature. These include role of rituximab in management of lupus-associated diffuse alveolar hemorrhages, lupus-induced retinal vasculitis [10], recurrent pancreatitis [11], refractory lupus nephritis [12], neuropsychiatric lupus, lupus-induced transverse myelitis [13], lupus-induced pulmonary hypertension [14], refractory cutaneous lupus [15], lupus-induced panniculitis [16], lupus myocarditis [17], and catastrophic antiphospholipid antibody (APLA) syndrome. Regarding lupus-induced hematological abnormalities, it has been well known that high-dose rituximab therapy can correct lupus-induced aplastic anemia [18], thrombotic thrombocytopenic purpura (TTP) [19], and refractory autoimmune hemolytic anemia [20].

However, regarding efficacy of low-dose (100 mg weekly, 4 doses) rituximab, very limited data are available. Only few studies have been conducted regarding the potential role of low-dose rituximab in SLE, and these are only about lupus-induced thrombocytopenia [21, 22]. As low-dose intravenous rituximab has played a role in inducing sustained remission of lupus-induced GI vasculitis and pancytopenia, as seen in our patient, therefore, it can be suggested that low-dose rituximab has added advantages of cost-effectiveness and limited side effect profile and can be utilized as an effective option for refractory systemic lupus and lupus-induced pancytopenia. However, this preposition needs further validation.

In several studies, the therapeutic role of plasmapheresis in SLE has been mentioned. The use of plasmapheresis has been proposed for the management of lupus-induced diffuse alveolar hemorrhages, retinal vasculitis [10], posterior reversible encephalopathy syndrome [23], refractory TTP [24], lupus cerebritis [25], and catastrophic APLA [26]. However, according to our knowledge, for refractory lupus-induced GI vasculitis, no role of plasmapheresis has been mentioned in the literature.

Several studies have mentioned improvement in clinical and laboratory parameters with steroids [3, 5], mycophenolate mofetil (MMF) [27], and cyclophosphamide [28] and have mentioned the potential role of tacrolimus [28] and rituximab for recurrent lupus enteritis [29]. Our patient had persistent abdominal pain in spite of high-dose steroids and MMF and even required opioid analgesics along with anesthetic medication. In one study, it has been suggested to undergo laparotomy for abdominal pain not responding to immunosuppressants [2]. However, after getting an insight about dramatic response to plasmapheresis in our patient, it can be proposed that plasmapheresis can be used as a last resort in lupus-induced gastrointestinal vasculopathy, refractory to conventional immunosuppressive therapy.

As mentioned, overall reported mortality of lupus enteritis was 53% [2]. The major contributing factors leading to the enhanced mortality rate are late diagnosis and initiation of immunosuppression. However, in Asian population, benign clinical course and excellent prognosis of this distressful disorder have been mentioned [30, 31]. Although the response to steroids and MMF has not been satisfactory in providing symptomatic relief to our patient, yet after commencement of plasmapheresis and later on low-dose rituximab, patient remained in complete remission even after one year of therapy.

Few studies have described about the risk factors which determine the likelihood of gastrointestinal recurrence, which includes preexisting positive antiphospholipid antibodies (APLA), bowel wall thickness of more than 9 mm on CT scan [2], low-dose or early steroid withdrawal [30], and even rituximab [29] and cyclophosphamide [31] free immunosuppression protocol, have been associated with early recurrence. Absence of APLA antibodies, administration of high-dose pulse steroids with gradual tapering, and subsequent rituximab administration reduced the possibility of recurrence of lupus enteritis, as seen in our patient. However, to validate these findings, further studies are needed.

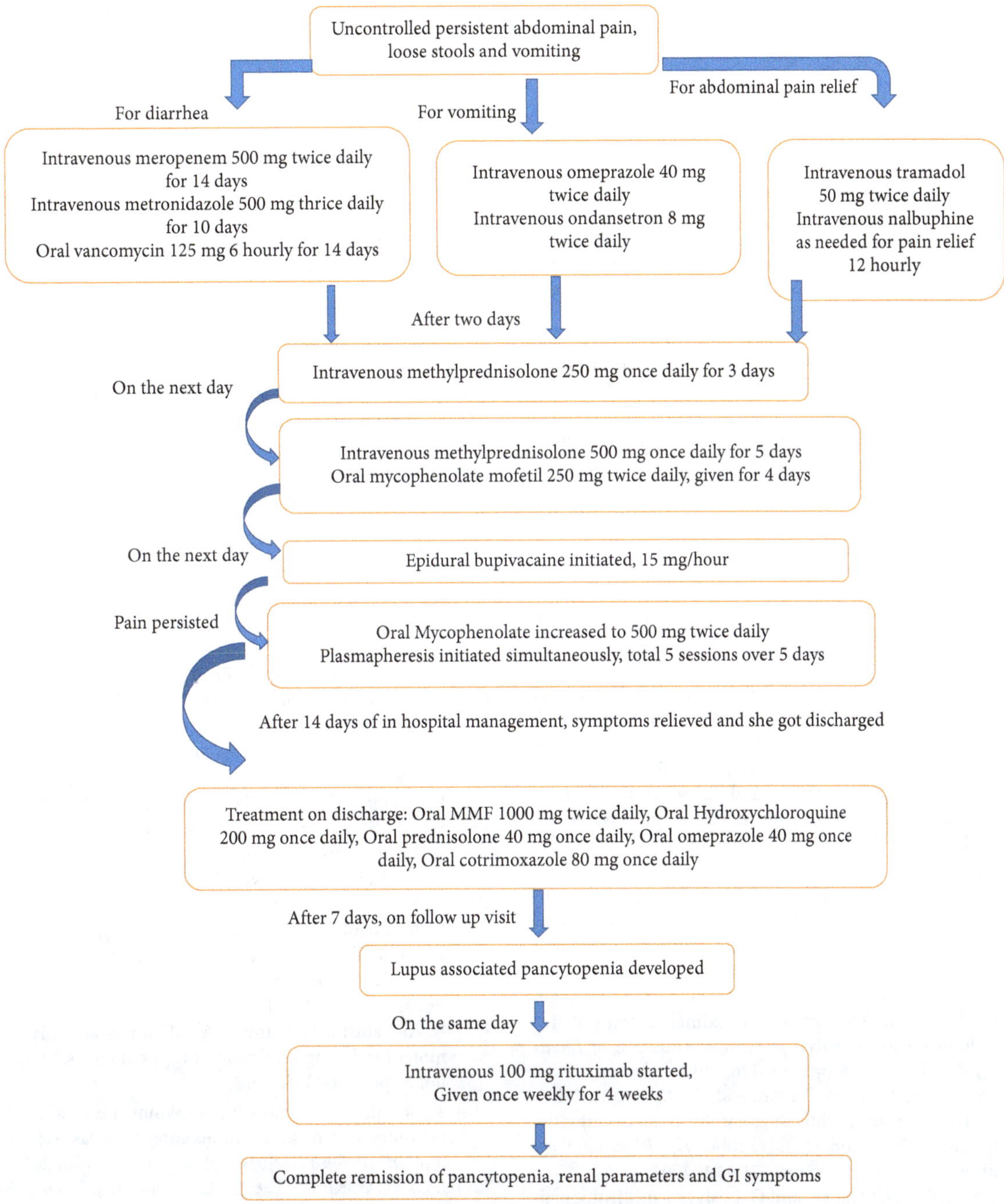

Figure 6: Summary of treatment received by the patient.

It can be concluded that in a young female with SLE and intractable abdominal pain, the possibility of lupus-associated abdominal vasculopathy must be kept in mind. Second, it is of utmost importance to diagnose early and manage this condition urgently in order to avoid life-threatening complications and surgical intervention. Third, as seen from this case, plasmapheresis can play a significant role in immediate correction of clinical and laboratory parameters in immunosuppressant refractory cases, thus precluding the immediate need for surgical intervention. Finally, low-dose rituximab can be tried in cases of nonresponding lupus-associated pancytopenia and can provide sustained remission of lupus-associated gastrointestinal vasculopathy as well. However, further studies are needed to validate these salient findings.

References

[1] R. Akitake, H. Nakase, S. Ueno, S. Miyamoto, N. Iehara, and T. J. D. Chiba, "Involvement of lupus enteritis in a patient with lupus cystitis and nephritis," *Digestion*, vol. 80, no. 3, pp. 160–4, 2009.

[2] H. Chng, B. Tan, C. The, and T. J. L. Lian, "Major gastrointestinal manifestations in lupus patients in Asia: lupus

enteritis, intestinal pseudo-obstruction, and protein-losing gastroenteropathy," *Lupus*, vol. 19, no. 12, pp. 1404–13, 2010.
[3] M. C. Abdulla and R. Mannarakkal, "Mannarakkal RJIJoS. Lupus Enteritis—an unusual cause for acute abdominal pain," *Indian Journal of Surgery*, vol. 83, pp. 1–3, 2020.
[4] R. B. Frittoli, J. F. Vivaldo, L. T. Costallat, and S. Appenzeller, "Gastrointestinal involvement in systemic lupus erythematosus," *A systematic review*, vol. 4, Article ID 100106, 2021.
[5] H. J. Na, Y.-r. Choi, D. H. Nam, C. H. Lee, S.-M. Park, and W. Kang, "A case of extensive involvement of lupus enteritis, from small bowel to rectum," *The Journal of the Korean Rheumatism Association*, vol. 14, no. 3, pp. 274–8, 2007.
[6] J. Bert and E. Gertner, "Lupus gastrointestinal tract vasculopathy: Lupus "Enteritis" Involving the entire gastrointestinal tract from esophagus to rectum," *Case Reports in Gastroenterology*, vol. 11, no. 1, pp. 48–53, 2017.
[7] P. Ungprasert, V. R. Chowdhary, M. D. Davis, A. J. L. Makol, and A. MAkol, "Autoimmune myelofibrosis with pancytopenia as a presenting manifestation of systemic lupus erythematosus responsive to mycophenolate mofetil," *Lupus*, vol. 25, no. 4, pp. 427–430, 2016.
[8] T. Iqbal, W. S. Baig, S. Arshad, and S. A. Awan, "Systemic Lupus Erythematosus associated refractory pancytopenia responding only to intravenous immunoglobulins," *European Journal of Medical Case Reports*, vol. 4, no. 4, pp. 123–125, 2020.
[9] Z. Almuwaqqat, J. W. Roberts, and Y. J. C. R. Bashtawi, "A rare and serious cause of pancytopenia in a patient with systemic lupus erythematosus: haemophagocytic lymphohistiocytosis," *BMJ case reports*, vol. 2018, 2018.
[10] N. Ali Dhirani, V. Ahluwalia, and S. Somani, "Case of combination therapy to treat lupus retinal vasculitis refractory to steroids," *Canadian Journal of Ophthalmology*, vol. 52, no. 1, pp. e13–e15, 2017.
[11] Z. S. Al-Musawi and U. J. Nabar, "Successful treatment of recurrent pancreatitis secondary to systemic lupus erythematosus with B-cell depletion therapy," *Archives of Iranian Medicineed*, vol. 14, no. 1, pp. 66–70, 2011.
[12] F. Alshaiki, E. Obaid, A. Almuallim, R. Taha, H. El-Haddad, and H. Almoallim, "Outcomes of rituximab therapy in refractory lupus: a meta-analysis," *European Journal of Rheumatologyol*, vol. 5, no. 2, pp. 118–126, 2018.
[13] D. J. Armstrong, M. T. McCarron, and G. D. Wright, "SLE-associated transverse myelitis successfully treated with Rituximab (anti-CD20 monoclonal antibody)," *Rheumatology International*, vol. 26, no. 8, pp. 771-772, 2006.
[14] S. Hennigan, R. N. Channick, and G. J. Silverman, "Rituximab treatment of pulmonary arterial hypertension associated with systemic lupus erythematosus: a case report," *Lupus*, vol. 17, no. 8, pp. 754–756, 2008.
[15] M. A. Penha, R. D. S. Liborio, and H. A. Miot, "Rituximab in the treatment of extensive and refractory subacute cutaneous lupus erythematosus," *Anais Brasileiros de Dermatologia*, vol. 93, no. 3, pp. 467–469, 2018.
[16] F. Moreno-Suarez and A. Pulpillo-Ruiz, "Rituximab for the treatment of lupus erythematosus panniculitis," *Dermatology and Therapy*, vol. 26, no. 5, pp. 415–418, 2013.
[17] P. Aggarwal, S. Singh, D. Suri, A. Rawat, N. Narula, and R. ManojKumar, "Rituximab in childhood lupus myocarditis," *Rheumatology International*, vol. 32, no. 6, pp. 1843-1844, 2012.
[18] G. H. Alishiri, A. Saburi, N. Bayat, A. R. Saadat, and E. Saburi, "The initial presentation of systemic lupus erythematosis with aplastic anemia successfully treated with rituximab," *Clinical rheumatology*, vol. 31, no. 2, pp. 381–384, 2012.
[19] M. Karimifar, "Thrombotic thrombocytopenic purpura treated with rituximab in systemic lupus erythematosus," *Journal of Renal Injury Prevention*, vol. 1, no. 2, pp. 53-54, 2012.
[20] M. Pavo-Blanco, M. Novella-Navarro, R. Caliz-Caliz, and M. A. Ferrer-Gonzalez, "Rituximab in refractory autoimmune hemolytic anemia in systemic lupus erythematosus," *Reumatología Clínica (English Edition)*, vol. 14, no. 4, pp. 248-249, 2018.
[21] C. Y. Wang, S. H. Guo, L. P. Wang, X. Y. Wang, and H. L. Shen, "Clinical efficacy of low-dose rituximab on hematological abnormalities in patients with connective tissue disease," *Int. Journal of Clinical Pharmacology and Therapeutics*, vol. 57, no. 10, pp. 500–505, 2019.
[22] O. Ilizaliturri-Guerra, R. Uriarte-Botello, R. A. Pineda-Sic et al., "Low-dose rituximab therapy in steroid-refractory thrombocytopenia due to systemic lupus erythematosus," *Rheumatology International*, vol. 40, no. 10, pp. 1717–1724, 2020.
[23] Z. I. Arslan, C. K. Turna, C. Y. Ozerdem, S. Yavuz, N. Baykara, and M. Solak, "Treatment of posterior reversible encephalopathy syndrome that occurred in a patient with systemic lupus erythematosus by plasmapheresis," *Turkish Journal of Anesthesia and Reanimation*, vol. 43, no. 4, pp. 291–294, 2015.
[24] W. Ma, W. Bai, X. Wu, J. Zhao, M. Li, and X. Zeng, "Successful treatment of refractory thrombotic thrombocytopenic purpura associated with systemic lupus erythematosus with combination of plasma exchange and low-dose rituximab," *Lupus*, vol. 29, no. 14, pp. 1961–1967, 2020.
[25] C. Magro-Checa, E. J. Zirkzee, T. W. Huizinga, and G. M. Steup-Beekman, "Management of neuropsychiatric systemic lupus erythematosus: current approaches and future perspectives," *Drugs*, vol. 76, no. 4, pp. 459–483, 2016.
[26] A. Kronbichler, B. Brezina, L. F. Quintana, and D. R. Jayne, "Efficacy of plasma exchange and immunoadsorption in systemic lupus erythematosus and antiphospholipid syndrome: a systematic review," *Autoimmunity Reviews*, vol. 15, no. 1, pp. 38–49, 2016.
[27] F. Al Balushi, F. Humby, A. Mahto et al., "Mycophenolate mofetil inducing remission of lupus enteritis," *Lupus*, vol. 21, no. 5, pp. 556–558, 2012.
[28] T. Shirai, Y. Hirabayashi, R. Watanabe et al., "The use of tacrolimus for recurrent lupus enteritis: a case report," *Journal of Medical Case Reports*, vol. 4, no. 1, p. 150, 2010.
[29] J. Oh, Y. G. Kim, S. Lee, C. K. Lee, and B. J. L. Yoo, "Successful treatment of recurrent lupus enteritis with rituximab," *Lupus*, vol. 19, no. 2, pp. 220–222, 2010.
[30] S.-K. Kwok, S.-H. Seo, J. Ju et al., "Lupus enteritis: clinical characteristics, risk factor for relapse and association with anti-endothelial cell antibody," *Lupus*, vol. 16, no. 10, pp. 803–809, 2007.
[31] T. Y. Lian, C. J. Edwards, S. P. Chan, and H. H. Chng, "Reversible acute gastrointestinal syndrome associated with active systemic lupus erythematosus in patients admitted to hospital," *Lupus*, vol. 12, no. 8, pp. 612–616, 2003.

5

A Case of Acute Esophageal Necrosis from Unruptured Thoracic Aortic Aneurysm

Abhishek Polavarapu,[1] Dhineshreddy Gurala ,[2] Bindu Mudduluru,[2] Pretty Sara Idiculla,[3] Jobin Philipose,[2] Magda Daoud,[4] Naureen Narula,[5] and Vivek Gumaste[1]

[1]*Gastroenterology and Hepatology, Staten Island University Hospital, Northwell Health, Staten Island, New York, USA*
[2]*Internal Medicine, Staten Island University Hospital, Northwell Health, Staten Island, New York, USA*
[3]*Medicine, Sree Gokulam Medical College and Research Foundation, Trivandrum, India*
[4]*Department of Pulmonary and Critical Care, Staten Island University Hospital, Northwell Health, Staten Island, New York, USA*
[5]*Department of Gastroenterology and Hepatology, Richmond University Medical Center, Staten Island, New York, USA*

Correspondence should be addressed to Dhineshreddy Gurala; dineshgurala@gmail.com

Academic Editor: Shiro Kikuchi

Acute esophageal necrosis (AEN), also known as black esophagus due to its appearance on endoscopy, classically involves the distal esophagus (97% of cases). AEN affecting the midesophagus with sparing of the distal esophagus is rare and usually occurs in patients with thoracic aortic aneurysmal (TAA) rupture or aortic dissection. Herein, we report a unique case of AEN in the midesophagus in a patient with an unruptured and undissected TAA.

1. Introduction

AEN is also known as the "black esophagus" caused predominantly by hypoperfusion of esophagus and characterized by diffuse, circumferential, black-appearing distal esophageal mucosa that stops at the gastro-esophageal junction (GEJ) but can extend proximally to various lengths on esophago-gastro-duodenoscopy (EGD) [1, 2]. It is a rare disease, and prevalence was 0.001% to 0.2% in a retrospective endoscopy case series [3]. It is more common in older men than women with a ratio of 4 : 1 and a mean age of 68. Its prevalence is higher in people with underlying medical conditions like hypertension, diabetes mellitus, renal insufficiency, Pulmonary diseases, and cardiac diseases [2]. The esophagus is an expandable muscular organ connecting the pharynx with the stomach with a diverse blood supply. The upper esophagus derives its blood supply from descending branches of the inferior thyroid artery. Midesophagus is supplied by the bronchial and esophageal branches of the thoracic aorta. The distal esophagus is supplied by the branches of the left gastric and left inferior phrenic artery and is the least vascular compared to the proximal and middle esophagus, which makes it slightly more watershed and more susceptible to ischemic injury [2]. The etiology of AEN is multifactorial and results from a combination of tissue hypoperfusion, impaired local defense barriers, and the massive influx of gastric contents that overwhelm the esophageal mucosa [2]. Hypoperfusion can arise from a variety of causes such as acute blood loss, trauma, shock, sepsis, and congestive heart failure, which makes the distal esophagus more vulnerable to injury. Other risk factors include infections, vascular diseases, diabetes mellitus, medications, advanced malignancies, and malnutrition [2, 4–6]. Proposed pathophysiology has two hypotheses: the initial event is the low-flow vascular state and defect in mucosal system repair (as seen in malnourished and debilitated physiological states) which predisposes the esophageal mucosa to a severe topical injury. Upper gastrointestinal (GI) bleed is the most common clinical presentation of AEN in approximately 90% of patients, with or without hemodynamic compromise. Other symptoms include epigastric pain, chest pain, dysphagia, and signs of sepsis, including tachycardia and hypotension [7]. We report a case of AEN in the midesophagus in a critically ill patient with unruptured and undissected TAA.

2. Case Description

A 79-year-old female presented to the emergency department with near syncope. She denied chest pain or gastrointestinal symptoms. She had a history of hypertension, atrial fibrillation on coumadin and TAA of 5.5 cm in size, diagnosed one month prior, and scheduled for repair. Her vital signs were stable with a blood pressure of 122/62 mmHg and a heart rate of 81 beats/minute, afebrile. Her initial laboratory studies were stable except for elevated d-dimer of 2029 and subtherapeutic international normalized ratio (INR) of 1.1. Physical examination was positive for bibasilar crackles on auscultation of lung fields. Computed tomography angiogram (CTA) of the chest revealed an acute bilateral pulmonary embolism (PE) with stable TAA and mural thrombus in descending thoracic aorta (Figure 1). Echocardiogram showed evidence of right heart strain, and she was started on heparin.

On day two, the patient went into acute hypoxemic respiratory failure due to PE requiring intubation. She subsequently developed shock and was started on norepinephrine for pressure support. On day five, she had melena, the bloody gastric residue was found in the nasogastric tube and hemoglobin dropped from 12.2 g/dL to 7.7 g/dL. Heparin was stopped, two units of blood were transfused, and an inferior venae cava (IVC) filter was placed. Upper endoscopy revealed extensive, circumferential deep ulceration in midesophagus with wall irregularity, friable, sloughy mucosa, and blackish discoloration of mucosa likely esophageal necrosis (Figures 2 and 3). Distal esophagus, gastro-esophagus junction, stomach, and duodenum appeared normal. Biopsies were not taken to avoid the risk of esophageal perforation. At this time, upon review, her prior CT chest showed a large TAA with mural thrombus causing compression in the midesophagus correlating with the area where on endoscopy was found to have a black esophagus. After consulting with the vascular surgery team, it was deemed that the patient is unstable to be considered for aneurysm repair or thrombectomy.

The patient was managed supportively with bowel rest, proton pump inhibitor (pantoprazole) infusion, IV fluids, antibiotics, and norepinephrine. While her hemoglobin was being stabilized, on day 23, due to the severity of the necrosis, deterioration of the overall condition, and persistent sepsis, she went into pulseless electrical activity and died after unsuccessful resuscitation.

3. Discussion

AEN, also referred to as "black esophagus" or "necrotizing esophagitis," was first described in 1990 by Goldenberg [8]. After that, several case reports have described this finding in critically ill patients with comorbidities. Even though distal esophageal necrosis is common due to its vasculature, midesophageal necrosis has also been reported usually due to compression by hematoma formed after TAA rupture or after its repair or aortic dissection.

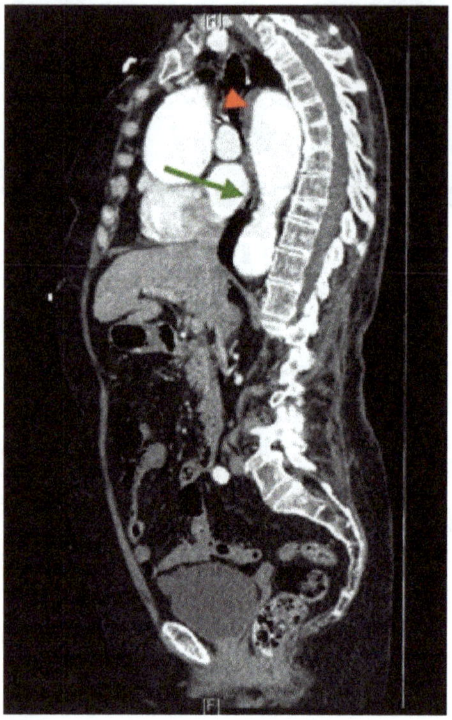

Figure 1: Sagittal section of CT angiogram of the chest showing thoracic aorta aneurysm of approx. 5.5 cm size causing extrinsic compression at midesophageal level (green arrow) along with intramural thrombus in the thoracic aorta (red arrowhead).

Watanabe et al. [9] described a case of esophageal necrosis secondary to ruptured thoracic aortic aneurysm resulting in mediastinal hematoma causing compression of the esophagus. Several other case reports of esophageal necrosis have been described after thoracic endovascular aortic repair (TEVAR) due to mediastinal hematoma (Tobisch et al. [10], Koizumi et al. [11], Abou-Al-Shaar et al. [12], Seto et al. [13]). In contrast to these cases, in our case, there was no evidence of rupture of TAA or mediastinal hematoma. The possible explanation for esophageal necrosis in our case is due to direct extrinsic esophageal compression secondary to enlarged aortic aneurysm (Figure 1), which can obliterate local venous return and arterial blood supply leading to infarction [14]. It is unlikely that a single etiological factor is responsible for this condition. The accepted hypothesis is a two-hit hypothesis. In our case, a decreased blood supply to the midesophagus by extrinsic compression of TAA is further exacerbated by low flow vascular state, hypotension from PE.

Endoscopy is the gold standard for diagnosing AEN. It appears as a circumferential black discoloration with underlying friable hemorrhagic tissue and a sharp transition to normal-appearing mucosa at the GEJ [5]. Although proximal involvement has been described, AEN usually involves the distal third of the esophagus, as it is the least vascular area in the esophagus. However, the involvement of midesophagus without distal esophagus is rare, which occurred in our case as a result of compression of TAA in the

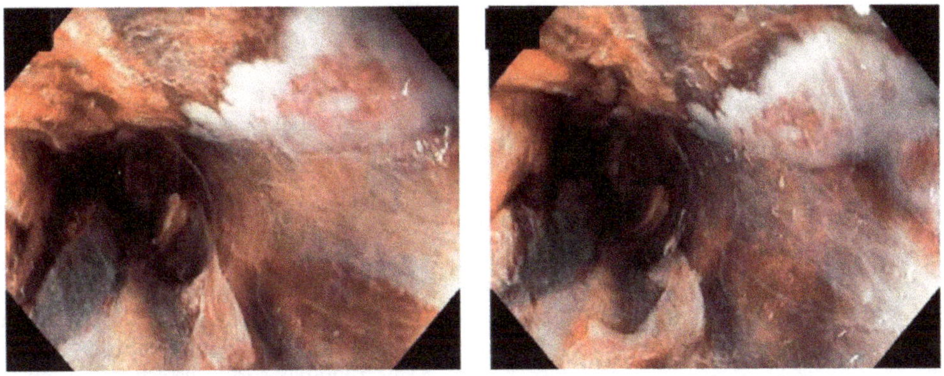

(a) (b)

Figure 2: Endoscopic images showing extensive circumferential esophageal ulcerations with blackish discoloration.

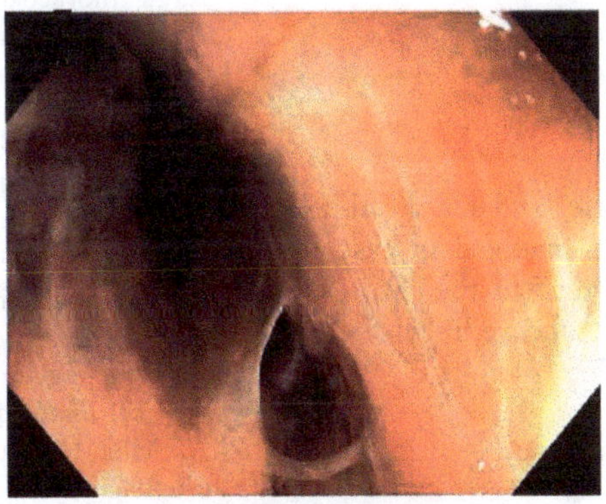

Figure 3: Endoscopic image showing friable esophageal mucosa, mucosal separation without active bleeding.

Table 1: Staging of AEN based on endoscopy findings.

Stage	Endoscopy findings
Stage 0	Prenecrotic viable esophagus
Stage 1	Diffuse, circumferential, black-appearing esophageal mucosa with occasional yellow exudates
Stage 2	Residual black areas in the esophagus, thick white exudates composed of necrotic debris covering friable pink mucosa
Stage 3	Normal endoscopic appearance, granulation tissue presents only microscopically

midesophagus and also decreased blood supply from esophageal arterial branches of the thoracic aorta due to mural thrombus in the TAA.

Staging of AEN based on endoscopy findings is mentioned in Table 1.

Biopsy differentiates AEN from other conditions such as malignant melanoma, acanthosis nigricans, coal dust deposition, pseudomelanosis, and melanocytosis of the esophagus [15, 16]. Biopsy is usually recommended but not required for the diagnosis [8].

AEN generally carries a poor prognosis with a mortality rate of 32% as these patients have multiple comorbidities like in our case. Esophageal perforation occurs as a complication in <7% of patients with AEN and requires urgent surgical intervention [2]. Other complications include mediastinitis and abscess formation. Esophageal stricture is a long-term complication likely to result from protective scar formation which has been reported in 25–40% of patients, common in stage 2 and 3 of AEN, and requires endoscopic dilatation [2].

Treatment mainly includes supportive care to increase organ perfusion with IV hydration, optimization of acid suppression using intravenous proton pump inhibitors, and treatment of underlying illness. Oral intake should be avoided for at least 24 hours, after which sucralfate suspension can be considered for its cryoprotective effects and its ability to bind pepsin and stimulate mucus secretion [17]. Empirical antibiotics should be initiated in suspected cases of esophageal perforation, unexplained fevers, rapid clinical decompensation, and immunocompromised individuals as in cirrhosis, AIDS, transplant recipient, and dialysis patients [18]. Surgical intervention in patients with AEN is reserved for perforated esophagus with resultant mediastinitis and abscess formation [19].

4. Conclusion

In summary, we described a case of esophageal necrosis as a result of a low flow state from PE (initial insult) that was exacerbated by compression from unruptured TAA in a critically ill patient and presented as upper GI bleed. AEN should be considered as one of the differential diagnosis of upper gastrointestinal bleed, especially in elderly patients with multiple comorbidities and hypotension in critically ill patients. Early diagnosis and management of AEN are necessary to prevent complications and to improve patient's outcome.

Disclosure

The abstract of this manuscript was presented as a poster at American College of Gastroenterology, (2017 https://www.eventscribe.com/2017/wcogacg2017/ajaxcalls/PosterInfo.asp?efp=S1lVTUxLQVozODMy&PosterID=116977&rnd=0.4019826).

Authors' Contributions

Dr. Polavarapu, Dr. Gurala, Dr. Philipose, and Dr. Mudduluru wrote the introduction and were involved in case description and discussion. Dr. Idiculla drafted the introduction, and Dr. Gumaste reviewed and edited the manuscript.

Acknowledgments

The authors thank Dr. Mansour for guiding them in choosing the radiological images.

References

[1] A. Sako, J. Kitayama, T. Inoue, S. Kaizaki, H. Nagawa, and H. Suzuki, "Black oesophagus—cause?" *Gut*, vol. 54, no. 2, p. 192, 2005.

[2] G. E. Gurvits, A. Shapsis, N. Lau, N. Gualtieri, and J. G. Robilotti, "Acute esophageal necrosis: a rare syndrome," *Journal of Gastroenterology*, vol. 42, no. 1, pp. 29–38, 2007.

[3] H. Khan, M. Ahmed, M. Daoud, J. Philipose, S. Ahmed, and L. Deeb, "Acute esophageal necrosis: a view in the dark," *Case Reports in Gastroenterology*, vol. 13, no. 1, pp. 25–31, 2019.

[4] M. Moretó, E. Ojembarrena, M. Zaballa, J. G. Tánago, and S. Ibánez, "Idiopathic acute esophageal necrosis: not necessarily a terminal event," *Endoscopy*, vol. 25, no. 8, pp. 534–538, 1993.

[5] M. Hoffman, E. Bash, S. A. Berger, M. Burke, and I. Yust, "Fatal necrotizing esophagitis due to *Penicillium chrysogenum* in a patient with acquired immunodeficiency syndrome," *European Journal of Clinical Microbiology & Infectious Diseases*, vol. 11, no. 12, pp. 1158–1160, 1992.

[6] Y.-H. Liu, Y.-S. Lin, H.-J. Chen, C.-Y. Tu, and W. Chen, "*Klebsiella pneumoniae* deep neck infection with acute necrotizing esophagitis," *South Medical Journal*, vol. 102, no. 2, p. 219, 2009.

[7] G. E. Gurvits and J. G. Robilotti, "Isolated proximal black esophagus: etiology and the role of tissue biopsy," *Gastrointestinal Endoscopy*, vol. 71, no. 3, p. 658, 2010.

[8] G. E. Gurvits, "Black esophagus: acute esophageal necrosis syndrome," *World Journal of Gastroenterology*, vol. 16, no. 26, pp. 3219–3225, 2010.

[9] S. Watanabe, R. Nagashima, Y. Shimazaki et al., "Esophageal necrosis and bleeding gastric ulcer secondary to ruptured thoracic aortic aneurysm," *Gastrointestinal Endoscopy*, vol. 50, no. 6, pp. 847–849, 1999.

[10] A. Tobisch, H. Ittrich, J. R. Izbicki, and A. M. Koenig, "Successful management of esophageal necrosis after endovascular repair of chronic type B aortic dissection," *The Annals of Thoracic Surgery*, vol. 98, no. 6, pp. 2209–2211, 2014.

[11] S. Koizumi, S. Yamaguchi, S. Asano, H. Fujita, T. Sueta, and S. Takeuchi, "Esophageal necrosis after endovascular repair for ruptured aortic dissection," *Asian Cardiovascular and Thoracic Annals*, vol. 25, no. 9, pp. 638–641, 2017.

[12] H. Abou-Al-Shaar, K. J. Zaza, M. A. Sharif, and S. Koussayer, "Free esophageal perforation following hybrid visceral debranching and distal endograft extension to repair a ruptured thoracoabdominal aortic aneurysm," *Vascular and Endovascular Surgery*, vol. 50, no. 7, pp. 502–506, 2016.

[13] T. Seto, D. Fukui, H. Tanaka et al., "Tracheo-bronchial obstruction and esophageal perforation after TEVAR for thoracic aortic rupture," *Annals of Vascular Diseases*, vol. 7, no. 4, pp. 421–425, 2014.

[14] A. Day and M. Sayegh, "Acute oesophageal necrosis: a case report and review of the literature," *International Journal of Surgery*, vol. 8, no. 1, pp. 6–14, 2010.

[15] R. Obermeyer, K. Kasirajan, V. Erzurum, and D. Chung, "Necrotizing esophagitis presenting as a black esophagus," *Surgical Endoscopy*, vol. 12, no. 12, pp. 1430–1433, 1998.

[16] A. Geller, H. Aguilar, L. Burgart, and C. J. Gostout, "The black esophagus," *The American Journal of Gastroenterology*, vol. 90, no. 12, pp. 2210–2212, 1995.

[17] M. Reichart, O. R. C. Busch, M. J. Bruno, and J. B. V. Lanschot, "Black esophagus: a view in the dark," *Diseases of the Esophagus*, vol. 13, no. 4, pp. 311–313, 2000.

[18] T. F. Mangan, A. T. Colley, and D. H. Wytock, "Antibiotic-associated acute necrotizing esophagitis," *Gastroenterology*, vol. 99, no. 3, p. 900, 1990.

[19] Y. H. Kim and S. Y. Choi, "Black esophagus with concomitant candidiasis developed after diabetic ketoacidosis," *World Journal of Gastroenterology*, vol. 13, no. 42, pp. 5662-5663, 2007.

6

Intraoperative Endoscopy in Transient Adult Jejunojejunal Intussusception

Takeshi Okamoto[1,2] **Hidekazu Suzuki**[2] **and Katsuyuki Fukuda**[1]

[1]*Department of Gastroenterology, St. Luke's International Hospital, 9-1 Akashicho, Chuo-ku, Tokyo 104-8560, Japan*
[2]*Department of Gastroenterology and Hepatology, Department of Internal Medicine, Tokai University School of Medicine, 143 Shimokasuya, Isehara, Kanagawa 259-1143, Japan*

Correspondence should be addressed to Takeshi Okamoto; tak@afia.jp

Academic Editor: Yoshihiro Moriwaki

Despite improvements in imaging modalities, causative lead points in adult intussusception may be difficult to diagnose. Such lead points can be malignant, causing recurrence or metastases if left unresected. We describe a case of transient adult jejunojejunal intussusception, in which intraoperative endoscopy was used to confirm the absence of a lead point. A 39-year-old woman with a history of laparoscopic oophorectomy presented with epigastric pain, nausea, and vomiting. Contrast computed tomography revealed jejunojejunal intussusception, with no visible lead point. Spontaneous reduction was confirmed during exploratory laparoscopy. After lysis of adhesions, intraoperative peroral jejunoscopy was performed with the surgeons' assistance. Endoscopy confirmed the absence of tumor, and bowel resection was avoided. No recurrence has been observed during 24 months of follow-up. Intraoperative endoscopy may provide additional reassurance for the absence of a lead point in cases where preoperative enteroscopy cannot be performed and no lead points can be identified on imaging.

1. Introduction

While intussusceptions in children are commonly idiopathic, adult intussusceptions (AI) generally have a causative lead point. Enteric intussusceptions, the most common type accounting for about 50% of AIs, have been reported to result from malignant tumors in 22.5% of cases, with metastatic carcinoma being the most common malignant lead point [1]. On the other hand, about 15% of AIs are idiopathic, with no apparent lead point.

One type of AI, classified as idiopathic by some authors, is caused by adhesions resulting from prior surgery [1–3]. Truly idiopathic AI may be caused by mechanisms such as bowel hyperactivity and be transient, causing chronic, intermittent, or nonspecific symptoms [4, 5]. While exploratory laparoscopy with bowel resection remains the most widely accepted treatment for AI, the need for such interventions has recently been brought into question [6, 7]. Almost 5% of AI patients were treated conservatively in a meta-analysis [1]. On the other hand, avoiding surgery may occasionally come at the cost of missing a malignant small bowel tumor, which may be undetected despite recent advances in imaging modalities [8–12]. Such an event may have various devastating results, including recurrence and metastatic disease.

Although not always possible preoperatively, enteroscopy offers an alternative to confirm the absence of a lead point without bowel resection. Herein, we report a case of intraoperative endoscopy performed on a patient with jejunojejunal AI which demonstrated the absence of tumor in the jejunum, providing additional reassurance that bowel resection could be avoided.

2. Case Presentation

A 39-year-old woman presented with epigastric pain, intermittent nausea, frequent vomiting, and loss of appetite over the last seven days. She denied weight loss. She could pass gas but had not passed stool over the last four days. She was able to tolerate a full meal the night before presenting to the hospital, but nausea and vomiting had resumed within several hours.

Her medical history was significant only for laparoscopic oophorectomy for a left ovarian cyst almost 20 years prior. She was taking no medications, herbal remedies, or nutritional supplements. She admitted to chronic alcohol abuse with frequent visits to the emergency department due to alcohol intoxication, but had never smoked cigarettes. She denied any recent sexual contact, overseas travel, raw food ingestion, or sick contacts.

Upon presentation, the patient appeared to be in moderate distress. Her respiratory rate was 24 breaths per minute, but vital signs were otherwise stable. She complained of discomfort on palpation of the epigastric region. The upper abdomen was soft but mildly distended. No mass was palpated. Small scars from previous laparoscopy were noted.

Laboratory results were only remarkable for a mildly elevated C-reactive protein of 0.44 mg/dL. Esophagogastroduodenoscopy (EGD) performed 20 hours after the patient's last meal revealed a mildly distended stomach with significant food residue in the esophagus and stomach (Figure 1). The patient vomited copious food residue during the procedure, precluding a thorough examination for fear of aspiration. No gross abnormalities were found up to the third part of the duodenum. Food residue and intraluminal air were suctioned to the extent possible at the end of the examination.

Despite the patient's ability to pass gas, an emergency computed tomography (CT) scan was conducted to rule out small bowel obstruction. CT without contract was largely unremarkable, with no visible signs of tumor or bowel obstruction (Figure 2(a)). However, CT with contrast taken several minutes later revealed the "target sign," a bowel-in-bowel configuration measuring 7 cm in the proximal jejunum with invaginated mesentery (Figure 2(b)). No lead point was identified. No proximal distension was observed, most likely as a result of vomiting and suction during EGD. The patient was diagnosed with jejunojejunal intussusception, most likely of a transient nature.

While the possibility of spontaneous reduction was explained, the patient wished to undergo exploratory laparoscopy due to the severity of her symptoms. The surgeons also agreed to exploratory laparoscopy in light of the severe obstructive symptoms, surgical history with possible adhesions, and possible recurrence if left untreated. Consent for intraoperative endoscopy was also obtained to evaluate the jejunum for a possible lead point, as the patient was not in a condition to undergo preoperative enteroscopy.

Exploratory laparoscopy was performed the next day. Severe jejunal hyperactivity was observed intermittently throughout the laparoscopy. However, no intussusception was observed, suggesting spontaneous reduction. Tumors and segmental edema in the proximal jejunum were also notably absent. Adhesions from previous laparoscopic oophorectomy were observed near a port placed in the right lower quadrant (Figure 3(a)). While adhesiotomy was performed, the adhesions were distant from the proximal jejunum and appeared as an unlikely cause of intussusception.

Intraoperative peroral jejunoscopy was performed with a long colonoscope (PCF-H290L, Olympus Corp., Tokyo, Japan) and carbon dioxide insufflation. A thorough laparoscopic exploration was completed prior to commencing intraoperative endoscopy, as endoscopic insufflation would hinder the laparoscopic view. The surgeons used laparoscopic grasping forceps to apply gentle pressure to the stomach to facilitate scope insertion (Figure 3(b)). When the endoscope reached the jejunum, the laparoscopic camera was pointed to a location in the jejunum believed to be distal to the reduced intussusception. Forceps were also gently placed at this location to facilitate insufflation (Figure 3(c)). The endoscope was inserted until light from the laparoscopic camera was visualized, confirming the absence of tumors or other lesions which may serve as a lead point for intussusception (Figure 4). Short bowel resection was therefore not performed. The patient was diagnosed with transient jejunojejunal intussusception, more likely associated with chronic alcoholism rather than adhesions from previous surgery.

The patient experienced complete resolution of her symptoms after the surgery. The postsurgical course was uneventful and the patient was discharged two days later, with instructions to stop drinking alcohol. No recurrence was observed during 24 months of follow-up.

3. Discussion

AI presents two problems for the patient: symptoms relating to bowel obstruction and a potentially malignant lead point.

AI can be difficult to diagnose due to its rarity and the chronic, nonspecific nature of its symptoms [1, 4]. In general, CT has a sensitivity of 83% in diagnosing the etiology of small bowel obstruction and of 82% in diagnosing small bowel tumors as the cause [13]. Helical CT-enteroclysis had particularly high pooled sensitivity (92.8%) and specificity (99.2%) for small bowel tumors in a meta-analysis [9]. On the other hand, only 52% of enteric AIs were recognized preoperatively in a study of 44 patients [7]. Another study of 318 patients found that AI patients presented with symptoms of complete and partial bowel obstruction in only 27% and 15% of cases, respectively [8]. CT failed to identify lead points in reports of jejunal AI caused by heterotopic gastric mucosa, laterally spreading tumor, and gastrointestinal stromal tumor [10–12].

While symptoms can be relieved by reduction or bowel resection, recurrence has been reported in about 6.5% of all AI cases [1]. This figure may be higher in enteric AI, as one

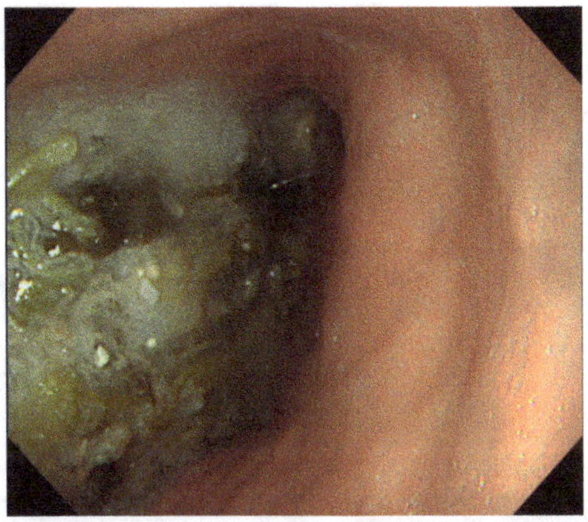

Figure 1: Esophagogastroduodenoscopy performed 20 hours after the patient's last meal revealed significant food residue in the esophagus and stomach, suggesting possible bowel obstruction.

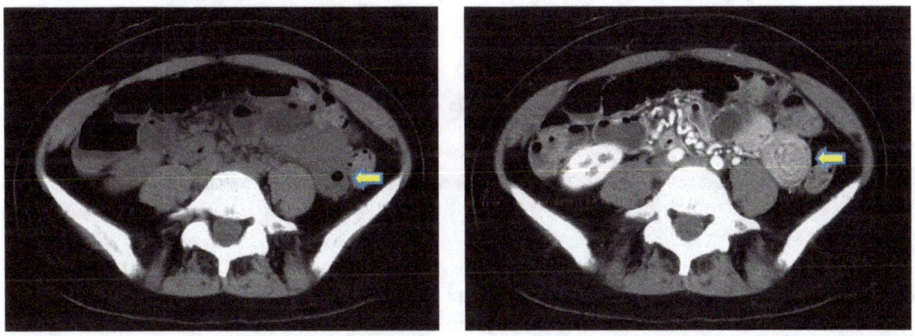

(a) (b)

Figure 2: (a) Computed tomography (CT) without contract was largely unremarkable, with no visible signs of tumor or bowel obstruction in the jejunum (arrow). (b) CT with contract taken several minutes later revealed a bowel-in-bowel configuration with invaginated mesentery, consistent with jejunojejunal intussusception (arrow). No mass was visualized.

report found recurrences in 21 of 230 enteric AI patients (9.1%) [8]. All recurrences occurred at the site of the initial AI and 63% required surgery. Recurrence occurs frequently in celiac disease, Crohn's disease, and polyposis syndromes such as Peutz–Jeghers syndrome due to their multifocal involvement [14–16]. Recurrence has also been reported in idiopathic enteric AI [17].

Transient intussusceptions with spontaneous reduction are very common in children as they are generally idiopathic in nature, particularly when the length of the intussusception is less than 3 cm [18, 19]. Similarly, intussusception length of less than 3.5 cm is an independent predictor for self-limiting AI [20]. The diagnosis of AI on CT may be more common than once believed, in part due to improvements in imaging technology. In a study of 37 CT diagnoses of AI, 31 were cared conservatively and none required surgery during a mean follow-up of 5.2 months [20]. Although we suspected transient AI based on the discrepancy between the plain and contrast CT scans in our case, exploratory laparoscopy was believed to be indicated due to the length of the intussusception (7 cm), severity of symptoms, possibility of recurrence, and the wishes of the patient.

As the adhesions observed during laparoscopy were distant from the site of intussusception, we suspect that bowel hyperactivity due to chronic alcoholism played a role in the pathogenesis of AI in our case. The effects of alcohol on small bowel motility depend on the alcohol concentration of consumed beverages and chronicity of alcohol use, with chronic consumption of large doses of alcohol accelerating small bowel transit [21, 22]. There is only one report of small bowel intussusception in a patient with chronic alcoholism, although various other factors such as malnutrition and brown bowel syndrome were also present in that case [23]. The role of alcohol use in transient AI has not been studied; the history of alcohol use is generally missing from case reports on AI. While alcohol is also associated with diarrhea due to inhibited water and sodium absorption as well as mucosal injury in the duodenum and upper jejunum, none of these findings were observed in our case [24]. The use of scopolamine during preoperative EGD may have temporarily reduced bowel hyperactivity, contributing to temporary resolution of AI before the CT scan.

Both antegrade enteroscopy and retrograde enteroscopy have been used to diagnose various types of lead points including gastrointestinal stromal tumor, inverted Meckel's diverticulum, inflammatory fibroid polyp, Peutz–Jeghers syndrome, heterotopic pancreatic mass, malignant melanoma, and mass-forming fibrogranulation from a healed

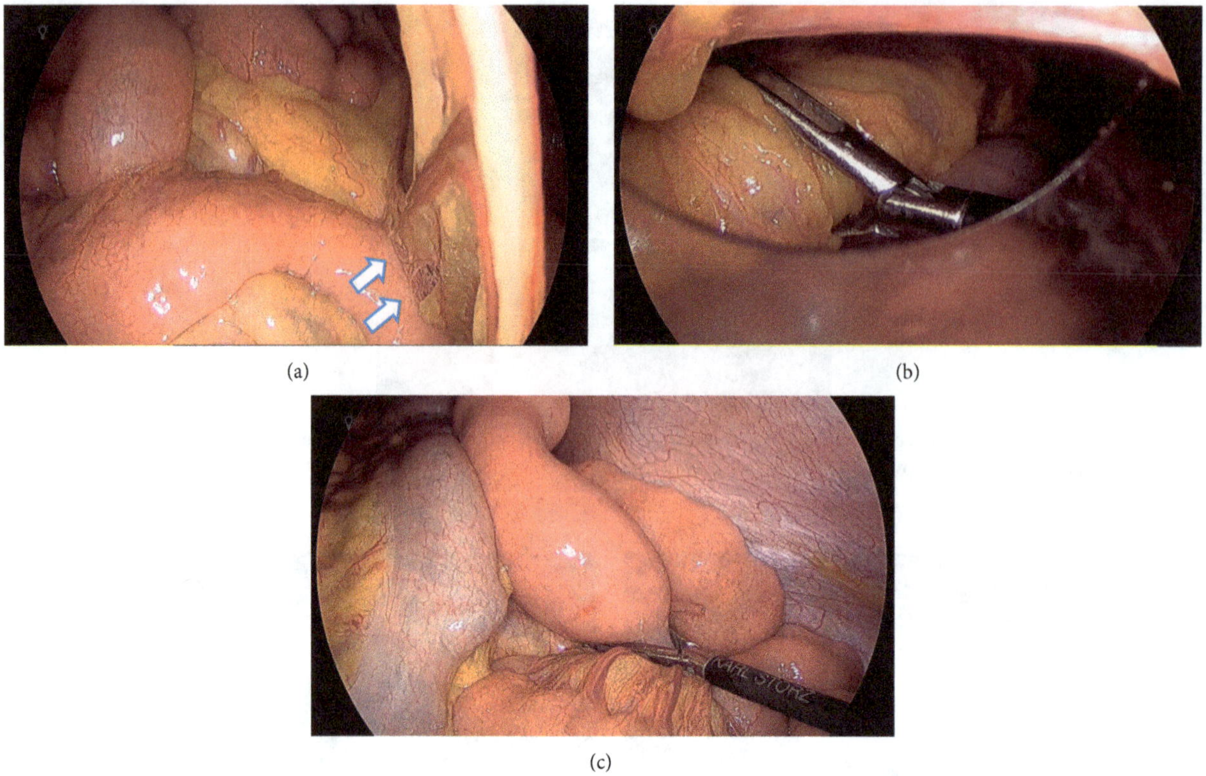

FIGURE 3: (a) Adhesions from previous laparoscopic oophorectomy observed near a port placed in the right lower quadrant (arrows). (b) The surgeons used laparoscopic grasping forceps to apply gentle pressure to the stomach to facilitate scope insertion during intraoperative peroral jejunoscopy. (c) When the endoscope reached the jejunum, the laparoscopic camera was pointed distal to the suspected location of the reduced intussusception to signal the desired destination for endoscopic viewing. Forceps were also gently placed at this location to facilitate insufflation.

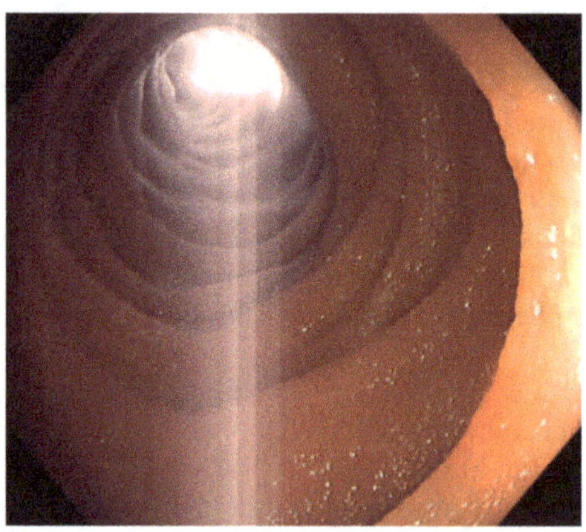

FIGURE 4: Light from the laparoscopic camera showing through the jejunal wall confirmed passage of the endoscope beyond the site of intussusception.

ulcer [25–31]. Preoperative enteroscopy can also identify signs of bowel ischemia, which occurs in about 15% of cases [1]. Furthermore, the balloon used in double-balloon enteroscopy has also been shown to be useful in achieving reduction of the intussusception [25, 28].

Endoscopy has been used in various surgical procedures such as laparoscopic endoscopic cooperative surgery, confirmation of anastomoses during gastrointestinal surgery, and in exploratory laparotomy for obscure gastrointestinal bleeding [32–34]. Intraoperative endoscopy can be performed via the peroral route, the transanal route, and enterotomies, achieving total small bowel visualization in 57–100% of cases [34]. Advantages over single-balloon or double-balloon enteroscopy include one-stage intervention when a tumorous lead point is discovered, the surgeon;s manual assistance during scope insertion, the use of enterotomies, and performance under general anesthesia in the operating theater [35, 36]. However, single-balloon enteroscopy and double-balloon enteroscopy have reduced the need for intraoperative endoscopy for diagnostic purposes, which is now only used when preoperative enteroscopy cannot be performed or when the diagnosis remains in question [37]. In our case, preoperative enteroscopy was not realistic without deep sedation and intubation, as copious vomiting, strong gag reflexes, and body movement were observed throughout the preoperative EGD. As the site of intussusception could be reached with a long colonoscope, we avoided the use of intraoperative double-balloon enteroscopy which would require additional time, cost, and preparation.

Reports of intraoperative endoscopy in the setting of AI are mainly limited to Peutz–Jeghers syndrome [38, 39]. There are isolated reports of intraoperative endoscopy for AI due to Meckel's diverticuli, cavernous hemangiomas, and duodenal pseudopolyps [40–42]. To the extent of our search, there are no reports in the literature on intraoperative endoscopy in suspected transient AI. However, it is difficult to be confident that there is no lead point, as CT scans can give false-negative results. Patients are often unable to tolerate preoperative enteroscopy, and capsule endoscopy is contraindicated in AI presenting with small bowel obstruction.

Insertion of the long colonoscope could be achieved without fluoroscopy with the surgeons' assistance. Although surgeons' hands in a laparotomy would be ideal, grasping forceps during laparoscopy provided helpful resistance during scope insertion in our case. The camera light clearly showed the planned destination for the enteroscopy in an otherwise uniform bowel. Intubation under general anesthesia allowed for a painless procedure with no risk of aspiration.

In conclusion, we report a case of transient jejunojejunal AI in which the absence of tumor was confirmed by intraoperative endoscopy. Intraoperative endoscopy may be helpful to assess the need for small bowel resection when no lead point can be identified on preoperative imaging and preoperative enteroscopy cannot be performed.

Acknowledgments

The authors would like to thank Dr. Shuntaro Hirose and Dr. Akihiro Suzuki, Department of Surgery, St. Luke's International Hospital for performing the laparoscopy.

References

[1] K. D. Hong, J. Kim, W. Ji, and S. D. Wexner, "Adult intussusception: a systematic review and meta-analysis," *Techniques in Coloproctology*, vol. 23, no. 4, pp. 315–324, 2019.

[2] M. G. Sarr, D. M. Nagorney, and D. C. McIlrath, "Postoperative intussusception in the adult," *Archives of Surgery*, vol. 116, no. 2, pp. 144–148, 1981.

[3] F. Agha, "Intussusception in adults," *American Journal of Roentgenology*, vol. 146, no. 3, pp. 527-531, 1986.

[4] O. Catalano, "Transient small bowel intussusception: CT findings in adults," *The British Journal of Radiology*, vol. 70, no. 836, pp. 805–808, 1997.

[5] T. E. Napora, K. E. Henry, T. J. Lovett, and M. S. Beeson, "Transient adult jejunal intussusception," *The Journal of Emergency Medicine*, vol. 24, no. 4, pp. 395–400, 2003.

[6] N. Aydin, A. Roth, and S. Misra, "Surgical versus conservative management of adult intussusception: case series and review," *International Journal of Surgery Case Reports*, vol. 20, pp. 142-146, 2016.

[7] M. Barussaud, N. Regenet, X. Briennon et al., "Clinical spectrum and surgical approach of adult intussusceptions: a multicentric study," *International Journal of Colorectal Disease*, vol. 21, no. 8, pp. 834–839, 2006.

[8] M. A. Amr, S. F. Polites, M. Alzghari, E. O. Onkendi, T. E. Grotz, and M. D. Zielinski, "Intussusception in adults and the role of evolving computed tomography technology," *The American Journal of Surgery*, vol. 209, no. 3, pp. 580–583, 2015.

[9] P. Soyer, M. Aout, C. Hoeffel, E. Vicaut, V. Placé, and M. Boudiaf, "Helical CT-enteroclysis in the detection of small-bowel tumours: a meta-analysis," *European Radiology*, vol. 23, no. 2, pp. 388–399, 2013.

[10] K. R. Ahn, J. S. Koo, H. I. Kim et al., "Endoscopic treatment of jejunal heterotopic gastric mucosa that caused recurrent intussusception," *Clinical Endoscopy*, vol. 50, no. 6, pp. 605–608, 2017.

[11] A. Ponte, R. Pinho, A. Rodrigues et al., "Sporadic jejunal lateral spreading tumor: a rare cause of recurrent jejunojejunal intussusception," *GE-Portuguese Journal of Gastroenterology*, vol. 24, no. 3, pp. 154-155, 2017.

[12] J. J. Sam, R. Mustard, G. Kandel et al., "Colonoscopy leads to a diagnosis of a jejunal gastrointestinal stromal tumour (GIST)," *Gastroenterology Research*, vol. 4, pp. 277–282, 2011.

[13] Z. Li, L. Zhang, X. Liu, F. Yuan, and B. Song, "Diagnostic utility of CT for small bowel obstruction: systematic review and meta-analysis," *PLoS One*, vol. 14, no. 12, Article ID e0226740, 2019.

[14] A. D. Beggs, A. R. Latchford, H. F. A. Vasen et al., "Peutz-Jeghers syndrome: a systematic review and recommendations for management," *Gut*, vol. 59, no. 7, pp. 975–986, 2010.

[15] T. A. Gonda, S.-U.-Z. Khan, J. Cheng, S. K. Lewis, M. Rubin, and P. H. R. Green, "Association of intussusception and celiac disease in adults," *Digestive Diseases and Sciences*, vol. 55, no. 10, pp. 2899–2903, 2010.

[16] S. M. Sainaba, A. S. Ganapath, A. Sivakumar, A. V. Gayathri, and I. P. Yadev, "Adult intussusception at a tertiary care center: a retrospective study," *Nigerian Journal of Surgery: Official Publication of the Nigerian Surgical Research Society*, vol. 26, pp. 63–65, 2020.

[17] N. Nkwam, A. Desai, and S. Radley, "Adult idiopathic jejuno-ileal intussusception," *Case Reports*, vol. 2010, Article ID bcr0520103050, 2010.

[18] A. Kornecki, A. Daneman, O. Navarro, B. Connolly, D. Manson, and D. J. Alton, "Spontaneous reduction of intussusception: clinical spectrum, management and outcome," *Pediatric Radiology*, vol. 30, no. 1, pp. 58–63, 2000.

[19] Q. Wang, M. Luo, X. Xie, Y. Wu, and B. Xiang, "Can intussusceptions of small bowel and colon be transient? A prospective study," *European Journal of Pediatrics*, vol. 178, no. 10, pp. 1537–1544, 2019.

[20] N. Lvoff, R. S. Breiman, F. V. Coakley, Y. Lu, and R. S. Warren, "Distinguishing features of self-limiting adult small-bowel intussusception identified at CT," *Radiology*, vol. 227, no. 1, pp. 68–72, 2003.

[21] S. Grad, L. Abenavoli, and D. Dumitrascu, "The effect of alcohol on gastrointestinal motility," *Reviews on Recent Clinical Trials*, vol. 11, no. 3, pp. 191–195, 2016.

[22] F. Izbéki, T. Wittmann, S. Csáti, E. Jeszenszky, and J. Lonovics, "Opposite effects of acute and chronic administration of alcohol on gastric emptying and small bowel transit in rat," *Alcohol and Alcoholism*, vol. 36, no. 4, pp. 304–308, 2001.
[23] W. M. Drake, T. A. Winter, S. K. Price, and S. J. O'Keefe, "Small bowel intussusception and brown bowel syndrome in association with severe malnutrition," *The American Journal of Gastroenterology*, vol. 91, pp. 1450–1452, 1996.
[24] C. Bode and J. Christian Bode, "Effect of alcohol consumption on the gut," *Best Practice & Research Clinical Gastroenterology*, vol. 17, no. 4, pp. 575–592, 2003.
[25] E. Rahimi, S. Guha, O. Chughtai, A. Ertan, and N. Thosani, "Role of enteroscopy in the diagnosis and management of adult small-bowel intussusception," *Gastrointestinal Endoscopy*, vol. 84, no. 5, pp. 863-864, 2016.
[26] Y. Kawasaki, S. Shinozaki, T. Yano et al., "Intussusception due to an inverted Meckel's diverticulum diagnosed by double-balloon enteroscopy," *Case Reports in Gastroenterology*, vol. 11, pp. 632–636, 2017.
[27] T. Miyata, H. Yamamoto, H. Kita et al., "A case of inflammatory fibroid polyp causing small-bowel intussusception in which retrograde double-balloon enteroscopy was useful for the preoperative diagnosis," *Endoscopy*, vol. 36, no. 4, pp. 344–347, 2004.
[28] Y. Miura, H. Yamamoto, K. Sunada et al., "Reduction of ileoileal intussusception by using double-balloon endoscopy in Peutz-Jeghers syndrome (with video)," *Gastrointestinal Endoscopy*, vol. 72, no. 3, pp. 658-659, 2010.
[29] T. Peeraphatdit, T. C. Smyrk, and G. L. Alexander, "Recurrent jejunal intussusception caused by heterotopic pancreas mass," *Clinical Gastroenterology and Hepatology*, vol. 15, no. 12, pp. e175–e176, 2017.
[30] K. Kouladouros, D. Gärtner, S. Münch, M. Paul, and M. R. Schön, "Recurrent intussusception as initial manifestation of primary intestinal melanoma: case report and literature review," *World Journal of Gastroenterology*, vol. 21, no. 10, pp. 3114–3120, 2015.
[31] T. Okamoto and K. Fukuda, "Ileocolic intussusception caused by mass-forming fibro-granulation from healed ulcer masquerading as small bowel lipoma," *Clinical Journal of Gastroenterology*, vol. 14, no. 2, pp. 522–530, 2021.
[32] M. Sakon, M. Takata, H. Seki, K. Hayashi, Y. Munakata, and N. Tateiwa, "A novel combined laparoscopic-endoscopic cooperative approach for duodenal lesions," *Journal of Laparoendoscopic & Advanced Surgical Techniques*, vol. 20, no. 6, pp. 555–558, 2010.
[33] Y. Sakanoue, K. Nakao, Y. Shoji, H. Yanagi, M. Kusunoki, and J. Utsunomiya, "Intraoperative colonoscopy," *Surgical Endoscopy*, vol. 7, no. 2, pp. 84–87, 1993.
[34] T. A. Bowden Jr., V. H. Hooks, and A. R. Mansberger Jr., "Intraoperative gastrointestinal endoscopy," *Annals of Surgery*, vol. 191, no. 6, pp. 680–687, 1980.
[35] S. Bonnet, R. Douard, G. Malamut, C. Cellier, and P. Wind, "Intraoperative enteroscopy in the management of obscure gastrointestinal bleeding," *Digestive and Liver Disease*, vol. 45, no. 4, pp. 277–284, 2013.
[36] V. Wadhwa, S. Sethi, S. Tewani et al., "A meta-analysis on efficacy and safety: single-balloon vs. double-balloon enteroscopy," *Gastroenterology Report*, vol. 3, no. 2, pp. 148–155, 2015.
[37] T. Voron, G. Rahmi, S. Bonnet et al., "Intraoperative enteroscopy," *Gastrointestinal Endoscopy Clinics of North America*, vol. 27, no. 1, pp. 153–170, 2017.
[38] R. G. Panos, F. G. Opelka, and J. J. Nogueras, "Peutz-Jeghers syndrome. A call for intraoperative enteroscopy," *The American Surgeon*, vol. 56, pp. 331–333, 1990.
[39] E. M. H. Mathus-Vliegen and G. N. J. Tytgat, "Intraoperative endoscopy: technique, indications, and results," *Gastrointestinal Endoscopy*, vol. 32, no. 6, pp. 381–384, 1986.
[40] M. Kopácová, J. Bures, L. Vykouril et al., "Intraoperative enteroscopy: ten years' experience at a single tertiary center," *Surgical Endoscopy*, vol. 21, pp. 1111–1116, 2007.
[41] Y. Wang, X. Zhao, and X. You, "Blue rubber bleb nevus syndrome coexisted with intestinal intussusception: a case report," *The Pan African Medical Journal*, vol. 17, p. 212, 2014.
[42] B. S. de Bakker, S. S. K. S. Phoa, M. Kara et al., "The vanishing duodenal polyp: mesenteric invagination presenting as duodenal pseudopolyp," *BMJ Case Reports*, vol. 2017, Article ID bcr2016214998, 2017.

A Novel Cause of Biliary Peritonitis after Endoscopic Retrograde Cholangiopancreatography: Case Report and Literature Review

Andrija Karačić,[1] Paula Batur,[2] Domagoj Štritof,[1] Taro Fukui,[3] Branko Bakula,[1] and Inka Kekez[4]

[1]*Department of General Surgery, Clinical Hospital Sveti Duh, Zagreb, Croatia*
[2]*School of Medicine, University of Zagreb, Zagreb, Croatia*
[3]*Department of Surgery, Saitama Medical Center, Jichi Medical University, Saitama, Japan*
[4]*Department of Radiology, Clinical Hospital Sveti Duh, Zagreb, Croatia*

Correspondence should be addressed to Andrija Karačić; karacic.andrija@gmail.com

Academic Editor: Olga I. Giouleme

Background. Endoscopic retrograde cholangiopancreatography (ERCP) can lead to several complications such as duodenal or bile duct perforation. The incidence of pneumoperitoneum post-ERCP is rarely seen (<1%) and is associated with perforations of the duodenum or common bile duct in therapeutic ERCP after sphincterotomy. In this case, we disclose a novel cause of biliary peritonitis after ERCP. *Case Presentation.* A 65-year-old man presented with abdominal pain and distended abdomen after uneventful ERCP with sphincterotomy. An abdominal computed tomography (CT) was performed whose finding indicated duodenal perforation. The patient was rushed to an emergency laparotomy where only a rupture of an otherwise normal subcapsular intrahepatic bile duct was found. The surrounding liver parenchyma was healthy. The cause of this condition was probably post-ERCP pneumobilia and the increase of pressure in the biliary tract. *Conclusions.* This is the first case in literature describing the rupture of a subcapsular healthy bile duct as cause of biliary peritonitis after ERCP. This case also suggests that in the management of post-ERCP complications, the cooperation of radiologists and surgeons is vital for the patient's wellbeing.

1. Background

Endoscopic retrograde cholangiopancreatography (ERCP) has, in its more than 50 years of clinical practice, been proven to be a relatively safe procedure not only in the diagnosis but also treatment of biliary and pancreatic diseases [1]. The main advantage of ERCP above its alternative, hepatobiliary surgery, is lower morbidity and mortality [2]. The most common complications of ERCP are infections such as cholangitis and pancreatitis, bleeding, or intestinal perforation [3]. Some therapeutic additional options, especially sphincterotomy, increase the risk of intestinal perforation [4]. Iatrogenic post-ERCP duodenal perforation is regarded as a common complication, while intrahepatic bile duct ruptures are rare and have been associated in case reports with surgically damaged liver tissue, liver metastasis, and abscesses [5, 6]. In our case report, the radiologist found the biliary peritonitis to be a consequence of duodenal perforation; however, the surgical team intraoperatively identified a ruptured, but otherwise, healthy subcapsular hepatic bile duct as the cause of the biliary peritonitis. A literature review was performed for similar cases, and no case of healthy hepatic bile duct rupture causing biliary peritonitis after ERCP has been reported. Written informed consent has been given by the patient. The following case report has been reported in line with the SCARE criteria [7].

2. Case Presentation

A 65-year-old male was referred to the gastroenterology department with obstructive icterus. His medical history was remarkable for arterial hypertension, gastric ulcer, and chronic gastritis, diverticulosis of the colon and sideropenic anemia. He presented with epigastric abdominal pain, nausea, and heartburn. His physical examination revealed icterus of the skin and conjunctiva. His bilirubin was found to be elevated (107 μmol/l). AST and ALT were 114 IU/l and 217 IU/l, respectively. The WBC count was 10.42×10^3/mm [3], and segments were 24.7%.

Ultrasound revealed an elongated gallbladder (10.5 cm) filled with sludge and tiny concrements, and the common bile duct was normal in diameter, without visible intraluminal substrate. The liver was slightly enlarged with hyperechogenic parenchyma diffusely. Computed tomography (CT) of the abdomen showed normal liver structure and an enlarged gallbladder without signs of pathological changes in the wall or lumen. MRCP showed choledocholithiasis, no signs of common bile duct dilation, and normal intrahepatic bile ducts (Figure 1).

He underwent ERCP for choledocholithiasis. Access to the major papilla next to a periampullar diverticulum was obtained, and a widened common bile duct was shown with small concrements prepapillary. A sphincterotomy and concrement extraction with a balloon was performed. The procedure passed without complications.

While waking up from the sedation, the patient immediately complained about abdominal pain. The gastroenterologist found the abdomen to be distended and referred the patient to an urgent CT of the abdomen. The WBC was 10.42×10^3/mm [3]. On CT, free air was found around the duodenum in level of the papilla in the retroperitoneum and around the liver equaling pneumoperitoneum and pneumoretroperitoneum (Figure 2). Postprocedural pneumobilia in the gallbladder, cystic duct, common bile duct, and intrahepatic bile ducts was found. Free contrast was found around the gastric fundus (Figure 3), paracolical, and pelvis, and the radiologist suspected duodenal perforation.

The patient was referred urgently to the general surgery department. The patient's abdomen was found to be distended with signs of peritonitis, no audible peristalsis. The patient was rushed to an emergency laparotomy. Intraoperative biliary peritonitis was found. After thorough exploration of the upper abdomen and kocherization of the duodenum and head of the pancreas, no perforation of the duodenum or common bile duct was found. Hence, retroperitoneal perforation as the source of the intraperitoneal biliary collection could be excluded. Only when removing the liver retractor on the anterior side of the III, liver segment ruptured, but otherwise, normally appearing bile duct was found with bile secretion into the peritoneal cavity (Figure 4). The defect was closed with sutures. A choledochotomy was performed, and a T-drainage positioned to facilitate the biliary drainage. Cholecystectomy, lymphadenectomy, and omentectomy were performed too. Since the site of the intrahepatic bile duct rupture was clearly seen, no indication for an intraoperative cholangiography was found; hence, the rupture of the intrahepatic bile duct was not confirmed radiologically during surgery. The procedure ran without complications.

The postoperative recovery was uneventful. A cholangiography was performed which excluded the presence of any aberrant intrahepatic bile ducts (Figure 5). The patient

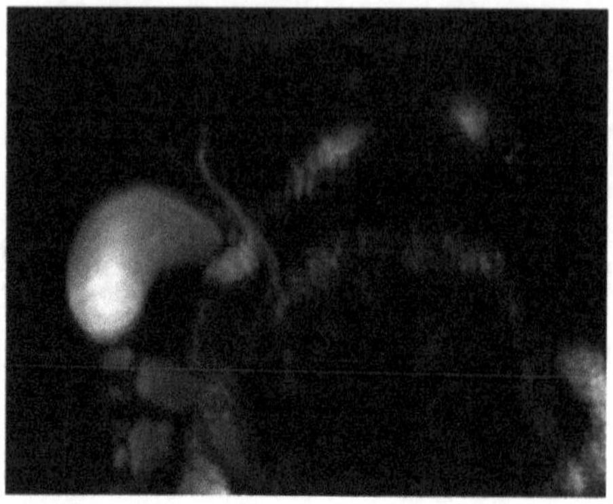

Figure 1: MRCP—choledocholithiasis; no signs of common bile duct dilation and normal intrahepatic bile ducts.

did not develop jaundice postoperatively. The patient was discharged on POD 15.

3. Discussion

The occurrence of duodenal and common bile duct perforations post-ERCP is overall rare (1%) [8], but it is most commonly the cause of biliary peritonitis and pneumoperitoneum post-ERCP [9].

In the context of post-ERCP intestinal perforations, duodenal perforations are regarded as a comparably common post-ERCP complication [10]. The perforations are mostly located in the duodenal wall or perivaterian and are most frequently caused by sphincterotomy or guide wire, less frequently by the endoscope itself or through stent placement [11]. Typical clinical signs of perforation are epigastric and back pain, tenderness with or without signs of peritoneal irritation, but can also be surgical emphysema, tachycardia, and fever [11]. Early diagnosis and prompt treatment is essential in the management of post-ERCP duodenal perforation [12]. Computed tomography has proven to be the most useful imaging method [13]. There are several classifications being used for this condition, but the most frequently used is the Stapfer classification [14], which besides the anatomical localization also includes the mechanism and severity of injury. The treatment can be conservative or surgical, although in recent times, endoscopic treatment has been more and more advocated [15]. The decision depends on the patient's condition, mechanism of injury, and localization of the perforation and degree of its containment [16]. Although, historically, the surgical approach was preferred [17], today, in the majority of cases, conservative treatment is being deployed which consists of nil per mouth, gastric decompression via a nasogastric or nasoduodenal tube, broad spectrum antibiotics, and frequent reevaluation [11]. The surgical management is based on two principles: control of sepsis and perforation repair with or without diversion [18]. Today, the mortality from this condition is around 6% [19] and when compared to earlier literature has almost halved.

On the other hand, the development of intrahepatic bile duct ruptures resulting in biliary peritonitis, and pneumoperitoneum is extremely rare [8]. In literature, the

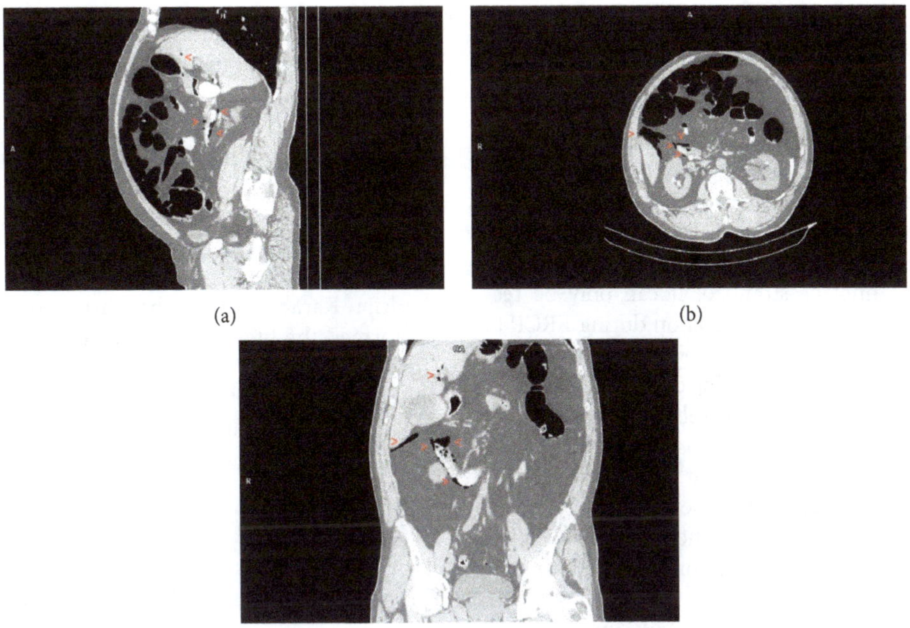

FIGURE 2: CT—free air around the duodenum in level of the papilla around the liver and visible retroperitoneum around the liver.

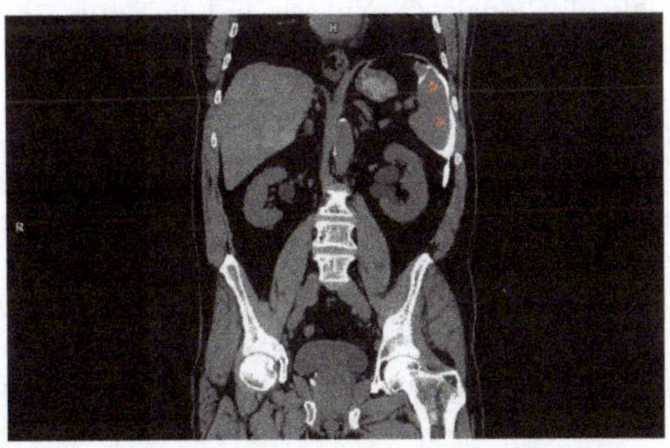

FIGURE 3: CT-free contrast around the gastric fundus and spleen.

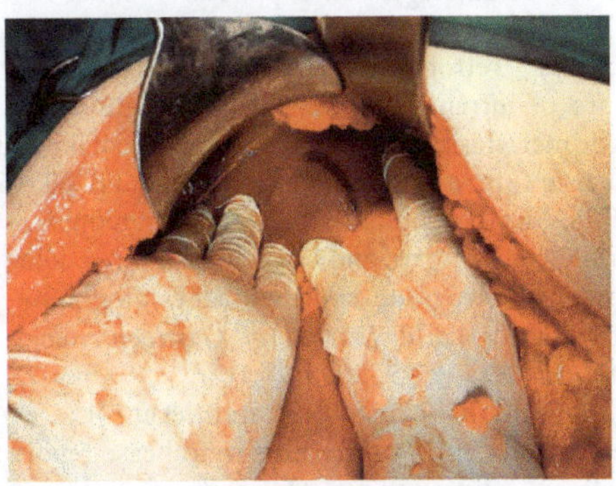

FIGURE 4: Intraoperative finding.

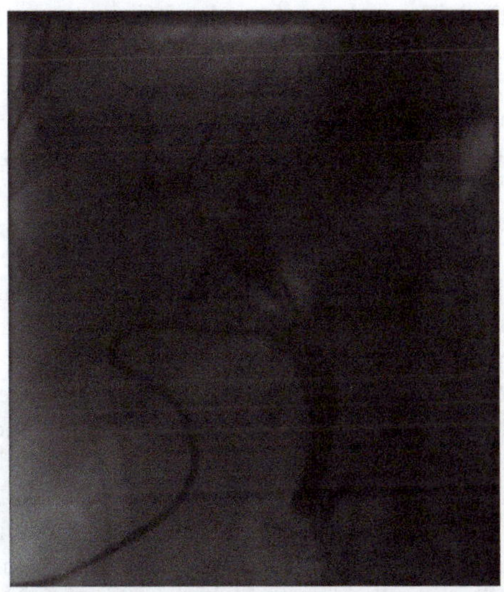

FIGURE 5: Cholangiography—no aberrant intrahepatic bile ducts are detected.

aforementioned condition has been scarcely reported, but its pathophysiology is associated with pathological changes in the liver parenchyma surrounding the ruptured bile duct: liver metastasis and abscesses [6, 20]. There is one case report by Fukui et al. [21] reporting a post-ERCP rupture of an intrahepatic duct, in otherwise, healthy liver parenchyma resulting in biliary peritonitis, but the rupture was associated with an innate anomaly identified as appendix fibrosa hepatis.

In the management of the above reported case, a substantial difference between the radiological and surgical diagnoses was observed. The clinical appearance (acute onset) and CT finding indicated duodenal perforation. The described pneumoperitoneum and especially pneumoretroperitoneum are anatomically associated with duodenal perforation and hence typical signs of it. But, intraoperatively, the duodenum, pancreas, and retroperitoneum were found to be intact, and the ruptured healthy hepatic bile duct was detected. It is curious though how no aberrant subcapsular hepatic bile duct or any other possible anatomic anomaly of the liver was found neither on MRCP, ERCP, or cholangiography. All this implies that our case report is the first in literature to describe a novel case of biliary peritonitis post-ERCP. Our case states that the rupture of a healthy subcapsular hepatic bile duct can lead to biliary peritonitis requiring immediate surgical treatment. The cause of this perforation was probably an excessive air insufflation during ERCP resulting in severe pneumobilia. Hence, the risk for the development of such a perforation cannot be stratified. It can only be recommended to avoid excessive air insufflation during ERCP to prevent this type of complication. Since the rupture of the bile duct in our case occurred probably during or immediately after ERCP, the insertion of an endoscopic nasobiliary drainage duct after ERCP would not have prevented this complication [22]. But our literature review has shown that carbon dioxide insufflation can reduce the incidence of post-ERCP complications such as pneumoperitoneum [23]; hence, its application could be recommended in the prevention of the aforementioned complication in our case.

Our case illustrates the need for a wholesome cooperation and coordination between radiologists and surgeons in the management of post-ERCP complications [9]. First, the radiological findings are essential in deciding between conservative and surgical management [24]. Correctly interpreting CT results enables the differentiation between intestinal perforation and other possible causes of pneumoperitoneum and can be essential for the execution of percutaneous interventions if available [25].

In the treatment of post-ERCP biliary peritonitis, there is no weighing, and immediate surgical treatment is required, no matter the cause being duodenal, common bile duct, or intrahepatic bile duct perforation [26]. In this case, on the other side, the radiological work-up, indicating the perforation site, can help in the planning of the adequate surgical treatment.

Based on our case, we would like to emphasize the diverse etiology of post-ERCP pneumoperitoneum and biliary peritonitis and the importance of good cooperation between radiologists and surgeons treating post-ERCP complications in order to decide for the correct treatment modality, plan adequate surgical procedures, and detect even extremely rare post-ERCP complications which can have fatal consequences [14].

4. Conclusions

We report a case of extremely rare etiology of post-ERCP pneumoperitoneum and biliary peritonitis which has never been reported in literature before. Based on the literature review and our case presentation, we conclude that the cooperation between radiologists and surgeon is vital for patients suffering from post-ERCP complications.

Abbreviations

ERCP: Endoscopic retrograde cholangiopancreatography
SCARE: Surgical case report guidelines
AST: Aspartate aminotransferase
ALT: Alanin aminotransferase
IU: International units
CT: Computed tomography
WBC: White blood cell count.
POD: Postoperative day.

Authors' Contributions

Andrija Karacic wrote the case report manuscript and performed the literature review. Paula Batur assisted in the literature review. Domagoj Stritof operated on the patient. Inka Kekez contributed the radiological images. Branko Bakula and Taro Fukui reviewed the article.

Acknowledgments

The authors thank Zarko Rasic (Professor and Chief of Department of General Surgery, University Hospital Sveti Duh).

References

[1] S. Köklü, E. Parlak, O. Yüksel, and B. Sahin, "Endoscopic retrograde cholangiopancreatography in the elderly: a prospective and comparative study," *Age and Ageing*, vol. 34, no. 6, pp. 572–577, 2005.
[2] L. K. Nathanson, N. A. O'Rourke, I. J. Martin et al., "Postoperative ERCP versus laparoscopic choledochotomy for clearance of selected bile duct calculi: a randomized trial," *Annals of Surgery*, vol. 242, no. 2, pp. 188–192, 2005.
[3] T. Z. Ong, J. L. Khor, D. S. Selamat, K. G. Yeoh, and K. Y. Ho, "Complications of endoscopic retrograde cholangiography in the post-MRCP era: a tertiary center experience," *World Journal of Gastroenterology*, vol. 11, pp. 5209–5212, 2005.
[4] T. H. Baron, "Complications of endoscopic biliary sphincterotomy: the first cut is the deepest," *Clinical Gastroenterology and Hepatology*, vol. 2, pp. 968–970, 2004.
[5] Z. Khan, U. Darr, M. Nawras et al., "Pneumoperitoneum after endoscopic retrograde cholangiopancreatography due to rupture of intrahepatic bile ducts and glisson's capsule in hepatic metastasis: a case report and review of literature," *Case Reports in Gastroenterology*, vol. 11, no. 3, pp. 603–609, 2017.
[6] S. F. Assimakopoulos, K. C. Thomopoulos, S. Giali, C. Triantos, D. Siagris, and C. Gogos, "A rare etiology of post-endoscopic retrograde cholangiopancreatography pneumoperitoneum," *World Journal of Gastroenterology*, vol. 14, no. 18, pp. 2917–2919, 2008.
[7] R. A. Agha, M. R. Borrelli, R. Farwana et al., "The SCARE 2018 statement: updating consensus surgical case report (SCARE) guidelines," *International Journal of Surgery*, vol. 60, pp. 132–136, 2018.
[8] S. Loperfido, G. Angelini, G. Benedetti et al., "Major early complications from diagnostic and therapeutic ERCP: a prospective multicenter study," *Gastrointestinal Endoscopy*, vol. 48, no. 1, pp. 1–10, 1998.
[9] H. K. Pannu and E. K. Fishman, "Complications of endoscopic retrograde cholangiopancreatography: spectrum of abnormalities demonstrated with CT," *RadioGraphics*, vol. 21, no. 6, pp. 1441–1453, 2001.

[10] S. Alfieri, F. Rosa, C. Cina et al., "Management of duodeno-pancreato-biliary perforations after ERCP: outcomes from an Italian tertiary referral center," *Surgical Endoscopy*, vol. 27, pp. 2005–2012, 2013.

[11] N. O. Machado, "Management of duodenal perforation post-endoscopic retrograde cholangiopancreatography. When and whom to operate and what factors determine the outcome? a review article," *Journal of the Pancreas*, vol. 13, pp. 18–25, 2012.

[12] N. S. Patil, N. Solanki, P. K. Mishra, B. C. Sharma, and S. S. Saluja, "ERCP-related perforation: an analysis of operative outcomes in a large series over 12 years," *Surgical Endoscopy*, vol. 34, no. 1, pp. 77–87, 2020.

[13] J. H. Wu, H. M. Tsai, C. Y. Chen, and Y. S. Wang, "Computed tomography classification of endoscopic retrograde cholangiopancreatography-related perforation," *The Kaohsiung Journal of Medical Sciences*, vol. 36, no. 2, pp. 129–134, 2020.

[14] M. Stapfer, R. R. Selby, S. C. Stain et al., "Management of duodenal perforation after endoscopic retrograde cholangiopancreatography and sphincterotomy," *Annals of Surgery*, vol. 232, no. 2, pp. 191–198, 2000.

[15] Y. J. Jin, S. Jeong, J. H. Kim et al., "Clinical course and proposed treatment strategy for ERCP-related duodenal perforation: a multicenter analysis," *Endoscopy*, vol. 45, pp. 806–812, 2013.

[16] M. E. Rabie, N. Mir, M. A. Skaini et al., "Operative and non-operative management of endoscopic retrograde cholangiopancreatography-associated duodenal injuries," *Annals of the Royal College of Surgeons of England*, vol. 95, no. 4, pp. 285–290, 2013.

[17] R. C. Bell, G. Van Stiegmann, J. Goff, M. Reveille, L. Norton, and N. W. Pearlman, "Decision for surgical management of perforation following endoscopic sphincterotomy," *The American Surgeon*, vol. 57, pp. 237–240, 1991.

[18] B. Koc, H. Y. Bircan, G. Adas et al., "Complications following endoscopic retrograde cholangiopancreatography: minimal invasive surgical recommendations," *PLoS One*, vol. 9, Article ID e113073, 2014.

[19] G. Zhu, F. Hu, and C. Wang, "Recent advances in prevention and management of endoscopic retrograde cholangiopancreatography-related duodenal perforation," *Videosurgery and Other Miniinvasive Techniques*, vol. 16, no. 1, pp. 19–29, 2021.

[20] I. Boškoski, A. Tringali, P. Familiari, and G. Costamagna, "An unusual post-ERCP pneumoperitoneum," *Digestive and Liver Disease*, vol. 43, p. 579, 2011.

[21] T. Fukui, T. Chochi, T. Maeda et al., "Biliary peritonitis caused by spontaneous bile duct rupture in the left triangular ligament of the liver after endoscopic sphincterotomy for choledocholithiasis," *Case Reports Gastroenterology*, vol. 15, no. 1, pp. 53–61, 2021.

[22] J. K. Lee, S. H. Lee, B. K. Kang et al., "Is it necessary to insert a nasobiliary drainage tube routinely after endoscopic clearance of the common bile duct in patients with choledocholithiasis-induced cholangitis? a prospective, randomized trial," *Gastrointestinal Endoscopy*, vol. 71, no. 1, pp. 105–110, 2010.

[23] H. Shi, S. Chen, G. Swar, Y. Wang, and M. Ying, "Carbon dioxide insufflation during endoscopic retrograde cholangiopancreatography: a review and meta-analysis," *Pancreas*, vol. 42, no. 7, pp. 1093–1100, 2013.

[24] M. S. Bray, A. J. Borgert, M. E. Folkers, and S. N. Kothari, "Outcome and management of endoscopic retrograde cholangiopancreatography perforations: a community perspective," *The American Journal of Surgery*, vol. 214, no. 1, pp. 69–73, 2017.

[25] R. P. Krishna, R. K. Singh, A. Behari, A. Kumar, R. Saxena, and V. K. Kapoor, "Post-endoscopic retrograde cholangiopancreatography perforation managed by surgery or percutaneous drainage," *Surgery Today*, vol. 41, no. 5, pp. 660–666, 2011.

[26] W. Kwon, J.-Y. Jang, J. K. Ryu et al., "Proposal of an endoscopic retrograde cholangiopancreatography-related perforation management guideline based on perforation type," *Journal of the Korean Surgical Society*, vol. 83, no. 4, pp. 218–226, 2012.

8

Adult Intestinal Intussusception Caused by the Gastrojejunostomy Tube: An Endoscopically Treatable Phenomenon

Kermit S. Zhang,[1] Jash Bansal,[2] Anmol Bansal,[3] and Vikas Chitnavis[2]

[1]*Virginia Tech Carilion School of Medicine, Roanoke, VA, USA*
[2]*Department of Gastroenterology, Carilion Clinic Memorial Hospital, Roanoke, VA, USA*
[3]*Department of Radiology, Carilion Clinic Memorial Hospital, Roanoke, VA, USA*

Correspondence should be addressed to Kermit S. Zhang; kzhang92@vtc.vt.edu

Academic Editor: Daniel C. Damin

Adult duodenoduodenal intussusception is extremely rare due to the retroperitoneal fixation of the second, third, and fourth parts of the duodenum. A majority of clinically significant intussusception with identifiable etiologies is typically neoplastic with more rare causes including retained food and indwelling enteral tubes, specifically with gastrojejunostomy (GJ) tubes. Herein, we discuss the case of a 23-year-old male who developed duodenoduodenal intussusception upon a PEGJ placement with associated gastroduodenal dilation and telescope phenomenon. To the best of our knowledge, there are no reports of intussusception found to be caused by GJ tubes in the adult population. The reported patient was found to have a 4-cm enteroenteric intussusception without obstruction or ischemia with bowel thickening proximal to the pathology. Although adult intussusception cases are typically managed surgically, we were able to reduce the intussusception via endoscopy due to rapid diagnosis upon presentation and intervention before the bowel wall could be compromised.

1. Introduction

Intussusception is the invagination of a distal segment of the small intestine into the proximal segment. By itself, this is a common phenomenon often disregarded within highly mobile segments of the jejunum. This condition is extremely rare in the duodenum due to the retroperitoneal fixation of the second, third, and fourth parts of the duodenum. In 80–90% of cases of clinically significant intussusception whose etiologies are identified, the lead point is typically neoplastic; this includes lesions such as Brunner's gland hamartomas, carcinomas, lipomas, and adenomas [1]. Additional causes of adult intussusception are polyps, strictures, and idiopathic and colonic diverticulum. While majority of cases self-resolve, those that do not can suffer compromised vascular flow and subsequent necrosis. The development of enteroenteric intussusception associated with indwelling enteral tubes is an extremely rare occurrence and is associated with substantial morbidity and mortality [2, 3]. Herein, we discuss the case of a 23-year-old male who developed duodenoduodenal intussusception upon a percutaneous gastrojejunostomy (PEGJ) and was with associated gastroduodenal dilation and telescope phenomenon.

2. Case Presentation

A 23-year-old male was hospitalized with generalized abdominal pain, nausea, and vomiting for 3 days. His medical history was significant for a traumatic cervical spinal injury six months prior with consequent paraplegia. He has been dependent on tracheostomy with ventilation and PEGJ placement since.

Vital signs on admission included a heart rate of 146 bpm, respiratory rate of 17, temperature of 99.8 F, and blood pressure of 89/51 mmHg. He was alert and oriented, but chronically-ill appearing with dry mucous membranes. His abdominal examination demonstrated a distended, diffusely tender abdomen with guarding and hypoactive bowel sounds. There was a bloody exudate at the ostomy site. Pertinent labs included a white blood cell count of 14,000/μL, hemoglobin of 17.3 g/dL, alkaline phosphatase 161 IU/L, and lactate of 0.6 mmol/L.

An abdominal plan radiograph revealed severe gaseous distension of the stomach and a large volume of stool in the colon (Figure 1). An abdominal computed tomography (CT) scan demonstrated the gastrojejunostomy (GJ) entering the gastric antrum, traversing the duodenum, and terminating in the midjejunum. A paucity of enteral fluid with a concentric soft tissue density surrounding the enteric catheter was shown at the junction of the second and third portions of the duodenum (Figure 2). This telescoping was interpreted by the radiologist as a 4 cm duodenoduodenal intussusception with the jejunostomy limb acting as a lead point. The jejunal and ileal loops appeared normal in caliber. There was no evidence of small bowel stranding, necrosis, ischemia, or perforation.

The gastroenterology service was consulted and planned for immediate reduction of the intussusception by removing the GJ. The endoscopy confirmed that the jejunostomy tube held traction on a segment of the distal bowel that had invaginated into the second portion of the duodenum (Figure 3). The tip of the endoscope was used to prevent the distal bowel from traveling proximally while the GJ removed and subsequently replaced with the gastrostomy tube. Postprocedural recovery was uncomplicated, and the patient's leukocytosis and lactate levels returned to the normal range within 24 hours.

3. Discussion

This report presents an adult case of duodenoduodenal intussusception and telescope phenomenon across the duodenal flexure caused by a GJ. There have been reports of cases in which a gastrostomy tube caused intussusception at the duodenal site related to improper fixation of the tube coupled with normal peristalsis. To our knowledge, few reports of intussusception have been found that it is caused by GJ tubes amongst adults, and the underlying mechanism for intussusception is not definitively understood. One theory by Wu et al. hypothesized it may be due to the tip of a jejunostomy limb inducing an inflammatory response causing mucosal hypertrophy leading to the formation of a lead point [4]. Similar to Wu et al., we believe that the PEG tube may not have been adequately sterilized between use allowing for inflammation surrounding the jejunostomy tip resulting in mucosal hypertrophy leading to this complication.

The successful management of intussusception depends on a reasonable degree of suspicion, early diagnosis, and prompt reduction. Treatment modalities for intussusception are variable. Amongst the 90% of adult intussusception cases that do not resolve spontaneously, surgery is often the intervention of choice due to the high likelihood of an associated pathologic lead point [5]. This is commonly employed in patients with symptomatic bowel obstruction and signs concerning for malignancy such as anorexia, unintended weight loss, and night sweats. Adults with

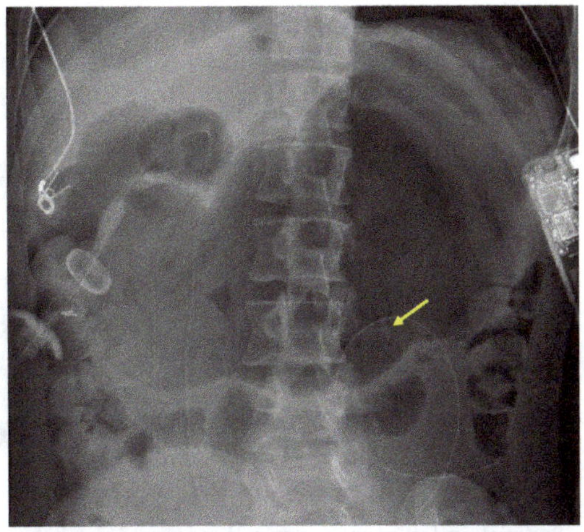

Figure 1: Abdominal X-ray demonstrating severe gaseous distention of the entire stomach with the balloon of presumed gastrostomy projecting over the right abdomen. The tip of a jejunostomy tube placed through the gastrostomy projects over the left midabdomen (yellow arrow). There is no gross evidence of free air noted given inherent limitations of this portable supine radiograph.

intussusception in the large intestine such as ileocolic and colocolic intussusception may also be candidates for surgery given the higher association for neoplasm [6]. Nonoperative management including endoscopic reduction and radiologic decompression are reasonable interventions amongst patients without such clinically severe features [3]. The current existing literature describes a high risk of perforation and recurrence after endoscopic intussusception reduction [7]. However, retrospective studies have demonstrated successful nonoperative and minimally invasive management in as many as 82% of radiographic intussusceptions even in the setting of gastrointestinal symptoms [6].

Given the nonspecific nature of the clinical presentation of intussusception in adults and the need to exclude other critical diagnoses, CT is the imaging modality of choice. Classic findings on CT include the "bulls-eye" or sausage-shaped concentric lesions created by the anatomic invagination of the affected enteric segments. Furthermore, CT can identify compromised vascular perfusion of the mesenteric vessels within the bowel lumen. Carucci et al. reported a series of four cases of jejunojejunal intussusception following a jejunostomy feeding tube with distinguishable radiographic findings while the feeding tube was still in place [8]. However, radiography has its diagnostic limitations as Kareem et al. reported a case of adult jejunojejunal intussusception secondary to GJ placement with no distinguishable findings on CT [9]. The findings in our patient's CT clearly demonstrated a telescope phenomenon surrounding the jejunostomy limb and were amenable to endoscopic reduction.

In our case, factors that contributed to successful endoscopic management were rapid diagnosis and intervention before bowel integrity could be compromised. This allowed for optimal conditions to treat the patient without undue burden of an operation in traditionally surgically managed patients as there was low concern for malignancy

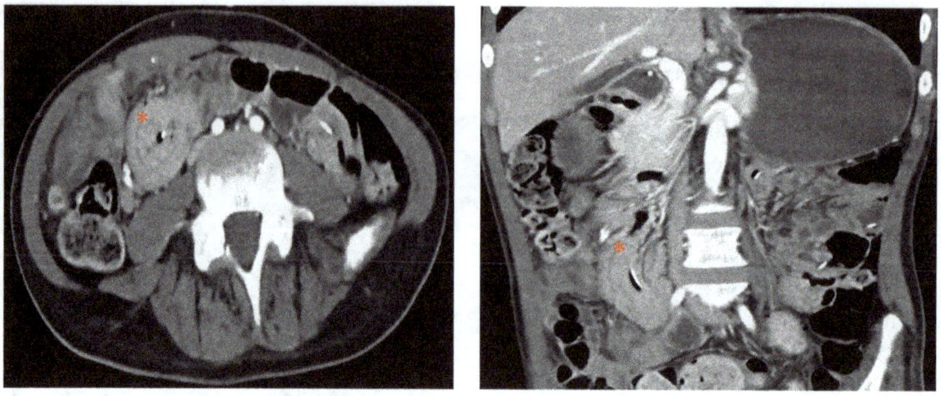

(a) (b)

Figure 2: Axial and coronal computed tomography of the (a) abdomen and (b) and pelvis (with contrast) demonstrating enteroenteric intussusception at the junction of the second and third portions of the duodenum (red asterick) with the jejunostomy limb acting as the presumed lead point.

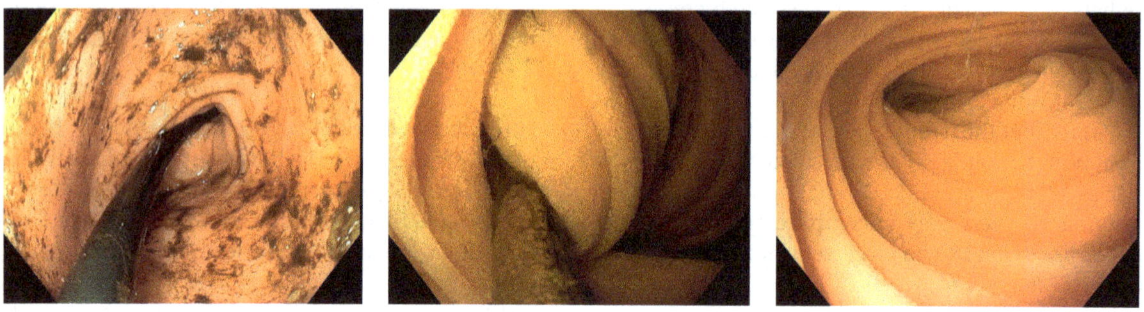

(a) (b) (c)

Figure 3: Esophagogastroduodenoscopy demonstrated retained semisolid food at the pyloric junction (a), significant bowel obstruction due to intussusception likely as a result of mucosal traction from the patient's jejunostomy limb tip at the second portion of the duodenum (b), and subsequent patent bowel following reduction in the intussuscepted bowel following reduction (c). The jejunostomy was also removed being replaced with a gastrostomy tube.

based on patient presentation and radiography. In an era of advancing endoscopy and a focus on minimally invasive procedures, adult intussusception without complications can be considered for endoscopic management.

Authors' Contributions

Kermit Zhang conceptualized the study, Kermit Zhang performed investigation, Jash Bansal supervised the work, Kermit Zhang and Jash Bansal performed visualization, Kermit Zhang wrote the original draft of the manuscript, and Kermit Zhang, Jash Bansal, Anmol Bansal, and Vikas Chitnavis reviewed and edited the manuscript.

References

[1] G. Lianos, N. Xeropotamos, C. Bali, G. Baltoggiannis, and E. Ignatiadou, "Adult bowel intussusception: presentation, location, etiology, diagnosis and treatment," *Il Giornale di chirurgia*, vol. 34, no. 9-10, pp. 280–3, 2013.

[2] P. Marsicovetere, S. J. Ivatury, B. White, and S. D. Holubar, "Intestinal intussusception: etiology, diagnosis, and treatment," *Clinics in Colon and Rectal Surgery*, vol. 30, no. 1, pp. 30–39, 2017.

[3] S. P. Schrag, R. Sharma, N. P. Jaik et al., "Complications related to percutaneous endoscopic gastrostomy (PEG) tubes. a comprehensive clinical review," *Journal of Gastrointestinal and Liver Diseases: JGLD*, vol. 16, no. 4, pp. 407–18, 2007.

[4] T.-H. Wu, C.-W. Lin, and W.-Y. Yin, "Jejunojejunal intussusception following jejunostomy," *Journal of the Formosan Medical Association*, vol. 105, no. 4, pp. 355–358, 2006.

[5] Y. H. Kim, M. A. Blake, M. G. Harisinghani et al., "Adult intestinal intussusception: CT appearances and identification of a causative lead point," *Radiographics*, vol. 26, no. 3, pp. 733–744, 2006.

[6] J. D. Rea, M. E. Lockhart, D. E. Yarbrough, R. R. Leeth, S. E. Bledsoe, and R. H. Clements, "Approach to management of intussusception in adults: a new paradigm in the computed tomography era," *The American Surgeon*, vol. 73, no. 11, pp. 1098–1105, 2007.

[7] F. Y. Chang, J. T. Cheng, and K. H. Lai, "Colonoscopic diagnosis of ileocolic intussusception in an adult. a case report," *South African Medical Journal = Suid-Afrikaanse Tydskrif Vir Geneeskunde*, vol. 77, no. 6, pp. 313-314, 1990.

[8] L. R. Carucci, M. S. Levine, S. E. Rubesin, I. Laufer, S. Assad, and H. Herlinger, "Evaluation of patients with jejunostomy tubes: imaging findings," *Radiology*, vol. 223, no. 1, pp. 241–247, 2002.
[9] T. S. Kareem and M. A. Abdi, "Jejunojejunal intussusception following jejunostomy closure: a case report," *International Journal of Surgery Case Reports*, vol. 76, pp. 446–449, 2020.

9

First Documented Case of Percutaneous Endoscopic Gastrostomy (PEG) Tube-Associated Bacterial Peritonitis due to *Achromobacter* Species with Literature Review

Nishant Tripathi,[1] **Niki Koirala**,[2] **Hirotaka Kato**,[1] **Tushi Singh**,[1] **Kishore Karri**,[1] **and Kshitij Thakur**[1]

[1]*Department of Internal Medicine, University of Kentucky, Lexington, KY, USA*
[2]*Department of Clinical Pharmacy, University of Kentucky, Lexington, KY, USA*

Correspondence should be addressed to Nishant Tripathi; nishant55@icloud.com

Academic Editor: Engin Altintas

Introduction. Achromobacter species (spp.) peritonitis has seldom been identified in medical literature. Scarce cases of *Achromobacter* peritonitis described previously have been correlated with peritoneal dialysis and more sparingly with spontaneous bacterial peritonitis. *Achromobacter* exhibits intrinsic and acquired resistance, especially in chronic infections, to most antibiotics. This article conducts a literature review of all previously reported *Achromobacter* spp. peritonitis and describes the first reported case of *Achromobacter* peritonitis as a complication of percutaneous endoscopic gastrostomy (PEG) tube placement. *Discussion. Achromobacter* peritonitis as a complication of PEG-tube placement has not been previously reported. In our patients' case, the recently placed PEG-tube with ascitic fluid leakage was identified as the most plausible infection source. Although a rare bacterial peritonitis pathogen, *Achromobacter* may be associated with wide antimicrobial resistance and unfavorable outcomes. *Conclusion.* No current guidelines provide significant guidance on treatment of PEG-tube peritonitis regardless of microbial etiology. Infectious Disease Society of America identifies various broad-spectrum antibiotics targeting nosocomial intra-abdominal coverage; some of these antimicrobial selections (such as cefepime and metronidazole combination) may yet be inadequate for widely resistant *Achromobacter* spp. Recognizably, the common antibiotics utilized for spontaneous bacterial peritonitis, i.e., third generation cephalosporins and fluoroquinolones, to which *Achromobacter* is resistant and variably susceptible, respectively, would be extensively insufficient. Piperacillin/tazobactam (P/T) and carbapenem were identified to provide the most reliable coverage *in vitro*; clinically, 5 out of the 8 patients who received either P/T or a carbapenem, or both, eventually experienced clinical improvement.

1. Introduction

Achromobacter species (spp.) are nonfermenting, oxidase positive, catalase positive, aerobic, and motile Gram-negative rods [1]. As environmental organisms, *Achromobacter* spp. are naturally distributed in aqueous surroundings including soil and water [2–4]. Similarly, they may contaminate fluids in the health care setting, and have been considered infectious etiologies in nosocomial infection outbreaks associated with contaminated fluids [5], pressure transducers [6], incubators [7], and disinfectants [7]. Although opportunistic organisms [8], *Achromobacter* spp. are deemed to be the etiology for a myriad of infectious diseases with significant morbidity and mortality such as biliary tract sepsis [9], meningitis [10], pneumonia [11], spontaneous bacterial peritonitis [12, 13], peritoneal dialysis associated peritonitis [5, 14], urinary tract infection [11], conjunctivitis [15], osteomyelitis [16], prosthetic knee infection [17], mesh infection [18], necrotizing pancreatitis [19], prosthetic valve endocarditis [20], bacteremia [6, 11, 21], and cystic fibrosis [4, 22], among others. While the majority of these diseases occur as a polymicrobial infection in immunocompromised states such as cancer [21], human immunodeficiency virus/acquired immunodeficiency syndrome [23], chronic renal failure or diabetes mellitus [20], a portion of them occur due to nosocomial outbreaks in immunocompetent hosts [11, 24].

The organism is highly resistant to commonly utilized antibiotics in intra-abdominal infections. Piperacillin/tazobactam (P/T) and carbapenems show activity *in vitro* and are considered the most active antimicrobials against *Achromobacter* spp. [2]. On the other hand, sulfamethoxazole/trimethoprim may be a reasonable non beta-lactam alternative [25]. Due to the extensive inherent and acquired resistance to significant number of antimicrobials, providing dual coverage for chronic infections may be prudent [25].

2. Case Summary

A 65-year-old Caucasian male with a history of chronic alcoholism (without cirrhosis or ascites), hypertension and prior tonsillar adenocarcinoma status post chemo-radiation presented to a regional hospital with progressive fatigue and jaundice, epigastric pain, and decreased appetite causing twenty-five-pound weight loss spanning over a month. Leukocytosis along with lactic acidosis was observed. Patient was treated empirically with P/T for biliary pancreatitis secondary to choledocolithiasis. Initial endoscopic retrograde cholangiopancreatography (ERCP) on day (D) 2 of hospitalization identified distal common bile duct stone; sphincterotomy was performed with 7- French 5 cm plastic common bile duct stent placement. Despite the interventions, liver enzymes continued to rise; antibiotic was altered to levofloxacin and metronidazole on D4 to cover intra-abdominal infections and a repeat ERCP was performed. Recently placed CBD stent, which appeared clogged with debris, was removed uneventfully with snare. Appropriate drainage from CBD and cystic duct was confirmed; however, gall bladder could not be visualized with contrast. Due to the development of pneumonia, antibiotics were switched to linezolid and doxycycline on D6 of hospitalization. On D11, due to poor nutritional status and emerging aspiration pneumonia, PEG-tube was inserted. Subsequently, developing and rapidly worsening ascites and ascitic fluid leakage around the PEG-tube insertion site was identified. Paracentesis was performed on D13 of hospitalization without evidence of peritonitis; however, antibiotics were escalated to meropenem and linezolid due to worsening clinical status. Due to thrombocytopenia, linezolid was discontinued, and antimicrobial therapy was narrowed to meropenem on D17. Due to worsening of ascitic fluid leakage around the PEG insertion site, and exacerbation of liver enzymes, the patient was transferred to our academic facility for further management, including possible cholecystectomy on D17.

Upon transfer, the patient was hemodynamically stable with a constellation of physical exam findings significant for leaking ascites, icterus, spider angioma, fine crackles throughout lung fields, and 3+ bilateral pitting edema; no evidence of encephalopathy was noted. The laboratory tests were remarkable for white blood cells 21,600/mcl, serum creatinine 0.55 mg/dl, aspartate aminotransferase 201 U/L, alanine transferase 74 U/L, alkaline phosphatase 458 U/L, total bilirubin 9.0 mg/dl, serum albumin 1.8 g/dl, and INR 1.5. Patient was further diagnosed with alcoholic cirrhosis decompensated by ascites with MELD-Na score of 23, and suspected alcoholic hepatitis with Maddrey's discriminant function of 28. Antibiotic therapy was held until further work-up due to previously negative cultures and extended duration of therapy prior to transfer. Interventional radiology guided paracentesis was performed on D22 of hospitalization as bedside procedure was unsuccessful. Ascitic fluid analysis revealed albumin of 0.3 gm/dL and polymorphonuclear neutrophil count of 1950 cells/mcl. PEG-tube was retained to allow for maturation of PEG-tube tract; P/T and vancomycin were initiated and continued for two days (D22-D23); therapy was empirically altered to cefepime, metronidazole, and vancomycin to prevent acute kidney injury secondary to concomitant vancomycin and P/T use, which was continued for four days (D24-27). Ascitic fluid cultures revealed P/T susceptible and cefepime resistant *Achromobacter xylosoxidans* as the infectious etiology (Isolate was identified by MALDI TOF: MALDI Biotyper CA system. Please refer to Table 1 for minimal inhibitory concentration values). Empiric regimen of cefepime, metronidazole, and vancomycin was narrowed to P/T on D27. Bronchoalveolar Lavage on D27 due to worsening respiratory failure also identified *A. xylosoxidans*. Following five days of treatment with P/T, however, his abdomen demonstrated peritoneal signs with increasing ascites. Repeat paracentesis confirmed worsening bacterial peritonitis, with additional findings of vancomycin resistant *Enterococcus* and *Candida glabrata*. Despite broadened antimicrobial coverage with meropenem and vancomycin for four days (D28–D31), the patient deteriorated with acute kidney injury and hypotension, and was deceased within twenty-four hours of intensive care unit transfer.

3. Discussion

3.1. Nomenclature. The taxonomic designation for *Achromobacter* spp. has been inconsistent due to the limited differentiating capability of previous identification methods [26, 27]. Solely multilocus sequence typing (MLST) and species identification via *nrdA* sequence analysis for *Achromobacter* genus have been deemed to be effective in differentiating between various *Achromobacter* spp. [26, 27]. Prior to utilization of these methods, various alternate *Achromobacter* species might have been misidentified as *Achromobacter xylosoxidans*; currently, reclassification of *Achromobacter* species has resulted from utilization of these techniques [26–31]. The ascitic culture in our patient case was assessed by MALDI TOF MS (Matrix Assisted Laser Desorption/Ionization Time of Flight Mass Spectrometry); thus, exact species identification might not have been accurate. As such, our literature review attempts to include all previously documented *Achromobacter* species peritonitis cases to ensure an inclusive analysis.

3.2. Antimicrobial Susceptibility Patterns. Achromobacter susceptibility profile identifies the organism as being extensively resistant among various classes of antimicrobials, including fluoroquinolones, aminoglycosides, and the majority of broad-spectrum β-lactam antibiotics [32]. The resistance-nodulation-cell division (RND)-type multidrug efflux pumps, AxyABM [33, 34] and AxyXY-OprZ [35] have been associated with innate resistance. Essentially, resistant to all cephalosporins, except

Table 1: All reported cases of *Achromobacter* spp. peritonitis-demographics, coinfection etiologies, and catheter or tube removal status.

Case	Year	Age/sex	PD catheter or PEG-tube removal	Coinfection microbes
			Bacterial peritonitis secondary to peritoneal dialysis	
1 [8]	1980	53/M	No	*Staphylococcus epidermidis*
2 [5]	1984	40/M	No	*Stenotrophomonas maltophilia*
3 [53]	1986	34/F	No	None
4 [54, 55]	1995	45/M	Yes. Day 48	None
5 [55]	1998	52/F	Yes. Day 10	None
7 [56]	Sep 2001	46/F	Yes. Day 6	None
8 [56]	Sep 2001	35/F	Yes. Day 8	None
10 [49]	2004	16/M	Yes. Day NR	None
11 [57]	2007	72/F	No	None
12 [58]	2010	51/F	Yes. Day 1	None
13 [59]	2011	74/F	Yes. Day 19	*Pseudomonas aeruginosa*
14 [60]	May 2012	82/F	No	*Achromobacter denitrificans*
15 [50]	Jul 2012	31/M	No	None
16 [51]	Jan 2014	60/F	No	None
17 [14]	2017	45/F	Removed prior to *Achromobacter* peritonitis	None
18 [52]	2018	27/F	Yes. Day NR. During third episode	None
			Sponteneous bacterial peritonitis	
6 [12]	2000	43/M	N/A	None
9 [13]	2001	54/M	N/A	Likely *Escherichia coli*
			Percutaneous endoscopic gastrostomy tube-associated peritonitis	
19	2018	65/M	No	*Enterococcus faecium* *Candida glabrata*

In case 7, PD catheter was replaced one-month postantibiotics. In case 8, catheter was replaced 6 weeks postantibiotics; PD catheter failed; subsequently, hemodialysis was initiated. Cases 11, 14, and 15 were reported as exit site infections. Case 16 was reported to be a tunnel infection. Abbreviations: PD = peritoneal dialysis, PEG = percutaneous endoscopic gastrostomy, NR = not reported, N/A = not applicable.

ceftazidime, due to the presence of AxyABM efflux system [29, 33], *Achromobacter* spp. may also contain AxyXY-OprZ efflux pump associated with aminoglycoside resistance [29, 35]. On the other hand, most isolates are typically susceptible to carbapenems, piperacillin, and P/T [29]. While a few acquired betalactamases have been described, overall acquired resistance mechanisms remain unknown [36–40].

3.3. PEG-Tube Associated Complications. This case report documents the first percutaneous endoscopic gastrostomy (PEG) tube-associated *Achromobacter* peritonitis. PEG-tube is a reliable source of enteral nutrition for patients with the inability to maintain oral nutrition on a long-term basis. Although minimally invasive, gastrostomy tubes have been associated with major complications such as peritonitis, major gastrointestinal bleeds, aspiration pneumonia, gastroenteric fistula, and gastrocolocutaneous fistula; minor complications include cellulitis, leakage around the tube, and granulation tissue at gastrostomy site [41–43]. In order to minimize these complications, the European Society for Clinical Nutrition and Metabolism guidelines on artificial enteral nutrition identifies a variety of contraindications to gastrostomy tubes including, serious coagulation disorders, INR greater than 1.5, platelets less than 50,000/mcl, marked peritoneal carcinomatosis, interposed organs (liver and colon), severe ascites, peritonitis, anorexia nervosa, severe psychosis, and discernibly limited life expectancy [44].

Specific risk factors for PEG-tube peritonitis include poor tissue healing, procedural, and technical issues, BMI over 30 kg/m2, albumin less than 2.5 g/dL, and dislodgement or reinsertion of tube [41, 42]. *Pseudomonas aeruginosa, Methicillin resistant Staphylococcus aureus,* and enteric Gram-negative rods are implicated as the most common infective etiologies of PEG site infections [45–47]. Abuksis et al. report 30-day mortality rate of 4.1–26% for stomal infections [48].

Despite the wide array of *Achromobacter* spp. infections previously reported, *Achromobacter* peritonitis is extremely rare and has been documented primarily in the setting of peritoneal dialysis. Despite the fact, *Achromobacter* infections in peritoneal dialysis are also exceptionally infrequent. Moreover, etiologies reported prior to *nrdA* sequencing might have been inaccurately identified as *A. xylosoxidans* and may rather represent *Achromobacter* spp. [11, 26–28]. In order to identify all reported and published cases of *Achromobacter* peritonitis, thorough PubMed (January 1st, 1966–April 7th, 2019) literature searches were conducted from March 20th, 2019 through April 7th, 2019, and October 10th, 2019 through October 21st, 2019 independently by both primary authors. Search terms that were used include "PEG or percutaneous endoscopic gastrostomy tube peritonitis" with no relevant results, "*Achromobacter* peritonitis" with four relevant results [49–52], and "*Alcaligenes* peritonitis" with additional 8 relevant results [12, 13, 53–58]. Five additional cases were identified through previously published case reports, and extensive search in PubMed with

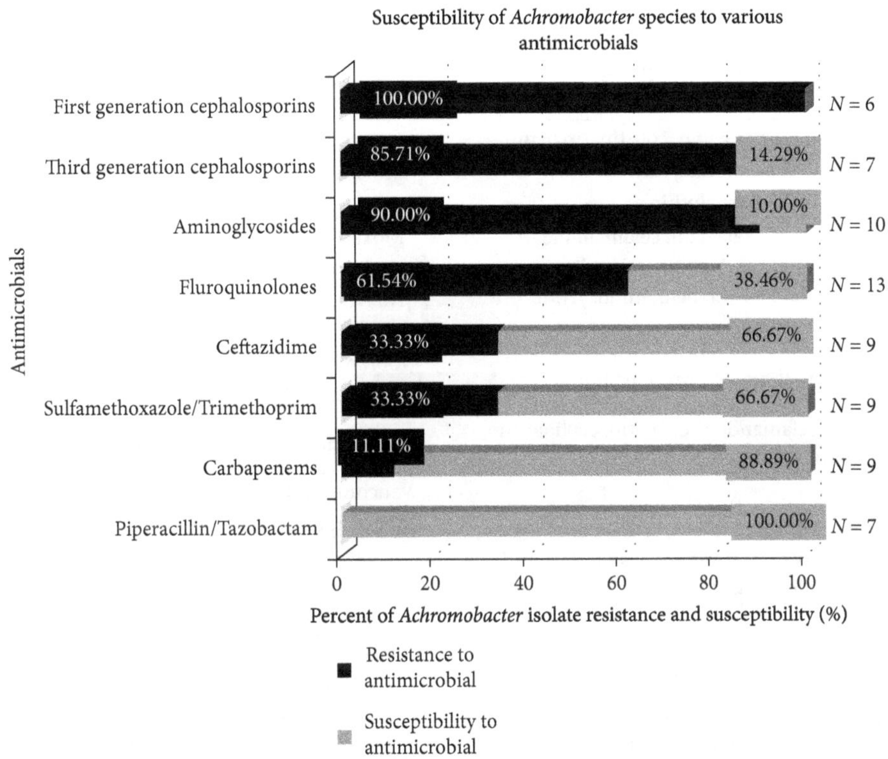

FIGURE 1: Susceptibility of *Achromobacter* spp. to various antimicrobials. Seven cases reported *Achromobacter* spp. sensitivity to piperacillin/tazobactam and all 7 isolates were susceptible to P/T. Similarly, 9 cases reported carbapenem sensitivity; 8 of 9 (88.89%) isolates were susceptible. SMZ/TMP and ceftazidime sensitivities were reported by 9 cases, of which 6 isolates (66.67%) were susceptible to each agent. On the other hand, 13 cases reported fluoroquinolones, of which, only 5 *Achromobacter* isolates (38.46%) were susceptible. Only 1 of 10 isolates (10%) were susceptible to aminoglycosides. None (0 out of 6) of the isolates were susceptible to first generation cephalosporins; and solely 1 out of 7 (14.29%) *Achromobacter* isolates were sensitive to third generation cephalosporins. Although *Achromobacter* susceptibility to other agents were also reported by most of the patient cases, sensitivity trends were not reported in this figure if data for at least five isolates could not be attained.

search terms "*Achromobacter xylosoxidans*", "*Achromobacter*", and "*Alcaligenes*" [5, 8, 14, 59, 60].

In totality, eighteen previous *Achromobacter* peritonitis cases were encountered; of which, two were diagnosed as spontaneous peritonitis [12, 13] while remaining sixteen cases of peritonitis were associated with peritoneal dialysis [5, 8, 14, 49–60]. No previous cases of PEG tube-associated *Achromobacter* peritonitis were discovered. Tables 1 and 2 summarize, in as much detail as could be obtained, the infectious diagnosis of each patient case, cultures, and sensitivities, antimicrobial therapies selected, and overall outcomes. Likewise, Figure 1 utilizes a bar graph to indicate the overall *in vitro* susceptibility profiles of the *Achromobacter* strains that were encountered in all nineteen cases of *Achromobacter* spp. peritonitis.

While 14 patients ultimately experienced clinical improvement, 4 patients were deceased. Patient responses to each antimicrobial group were assessed. P/T and carbapenem were identified to provide the most reliable coverage *in vitro*; clinically, 5 out of the 8 patients who received P/T or a carbapenem, or both, eventually experienced clinical improvement. Of the three patients who did not, patient in case nine was administered P/T but patient was deceased very shortly after presentation. Patient likely presented with high disease severity; thus, overall outcome may not reflect utility of the treatment. Likewise, patient in case thirteen was initiated on amikacin upon presentation, which was continued for seven days without confirmed susceptibility; the case report identified susceptible agents, which did not include any aminoglycosides. Following seven days of likely inadequate treatment, therapy was escalated to imipenem and P/T dual-therapy, which was narrowed to imipenem. Despite the eventual initiation of antimicrobials with verified susceptibility, patient failed to respond to therapy despite over 30 days of carbapenem therapy. Such response may have been due to delayed removal of peritoneal dialysis catheter as well as delayed initiation of adequate antimicrobial coverage. Finally, patient described in this case report was initiated on P/T and vancomycin; empirically, therapy was altered to cefepime, metronidazole and vancomycin for four days to prevent acute kidney injury. Unfortunately, the ascitic fluid culture resulted cefepime-resistant but P/T sensitive *Achromobacter* spp. Despite definitive treatment with P/T for five days and meropenem for four additional days, no recovery was observed. Such outcome may have resulted due to interruption of appropriate treatment as well as retention of PEG-tube despite multiple positive ascitic fluid cultures. No trend in antibiotic selection was observed among nine additional patients with clinical recovery who received agents other than carbapenems and P/T. While the International Society for Peritoneal Dialysis

Table 2: All reported cases of *Achromobacter* spp. peritonitis-bacterial sensitivities, antibiotics selection with duration, and outcomes.

Case	Antimicrobial sensitivities	Antibiotics utilized	Antibiotic duration	Outcomes
	Bacterial peritonitis secondary to peritoneal dialysis			
1 [8]	S: ampicillin, carbenicillin, colistin, smz/tmp R: AG, tetracycline I: cephalothin	Carbenicillin IV	NR	Cure
2 [5]	S: colistin, moxalactam, cefamandole R: piperacillin, azlocillin, ceftazidime, cefoperazone, novobiocin, minocycline I: rifampin, rosoxacin	Moxalactam* Noxytiolin IP	Likely 15 days	Deceased
3 [53]	S: smz/tmp, AG, carbenicillin R: ampicillin, cefamandole, cefoxitin, cephalothin, tetracycline, chloramphenicol	Tobramycin IP Cephalothin IP smz/tmp IP	3 days 10 days	Relapse Cure
4 [54, 55]	R: AG *Complete sensitivity profile was not available. Initial response to gentamicin was documented by El-Shahawy, et al. [46].*	Vancomycin IP Gentamicin IP Gentamicin IP Ciprofloxacin PO Piperacillin IV	1 dose NR 7 days	Deterioration Deterioration Cure
5 [55]	S: ofloxacin R: AG, aztreonam, cefazolin, cefotaxime, cefoxitin, ceftriaxone, ceftazidime, cefuroxime, ciprofloxacin, imipenem, piperacillin, smz/tmp	Vancomycin IP Ceftazidime IV Ceftazidime IV Ofloxacin PO	3 days 14 days	Cure
7 [56]	S: P/T R: ampicillin, cephalothin, ceftriaxone, AG, ciprofloxacin, smz/tmp	Cefazolin IP Tobramycin IP Amikacin IP Ceftazidime IP P/T IV	3 days 3 days 21 days	Cure
8 [56]	S: piperacillin, ticarcillin, ceftriaxone, ceftazidime, smz/tmp R: AG	Cefazolin IP Tobramycin IP Amikacin IP Ceftazidime IP P/T IV	3 days 5 days 21 days	Cure
10 [49]	S: ciprofloxacin, imipenem R: ceftazidime, smz/tmp	Vancomycin IP Ceftazidime IP Ciprofloxacin PO Ceftazidime IP Amikacin IP smz/tmp PO Imipenem IP Ciprofloxacin PO	NR	Cure
11 [57]	S: imipenem, P/T R: cefotaxime, AG I: ciprofloxacin	Ceftazidime IP Cefazolin IP Ciprofloxacin PO Imipenem IV Imipenem IP Ciprofloxacin PO	1 dose NR 3 doses 30 days 10 days	Cure
12 [58]	*Complete sensitivity profile was not reported but ampicillin/sulbactam, ciprofloxacin and cefepime were definitive therapies*	Ceftazidime IV Cefazolin IV amp/sulb IV Ciprofloxacin* Cefepime*	NR 7 days 2 days 7 days	Cure

TABLE 2: Continued.

Case	Antimicrobial sensitivities	Antibiotics utilized	Antibiotic duration	Outcomes
13 [59]	S: ceftazidime, imipenem, meropenem, levofloxacin, piperacillin	Vancomycin IP Amikacin IP	7 days	Deterioration
		Imipenem/cil IP P/T IP	7 days	
	R: NR	Ceftazidime Cefazolin Imipenem/cil Vancomycin	NR	Deceased
		Imipenem/cil IP Vancomycin IP	NR	
		Imipenem/cil IV Vancomycin IV	29 days	
14 [60]	S: ceftazidime, cefepime, sulfonamide, quinolones, carbapenem, P/T R: NR	Ciprofloxacin PO	14 days	Cure
15 [50]	*Unable to obtain due to lack of article access*	Cefazolin IP Ceftazidime IP	3 days	Cure
		Ceftazidime IP	4 days	
16 [43]	S: ciprofloxacin, others NR R: NR	Ciprofloxacin*	NR	Cure
17 [14]	S: amp/sulb, smz/tmp, carbapenem, cephoperazone/ sulbactam, ceftazidime, P/T, tigecycline	Cephalosporin PO	14 days	Relapse
	R: 1st generation cephalosporin, ciprofloxacin	Cefazolin IP Ceftazidime IP	7 days	Cure
		amp/sulb PO	14 days	
18 [52]	S: P/T, ceftazidime, imipenem	Ceftazidime IP Cefazolin IP	NR	Replase
		Imipenem/cil*	14 days	
	R: ciprofloxacin, cefepime	Imipenem IV Ceftazidime IV	14 days	Replase
		Imipenem IV Ceftazidime IV	14 days	Cure
	Sponteneous bacterial peritonitis			
6 [12]	S: amox/clav, ceftazidime, P/T, imipenem, meropenem, cotrimoxazole I: cefotaxime, ceftriaxone, ofloxacin, ciprofloxacin R: AG, aztreonam, cefazolin, cefuroxime	Ceftriaxone IV	10 days	Cure
9 [13]	S: NR R: cefotaxime, aztreonam, AG, ciprofloxacin	P/T IV	Few hours	Deceased (few hours later)

Table 2: Continued.

Case	Antimicrobial sensitivities	Antibiotics utilized	Antibiotic duration	Outcomes
	Percutaneous endoscopic gastrostomy tube-associated peritonitis			
	S: P/T (≤2/4), smz/tmp (≤0.5/9.5), meropenem (0.25)	P/T IV	4 days	Deterioration
	R: aztreonam (16), cefepime (16), gentamicin (8)	Levofloxacin IV Metronidazole IV	2 days	Deterioration
		Linezolid IV Doxycycline IV	7 days	Deterioration
		Meropenem IV Linezolid IV	4 days	Adverse reaction
19		Meropenem IV	2 days	Transferred to UK
	I: amikacin (32), levofloxacin (4), tobramycin (8)	P/T IV Vancomycin IV	2 days	Adverse reaction
		Cefepime IV Vancomycin IV Metronidazole IV	4 days	Deterioration
		P/T IV	5 days	Deterioration
		Meropenem IV Vancomycin IV	4 days	Deceased

In case 2, the duration of treatment was not clearly reported but was likely 15 days; route of moxalactam was unreported. Case 12 did not report route of ciprofloxacin and cefepime; total of 20 days of antibiotics were administered as patient had presented with 5th episode of peritonitis; subsequently, hemodialysis was initiated. Case 13 reported total of 48 days of antimicrobial treatment. Case 16 did not report full culture and sensitivities, route of ciprofloxacin and total duration of the treatment. Case 18 does not report route of imipenem/cilastatin. Abbreviations: S = Sensitive, R = resistant, I = intermediate, smz/tmp = sulfamethoxazole/ trimethoprim, P/T = piperacillin/tazobactam, amp/sulb = ampicillin/sulbactam, amox/clav = amoxicillin/clavulanate, cil = cilastatin, AG = aminoglycosides, IV = intravenous, IP = intraperitoneal, PO = oral, NR = not reported.

(ISPD) guideline suggests structurally similar *Pseudomonas* associated peritonitis treatment with dual antibiotic regimen, the guideline makes no specific recommendations for *Achromobacter* treatment [43]. Per *in vitro* and in vivo data collected in this article and through numerous studies, P/T and carbapenems yield the most preferable clinical outcomes in *Achromobacter* peritonitis [2, 24, 25, 34].

PD catheter was removed in 9 out of 14 non-SBP patients with clinical cure. All patients with resolved infection received at least seven days of antimicrobial treatment. Five patients received seven to ten days; four patients received fourteen days; two patients received twenty-one days, and one patient received over 30 days of antibiotics. Glucose containing peritoneal dialysate and aqueous environment foster *Achromobacter* proliferation and associated infection. Moreover, *Achromobacter* colonies may have the ability to surround the PD catheter with biofilm [14, 52, 61, 62]. Bacteria in biofilms in vivo are significantly less susceptible to antimicrobials identified to have adequate coverage through laboratory testing *in vitro* [43]. This fact may further clarify the treatment failures, relapses, and patient deaths resulting in patients who received P/T or carbapenems in these case reports. In addition to appropriate antimicrobial therapy, case seventeen also highlights the importance of timely removal of peritoneal dialysis catheter. Donderski et al. [52] report multiple peritonitis relapse associated readmissions; fortunately, no further episodes were reported following PD catheter removal and a course of adequate antimicrobial regimen. Thus, multiple case studies highlight the importance of timely removal of *Achromobacter* infected PD catheters; Donderski et al. [52] identify catheter removal as the most preferred treatment method. ISPD Peritonitis Recommendations: 2016 Update on Prevention and Treatment identifies peritonitis as a common and serious complication of PD [43]. Severe or prolonged peritonitis can induce functional and structural deformations resulting in membrane failure. Gram-negative peritonitis presents higher risks of catheter loss and death compared to Gram-positive infections [63–67]. ISPD guideline recommends removal of PD catheter in cases of recurrent, relapsed, and refractory (lack of clearance of ascitic fluid despite 5 days of appropriate antimicrobial treatment) peritonitis in order to protect the peritoneal membrane [43]. Timely catheter removal is essential in recurrent episodes. Nonetheless, PD catheter or PEG-tube removal within ten days to four weeks of insertion may not allow respective insertion tracts to mature causing further leakage and complications [44, 68–70].

Additionally, ISPD suggests at least 3 weeks of treatment in nonpseudomonas Gram-negative, and polymicrobial PD peritonitis [43]. No current guidelines provide significant direction on treatment of PEG tube peritonitis regardless of microbial etiology. Nevertheless, clinical practice guidelines for antimicrobial prophylaxis in surgery strongly recommends prophylactic antibiotic use to significantly reduce the risk of peristomal wound infection associated with PEG-tube insertion [71]. ASPEN guidelines recommend gastropexy using temporary sutures or T-fasteners to secure the stomach to the abdominal wall [72]. These techniques allow for appropriate attachment of tube, minimizing potential for peritoneal leakage, and reducing difficulty and challenges associated with tube replacement, if indicated [72]. Upon development of peritonitis, tube feeds should be held with initiation of broad-spectrum antibiotics. Evidence of perforation should be assessed via abdominal imaging; potential for wound should be evaluated. Surgical consult to perform laparotomy should be obtained. As misplaced tube may cause peritonitis and death, test must be performed to detect misplacement of tube at exchange. In instances of early inadvertent gastrostomy tube removal, parenteral broad-spectrum antibiotics and monitoring for peritonitis signs are indicated [72]. Although recommendations for total duration of antibiotics for treatment of PEG-tube peritonitis could not be encountered in current literature, in case of suspected peritonitis, clinical knowledge extrapolated from similar gastrointestinal perforations suggests that antibiotics may be discontinued after seven days if peritonitis is not observed [70]. Longer duration of treatment may be required in cases of confirmed PEG-tube peritonitis, particularly in cases without adequate source control [70]. Due to the lack of data to guide treatment of PEG tube-associated *Achromobacter* peritonitis, we attempted to draw similarities between *Achromobacter* peritonitis due to PEG-tube and PD. Nonetheless, the authors acknowledge that one of the major differences between the two insertions is the accessibility of the peritoneal cavity; while PD catheter readily allows for diagnosis as well as intraperitoneal treatment of peritonitis, PEG tubes should ideally not provide direct access to the peritoneal cavity.

Multiple risk factors for PEG tube related complications could be identified in the patient presented in our case study. Undiagnosed advanced liver disease, severe ascites, hypoalbuminemia, prolonged hospitalization, and immunocompromise secondary to liver cirrhosis, all place the patient is at high risk for PEG-tube related complications. Polymicrobial nature of the patient's peritonitis also portends adverse outcomes; likewise, patient's ultimate demise indicates the severity of the disease.

4. Conclusion

Achromobacter spp. peritonitis as a complication of PEG-tube placement has not been previously reported. In our patients' case, the recently placed PEG-tube with ascitic fluid leakage was identified as the most plausible infection source. Although a rare bacterial peritonitis pathogen, *Achromobacter* spp. may be associated with wide antimicrobial resistance and unfavorable outcomes. Thus, clinicians should consider broad empirical antimicrobial regimen, with *Achromobacter* coverage, such as P/T or a carbapenem, if any concern for *Achromobacter* spp. secondary peritonitis associated with PEG placement exists, as they may not always represent clinical sample contamination. While the management of *secondary* peritonitis involving biliary stent and PEG-tube would generally include surgical intervention for infection source control with broad spectrum antibiotics targeting nosocomial coverage per Infectious Disease Society of America, some of antimicrobial selections (such as cefepime and metronidazole combination) may yet be inadequate for widely resistant *Achromobacter* species. Recognizably, the common antibiotics for *spontaneous* bacterial peritonitis, i.e., third generation cephalosporins and fluoroquinolones, to which *Achromobacter* is resistant and variably susceptible, respectively, would be extensively insufficient. Moreover, repeat ascitic fluid culture may be beneficial in verifying continued susceptibility of selected definitive antibiotics. In addition, as these pathogens are generally identified in polymicrobial infections, their presence may serve as a surrogate marker of unfavorable outcomes. Due to the high disease severity, delay or interruption in efficacious therapy may lead to increased mortality rates.

Authors' Contributions

Nishant Tripathi and Niki Koirala developed the concept and design of the literature review; Hirotaka Kato and Nishant Tripathi developed the concept of case report; Nishant Tripathi, Niki Koirala, Hirotaka Kato, Tushi Singh, Kishore Karri, and Kshitij Thakur performed acquisition of clinical information regarding the patient case. Nishant Tripathi and Niki Koirala each independently conducted PubMed searches to gather relevant articles for the literature review. Nishant Tripathi and Niki Koirala acquired relevant data from the gathered articles, analyzed, and interpreted the data. Nishant Tripathi, Niki Koirala, and Hirotaka Kato drafted the manuscript. All authors revised the manuscript critically, approved the final draft of the manuscript to be published, and agree to be accountable for all aspects of the work.

References

[1] E. Yabuuchi and A. Oyama, "*Achromobacter xylosoxidans* n. sp. from human ear discharge," *Japanese Journal of Microbiology*, vol. 15, no. 5, pp. 477–481, 1971.

[2] V. Waters, "New treatments for emerging cystic fibrosis pathogens other than *Pseudomonas*," *Current Pharmaceutical Design*, vol. 18, no. 5, pp. 696–725, 2012.

[3] L. Amoureux, J. Bador, S. Fardeheb et al., "Detection of *Achromobacter xylosoxidans* in hospital, domestic, and outdoor environmental samples and comparison with human clinical isolates," *Applied Environmental Microbiology*, vol. 79, no. 23, pp. 7142–7149, 2013.

[4] A. Lambiase, M. R. Catania, M. Del Pezzo et al., "*Achromobacter xylosoxidans* respiratory tract infection in cystic fibrosis patients," *European Journal of Clinical Microbiology & Infectious Diseases*, vol. 30, no. 8, pp. 973–980, 2011.

[5] M. E. Reverdy, J. Freney, J. Fleurette et al., "Nosocomial colonization and infection by *Achromobacter xylosoxidans*," *Journal of Clinical Microbiology*, vol. 19, no. 2, pp. 140–143, 1984.

[6] J. Gómez-Cerezo, I. Suárez, J. J. Ríos et al., "*Achromobacter xylosoxidans* bacteremia: a 10-year analysis of 54 cases," *European Journal of Clinical Microbiology and Infectious Diseases*, vol. 22, no. 6, pp. 360–363, 2003.

[7] J. Molina-Cabrillana, C. Santana-Reyes, A. González-García, A. Bordes-Benítez, and I. Horcajada, "Outbreak of *Achromobacter xylosoxidans* pseudobacteremia in a neonatal care unit related to contaminated chlorhexidine solution," *European Journal of Clinical Microbiology & Infectious Diseases*, vol. 26, no. 6, pp. 435–437, 2007.

[8] Y. Igra-Siegman, H. Chmel, and C. Cobbs, "Clinical and laboratory characteristics of *Achromobacter xylosoxidans*

infection," *Journal of Clinical Microbiology*, vol. 11, no. 2, pp. 141–145, 1980.

[9] S. O. Teng, T. Y. Ou, Y. C. Hsieh, W. C. Lee, Y. C. Lin, and W. S. Lee, "Complicated intra-abdominal infection caused by extended drug-resistant *Achromobacter xylosoxidans*," *Journal of Microbiology, Immunology and Infection*, vol. 42, no. 2, pp. 176–180, 2009.

[10] F. Bellissimo, M. R. Pinzone, S. Tosto, G. Nunnari, and B. Cacopardo, "*Achromobacter xylosoxidans* meningitis in an immunosuppressed patient," *An International Journal of Medicine*, vol. 107, no. 1, pp. 65–66, 2014.

[11] K. Marion-Sanchez, K. Pailla, C. Olive, X. Le Coutour, and C. Derancourt, "*Achromobacter* spp. healthcare associated infections in the French West Indies: a longitudinal study from 2006 to 2016," *BMC Infectious Diseases*, vol. 19, no. 1, p. 795, 2019.

[12] C. Palmero Palmero, A. Giráldez Gallego, S. García Morillo, and M. L. Miranda Guisado, "Spontaneous bacterial peritonitis caused by *Alcaligenes xylosoxidans*," *Medicina Clinica*, vol. 115, no. 1, pp. 36–37, 2000.

[13] J. Castellote, G. Tremosa, S. L. Ben, and S. Vazguez, "Spontaneous bacterial peritonitis due to *Alcaligenes xylosoxidans*," *The American Journal of Gastroenterology*, vol. 96, no. 5, pp. 1650–651, 2001.

[14] J. L. Tsai and S. F. Tsai, "Case report: the first case of *Achromobacter xylosoxidans*-related tunnel infection in a patient receiving peritoneal dialysis," *Medicine (Baltimore)*, vol. 96, no. 16, p. e6654, 2017.

[15] J. I. Arshad, A. Saud, D. E. White, N. A. Afshari, and R. R. Sayegh, "Chronic conjunctivitis from a retained contact lens," *Eye Contact Lens*, 2019.

[16] T. Shinha and I. C. Oguagha, "Osteomyelitis caused by *Achromobacter xylosoxidans*," *IDCases*, vol. 2, no. 1, pp. 11–12, 2015.

[17] P. Taylor and L. Fischbein, "Prosthetic knee infection due to *Achromobacter xylosoxidans*," *The Journal of Rheumatology*, vol. 19, no. 6, pp. 992–993, 1992.

[18] V. Gupta, S. Nirkhiwale, P. Gupta, and S. Phatak, "*Achromobacter xylosoxidans* mesh related infection: a case of delayed diagnosis and management," *Journal of Infection*, vol. 64, no. 3, pp. 1–5, 2012.

[19] V. K. Eshwara, C. Mukhopadhyay, S. Mohan, R. Prakash, and G. Pai, "Two unique presentations of *Achromobacter xylosoxidans* infections in clinical settings," *The Journal of Infection in Developing Countries*, vol. 5, no. 2, pp. 138–141, 2011.

[20] M. S. Ahmed, C. Nistal, R. Jayan, M. Kuduvalli, and H. K. Anijeet, "*Achromobacter xylosoxidans*, an emerging pathogen in catheter-related infection in dialysis population causing prosthetic valve endocarditis: a case report and review of literature," *Clinical Nephrology*, vol. 71, no. 3, pp. 350–354, 2009.

[21] G. Aisenberg, K. V. Rolston, and A. Safdar, "Bacteremia caused by *Achromobacter* and *Alcaligenes* species in 46 patients with cancer (1989–2003)," *Cancer*, vol. 101, no. 9, pp. 2134–2140, 2004.

[22] L. Amoureux, J. Bador, E. Siebor, N. Taillefumier, A. Fanton, and C. Neuwirth, "Epidemiology and resistance of *Achromobacter xylosoxidans* from cystic fibrosis patients in Dijon, Burgundy: first French data," *Journal of Cystic Fibrosis*, vol. 12, no. 2, pp. 170–176, 2013.

[23] R. Manfredi, A. Nanetti, M. Ferri, and F. Chiodo, "Bacteremia and respiratory involvement by *Alcaligenes xylosoxidans* in patients infected with the human immunodeficiency virus," *European Journal of Clinical Microbiology and Infectious Diseases*, vol. 16, no. 12, pp. 933–938, 1997.

[24] S. L. Claassen, J. M. Reese, V. Mysliwiec, and S. D. Mahlen, "*Achromobacter xylosoxidans* infection presenting as a pulmonary nodule mimicking cancer," *Journal of Clinical Microbiology*, vol. 49, no. 7, pp. 2751–2754, 2011.

[25] I. J. Abbott and A. Y. Peleg, "*Stenotrophomonas Achromobacter*, and nonmelioid *Burkholderia* species: antimicrobial resistance and therapeutic strategies," *Seminars in Respiratory and Critical Care Medicine*, vol. 36, no. 1, pp. 99–110, 2015.

[26] T. Spilker, P. Vandamme, and J. J. Lipuma, "Identification and distribution of *Achromobacter* species in cystic fibrosis," *Journal of Cystic Fibrosis*, vol. 12, no. 3, pp. 298–301, 2013.

[27] T. Spilker, P. Vandamme, and J. J. LiPuma, "A multilocus sequence typing scheme impliespopulation structure and reveals several putative novel *Achromobacter* species," *Journal of Clinical Microbiology*, vol. 50, pp. 3010–3015, 2012.

[28] P. A. Vandamme, C. Peeters, E. Inganäs et al., "Taxonomic dissection of *Achromobacter* denitrificans Coenye et al. 2003 and proposal of *Achromobacter* agilis sp. nov., nom. rev., *Achromobacter* pestifer sp. nov., nom. rev., *Achromobacter* kerstersii sp. nov. and *Achromobacter* deleyi sp. nov," *International Journal of Systematic and Evolutionary Microbiology*, vol. 66, no. 9, pp. 3708–3717, 2016.

[29] L. Amoureux, J. Bador, T. Verrier, H. Mjahed, C. De Curraize, and C. Neuwirth, "*Achromobacter xylosoxidans* is the predominant *Achromobacter* species isolated from diverse non-respiratory samples," *Epidemiology Infection*, vol. 144, no. 16, pp. 3527–3530, 2016.

[30] P. Vandamme, E. R. B. Moore, M. Cnockaert et al., "*Achromobacter* animicus sp. nov., *Achromobacter* mucicolens sp. nov., *Achromobacter* pulmonis sp. nov. and *Achromobacter* spiritinus sp. nov., from human clinical samples," *Systematic and Applied Microbiology*, vol. 36, pp. 1–10, 2013.

[31] P. Vandamme, E. R. B. Moore, M. Cnockaert et al., "Classification of *Achromobacter* genogroups 2, 5, 7 and 14 as *Achromobacter* insuavis sp.nov., *Achromobacter* aegrifaciens sp. nov., *Achromobacter* anxifer sp. nov. and *Achromobacter* dolens sp. nov., respectively," *Systematic and Applied Microbiology*, vol. 36, pp. 474–482, 2013.

[32] M. Almuzara, A. Limansky, V. Ballerini, L. Galanternik, A. Famiglietti, and C. Vay, "*In vitro* susceptibility of *Achromobacter* spp. isolates: comparison of disk diffusion, Etest and agar dilution methods," *International Journal of Antimicrobial Agents*, vol. 35, no. 1, pp. 68–71, 2010.

[33] J. Bador, L. Amoureux, J. M. Duez et al., "First description of an RND-type multidrug efflux pump in *Achromobacter xylosoxidans*, AxyABM," *Antimicrobial Agents and Chemotherapy*, vol. 55, no. 10, pp. 4912–4914, 2011.

[34] J. Bador, L. Amoureux, E. Blanc, and C. Neuwirth, "Innate aminoglycoside resistance of *Achromobacter xylosoxidans* is due to AxyXY-OprZ, an RND-type multidrug efflux pump," *Antimicrobial Agents and Chemotherapy*, vol. 57, no. 1, pp. 603–605, 2013.

[35] J. Bador, C. Neuwirth, P. Liszczynski et al., "Distribution of innate efflux-mediated aminoglycoside resistance among different *Achromobacter* species," *New Microbes New Infections*, vol. 12, no. 10, pp. 1–5, 2015.

[36] S. Iyobe, H. Kusadokoro, A. Takahashi et al., "Detection of a variant metallo-beta-lactamase, IMP-10, from two unrelated strains of *Pseudomonas aeruginosa* and an *Alcaligenes xylosoxidans* strain," *Antimicrobial Agents and Chemotherapy*, vol. 46, no. 6, pp. 2014–2016, 2002.

[37] M. L. Riccio, L. Pallecchi, R. Fontana, and G. M. Rossolini, "In70 of plasmid pAX22, a bla(VIM-1)-containing integron carrying a new aminoglycoside phosphotransferase gene cassette," *Antimicrobial Agents and Chemotherapy*, vol. 45, no. 4, pp. 1249–1253, 2001.

[38] K. S. Shin, K. Han, J. Lee et al., "Imipenem-resistant *Achromobacter xylosoxidans* carrying blaVIM-2-containing class 1 integron," *Diagnostic Microbiology and Infectious Disease*, vol. 53, no. 3, pp. 215–220, 2005.

[39] C. Neuwirth, C. Freby, A. Ogier-Desserrey et al., "VEB-1 in *Achromobacter xylosoxidans* from cystic fibrosis patient France," *Emerging Infectious Diseases*, vol. 12, no. 11, pp. 1737–1739, 2006.

[40] A. El Salabi, P. S. Borra, M. A. Toleman, Ø. Samuelsen, and T. R. Walsh, "Genetic and biochemical characterization of a novel metallo-β-lactamase, TMB-1, from an *Achromobacter xylosoxidans* strain isolated in Tripoli, Libya," *Antimicrobial Agents and Chemotherapy*, vol. 56, no. 5, pp. 2241–2245, 2012.

[41] R. D. Shah, N. Tariq, C. Shanley, J. Robbins, and R. Janczyk, "Peritonitis from peg tube insertion in surgical intensive care unit patients: identification of risk factors and clinical outcomes," *Surgical Endoscopy*, vol. 23, no. 11, pp. 2580–2586, 2009.

[42] W. Luman, K. R. Kwek, K. L. Loi, M. A. Chiam, W. K. Cheung, and H. S. Ng, "Percutaneous endoscopic gastrostomy–indications and outcome of our experience at the Singapore general hospital," *Singapore Medical Journal*, vol. 42, no. 10, pp. 460–465, 2001.

[43] P. K. Li, C. C. Szeto, B. Piraino et al., "ISPD peritonitis recommendations: 2016 update on prevention and treatment," *Peritoneal Dialysis International*, vol. 36, no. 5, pp. 481–508, 2016.

[44] C. Löser, G. Aschl, X. Hébuterne et al., "ESPEN guidelines on artificial enteral nutrition–percutaneous endoscopic gastrostomy (PEG)," *Clinical Nutrition*, vol. 24, no. 5, pp. 848–861, 2005.

[45] S. Krishna, S. Singh, K. R. Dinesh, R. Kp, I. Siyad, and S. Karim, "Percutaneous endoscopic gastrostomy (PEG) site infections: a clinical and microbiological study from university teaching hospital, India," *Journal of Infection Prevention*, vol. 16, no. 3, pp. 113–116, 2015.

[46] K. A. Chaudhary, O. J. Smith, P. G. Cuddy, and W. K. Clarkston, "PEG site infections: the emergence of methicillin resistant *Staphylococcus aureus* as a major pathogen," *The American Journal of Gastroenterology*, vol. 97, no. 7, pp. 1713–1716, 2002.

[47] G. G. Rao, M. Osman, L. Johnson, D. Ramsey, S. Jones, and H. Fidler, "Prevention of percutaneous endoscopic gastrostomy site infections caused by methicillin-resistant *Staphylococcus aureus*," *Journal of Hospital Infection*, vol. 58, no. 1, pp. 81–83, 2004.

[48] G. Abuksis, M. Mor, N. Segal et al., "Percutaneous endoscopic gastrostomy: high mortality rates in hospitalized patients," *The American Journal of Gastroenterology*, vol. 95, no. 1, pp. 128–132, 2000.

[49] M. Melgosa, O. Espinazo, A. Alonso, Perea A. García, and M. Navarro, "Dialysis-associated *Alcaligenes xylosoxidans* peritonitis: a pediatric case," *Peritoneal Dialysis International*, vol. 24, no. 1, pp. 72–75, 2004.

[50] G. Koçak, A. Azak, B. Huddam, S. Yanik, and M. Duranay, "Continuous ambulatory peritoneal dialysis-related peritonitis in an uremic outpatient: *Achromobacter xylosoxidans*," *Blood Purification*, vol. 34, no. 1, pp. 1–2, 2012.

[51] E. Cankaya, M. Keles, E. Gulcan, A. Uyanik, and H. Uyanik, "A rare cause of peritoneal dialysis-related peritonitis: *Achromobacter* denitrificans," *Peritoneal Dialysis International*, vol. 34, no. 1, pp. 135–137, 2014.

[52] R. Donderski, M. Grajewska, A. Mikucka, B. Sulikowska, E. Gospodarek-Komkowska, and J. Manitius, "*Achromobacter xylosoxidans* relapsing peritonitis and *Streptococcus suis* peritonitis in peritoneal dialysis patients: a report of two cases," *Case Reports in Nephrology*, vol. 2018, Article ID 9454520, 5 pages, 2018.

[53] A. J. Morrison Jr. and K. Boyce, "4th Peritonitis caused by *Alcaligenes* denitrificans subsp. *xylosoxydans*: case report and review of the literature," *Journal of Clinical Microbiology*, vol. 24, no. 5, pp. 879–881, 1986.

[54] S. S. Haqqie, M. Roth, and G. R. Bailie, "Unsuccessful treatment of CAPD peritonitis caused by *Alcaligenes xylosoxidans* subsp. denitrificans," *Renal Failure*, vol. 17, no. 5, pp. 611–614, 1995.

[55] M. A. El-Shahawy, D. Kim, and M. F. Gadallah, "Peritoneal dialysis-associated peritonitis caused by *Alcaligenes xylosoxidans*," *American Journal of Nephrology*, vol. 18, no. 5, pp. 452–455, 1998.

[56] S. Tang, C. C. Cheng, K. C. Tse et al., "CAPD-associated peritonitis caused by *Alcaligenes xylosoxidans* sp. *xylosoxidans*," *American Journal of Nephrology*, vol. 21, no. 6, pp. 502–506, 2001.

[57] S. G. Ledger and P. Cordy, "Successful treatment of *Alcaligenes xylosoxidans* in automated peritoneal dialysis-related peritonitis," *Peritoneal Dialysis International*, vol. 27, no. 5, pp. 596–598, 2007.

[58] S. F. Tsai and K. H. Shu, "CAPD peritonitis caused by *Alcaligenes xylosoxidans* in a diabetic cirrhosis patient," *Renal Failure*, vol. 32, no. 7, pp. 899–901, 2010.

[59] T. G. Oh, J. H. Baek, S. J. Jeong et al., "Continuous ambulatory peritoneal dialysis-associated peritonitis caused by *Achromobacter xylosoxidans*: a case report and comprehensive literature review," *Infection Chemotherapy*, vol. 43, no. 3, pp. 275–278, 2011.

[60] M. T. Tsai, W. C. Yang, and C. C. Lin, "Continuous ambulatory peritoneal dialysis-related exit-site infections caused by *Achromobacter* denitrificans and *A. xylosoxidans*," *Peritoneal Dialysis International*, vol. 32, no. 3, pp. 362–363, 2012.

[61] R. H. Pereira, R. S. Leão, A. P. Carvalho-Assef et al., "Patterns of virulence factor expression and antimicrobial resistance in *Achromobacter xylosoxidans* and *Achromobacter* ruhlandii isolates from patients with cystic fibrosis," *Epidemiology Infection*, vol. 145, no. 3, pp. 600–606, 2017.

[62] S. K. Tom, Y. C. Yau, T. Beaudoin, J. J. LiPuma, and V. Waters, "Effect of high-dose antimicrobials on biofilm growth of *Achromobacter* species isolated from cystic fibrosis patients," *Antimicrobial Agents and Chemotherapy*, vol. 60, no. 1, pp. 650–652, 2015.

[63] E. M. Jarvis, C. M. Hawley, S. P. McDonald et al., "Predictors, treatment, and outcomes of nonPseudomonas Gram-negative peritonitis," *Kidney International*, vol. 78, no. 4, pp. 408–414

[64] J. Valdés-Sotomayor, A. Cirugeda, M. A. Bajo et al., "Increased severity of *Escherichia coli* peritonitis in peritoneal dialysis

patients independent of changes in in vitro antimicrobial susceptibility testing," *Peritoneal Dialysis International*, vol. 23, no. 5, pp. 450–455, 2003.

[65] N. Prasad, A. Gupta, R. K. Sharma, K. N. Prasad, S. Gulati, and A. P. Sharma, "Outcome of Gram-positive and Gram-negative peritonitis in patients on continuous ambulatory peritoneal dialysis: a single-center experience," *Peritoneal Dialysis International*, vol. 23, no. 2, pp. 144–147, 2003.

[66] C. C. Szeto, V. C. Chow, K. M. Chow et al., "Enterobacteriaceae peritonitis complicating peritoneal dialysis: a review of 210 consecutive cases," *Kidney International*, vol. 69, no. 7, pp. 1245–1252, 2006.

[67] A. Zurowska, R. Feneberg, B. A. Warady et al., "Gram-negative peritonitis in children undergoing long-term peritoneal dialysis," *American Journal of Kidney Diseases*, vol. 51, no. 3, pp. 455–462, 2008.

[68] S. A. Galat, K. D. Gerig, J. A. Porter, and F. A. Slezak, "Management of premature removal of the percutaneous gastrostomy," *The American Surgeon*, vol. 56, no. 11, pp. 733–736, 1990.

[69] Y. Al-Abboodi, A. Ridha, M. Fasullo, and T. H. Naguib, "Risks of PEG tube placement in patients with cirrhosis-associated ascites," *Clinical and Experimental Gastroenterology*, vol. 10, pp. 211–214, 2017.

[70] M. R. Taheri, H. Singh, and D. R. Duerksen, "Peritonitis after gastrostomy tube replacement: a case series and review of literature," *Journal of Parenteral and Enteral Nutrition*, vol. 35, no. 1, pp. 56–60, 2011.

[71] M. C. Allison, J. A. Sandoe, R. Tighe, I. A. Simpson, R. J. Hall, and T. S. Elliott, "Antibiotic prophylaxis in gastrointestinal endoscopy," *Gut*, vol. 58, no. 6, pp. 869–880, 2009.

[72] J. I. Boullata, A. L. Carrera, L. Harvey et al., "ASPEN Safe practices for enteral nutrition therapy," *Journal of Parenteral and Enteral Nutrition*, vol. 41, no. 1, pp. 15–103, 2017.

10

A Case of Heterotopic Pancreatic Tissue Discovered in the Distal Esophagus

Dema Shamoon[1] **Vanessa Sostre**[1] **Varun Patel**[2] **and Ariy Volfson**[2]

[1]*Department of Medicine, St. Joseph's University Medical Center, Paterson, NJ, USA*
[2]*Division of Gastroenterology and Hepatology, St. Joseph's University Medical Center, Paterson, NJ, USA*

Correspondence should be addressed to Dema Shamoon; demamoon@gmail.com

Academic Editor: Hideto Kawaratani

Heterotopic pancreas (HP) is a congenital abnormality that represents ectopic pancreatic tissue that does not have anatomic, vascular, or ductal continuity. The prevalence of HP is 0.55% to 13.7% on autopsy, 0.2% to 0.5% of abdominal operations, and 0.9% of gastrectomies. It is commonly found in the stomach, duodenum, and proximal jejunum. Only 15 cases have been reported in the medical literature regarding involvement of the esophagus. Treatment depends on symptoms and location. In asymptomatic patients, simple observation may be sufficient; however, in those who are symptomatic, surgery may be warranted. We present a case of a 70-year-old male with heartburn, nausea, and abdominal bloating who underwent a diagnostic esophagogastroduodenoscopy (EGD) and was found to have HP on histology in the distal esophagus. In our case, symptoms were treated conservatively and successfully with a proton pump inhibitor (PPI).

1. Introduction

A heterotopic pancreas (HP) is a congenital anomaly that is anatomically separate yet histologically the same as the pancreas [1, 2]. This anomaly is also known as ectopic, aberrant, or as an accessory pancreas as it does not have anatomic, vascular, or ductal continuity [1, 2]. Cases are most commonly seen in the upper gastrointestinal tract (GIT) such as the stomach, duodenum, and proximal jejunum [2–4]. Although less common, HP may also be seen in the esophagus, ileum, Meckel diverticulum, and biliary tree [2]. HP affects males two times more than females and typically is not discovered until the fifth to sixth decade of life despite a few cases in children and young adults [5]. HP presenting in the esophagus is uncommon with approximately fifteen adult cases reported in the medical literature [1, 3, 5–19]. We present a case of a 70-year-old male who was incidentally found to have HP located in the distal esophagus on EGD after reported complaints of heartburn, nausea, and abdominal bloating.

2. Presentation

This is a case of a 70-year-old male with a medical history significant for hypertension, hypercholesterolemia, melanoma, and atrial fibrillation who presented with complaints of heartburn, nausea, and abdominal bloating. Patient reported to also have hiccups along with nausea but no episodes of vomiting. Patient endorsed mild abdominal distention. He denied abdominal pain, hematochezia, melena, hematemesis, change in bowel movements, or weight loss. Physical exam did not reveal any abnormalities. Routine blood work was unremarkable. Initially, our patient was treated for dyspepsia with a trial of PPI. He was scheduled for an EGD, which revealed an incidental 5 mm polypoid appearing lesion in the distal esophagus above the gastroesophageal junction (Figures 1 and 2). Biopsy results revealed squamous mucosa with active esophagitis and associated cardiac-type mucosa with focal pancreatic heterotopia and chronic inflammation in the distal esophagus (Figures 3–5). Given the relatively small size of the lesion, it

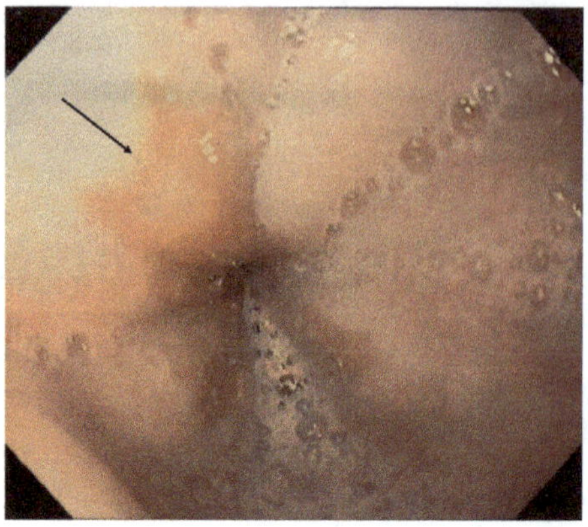

FIGURE 1: Endoscopic image of a polypoid lesion in the distal esophagus above the gastroesophageal junction.

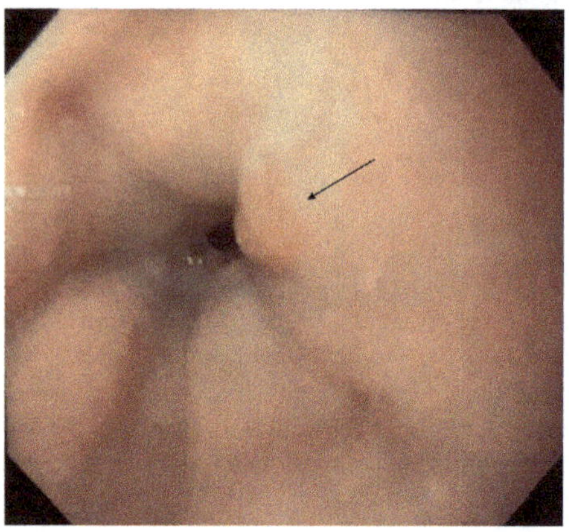

FIGURE 2: Another endoscopic image of a polypoid lesion in the distal esophagus above the gastroesophageal junction.

was resected endoscopically. The patient was treated conservatively with supportive with PPI for his gastric inflammation and symptoms. Patient is to be followed in one year for surveillance of the lesion with biopsy. Patient may need an endoscopic ultrasound (EUS) depending on his surveillance EGD results.

3. Discussion

Heterotopic pancreatic tissue is an uncommon congenital malformation that typically is found incidentally due to its nonspecific nature [4]. The incidence is hard to determine; however, the prevalence of HP is 0.55% to 13.7% on autopsy, 0.2% to 0.5% of abdominal operations, and 0.9% of gastrectomies [2–4].

The pathogenesis of the pancreas involves the fusion of the ventral and dorsal outpouchings of the foregut with detachment of branching pancreatic buds [3]. The embryologic basis of HP is unknown, but the theory of misplacement describes how pancreatic tissue is deposited in developing areas of the GIT [2]. Two additional theories are described in the literature [2]. The metaplasia theory depicts the migration of endodermal cells to the mucosa and subsequent change to pancreatic tissue during the time of embryogenesis [2]. The totipotent cell theory involves differentiation of cells that line the gut [2].

While HP does not have anatomic, vascular, and ductal continuity to the pancreas, it may still function similarly if it consists of acini, ducts, and islets of Langerhans [3, 15]. Acini, which are responsible for the exocrine function of the pancreas, permit the secretion of enzyme-rich serous fluid into the duct lumen due to its membrane-bound zymogen granules [3]. Leakage of proteolytic enzymes may lead to tissue breakdown and activation of the coagulation cascade [5]. Consequently, this event could lead to formation of small fibrin thrombi and secondary ischemic damage [5]. A secondary inflammatory response occurs from the release of lipase and phospholipase causing fat necrosis [5]. This is compounded by the release of proteases that digest protein substrates and further worsen the inflammatory response [5]. As seen in our case's histopathology, the chronic inflammation of the distal esophagus places him at higher risk for development of an inflammatory mass [5]. With the persistent inflammation and release of enzymes from cell breakdown, it may similarly present as chronic pancreatitis. Possible complications of ectopic tissue include benign or malignant transformation of tissue, pseudocyst or cyst formation, pancreatitis, gastrointestinal bleeding, ulceration, gastric outlet obstruction, or intussusception [2, 3, 15]. Table 1 exhibits the cases of HP found in literature with specific characteristics such as age, sex, location, presentation, and complications as well as treatment and follow-up.

Differentiating malignancy and HP can prevent unnecessary surgical intervention [2]. Most of the information available is related to HP in the stomach. Three criteria were reported by Guillou et al. that explain how malignancy may result from HP [8, 19, 20]. The first criteria states that the tumor must be found within or close in proximity to the lesion [8, 19, 20]. The second is when a clear evolution is seen between the carcinoma and pancreatic structures such as ductal cell dysplasia or carcinoma in situ [8, 19, 20]. The last criteria states that the nonneoplastic HP includes fully developed acini and ductal structures [8, 19, 20]. Our histology did not show malignant morphology and mainly pancreatic acini. The risk of pursuing surgical intervention immediately outweighs the risk of observation in this patient. The risk of malignancy from HP is rare and rather than subject an elderly patient with comorbidities to surgery, yearly observation seems appropriate [8]. Our patient presented with nausea and hiccups, but no other symptoms alarming for malignancy. If our patient develops symptoms of dysphagia, obstruction, upper GI bleed, pain, weight loss, nausea, or vomiting, it is important at that time to reassess as it could represent alarm symptoms for malignancy [2, 3, 5]. A feasible option is to also utilize EUS and fine needle aspiration (FNA) to further assess the depth of the lesion in comparison to the layers of the wall upon next evaluation. Of the fifteen cases of HP, two were found to be malignant and those patients had symptoms of weight loss, dysphagia, and epigastric pain [8, 9].

On CT, HP may appear as a small oval intramural mass with microlobulated margins and an endoluminal growth pattern [2]. Contrast enhancement and homogeneity are

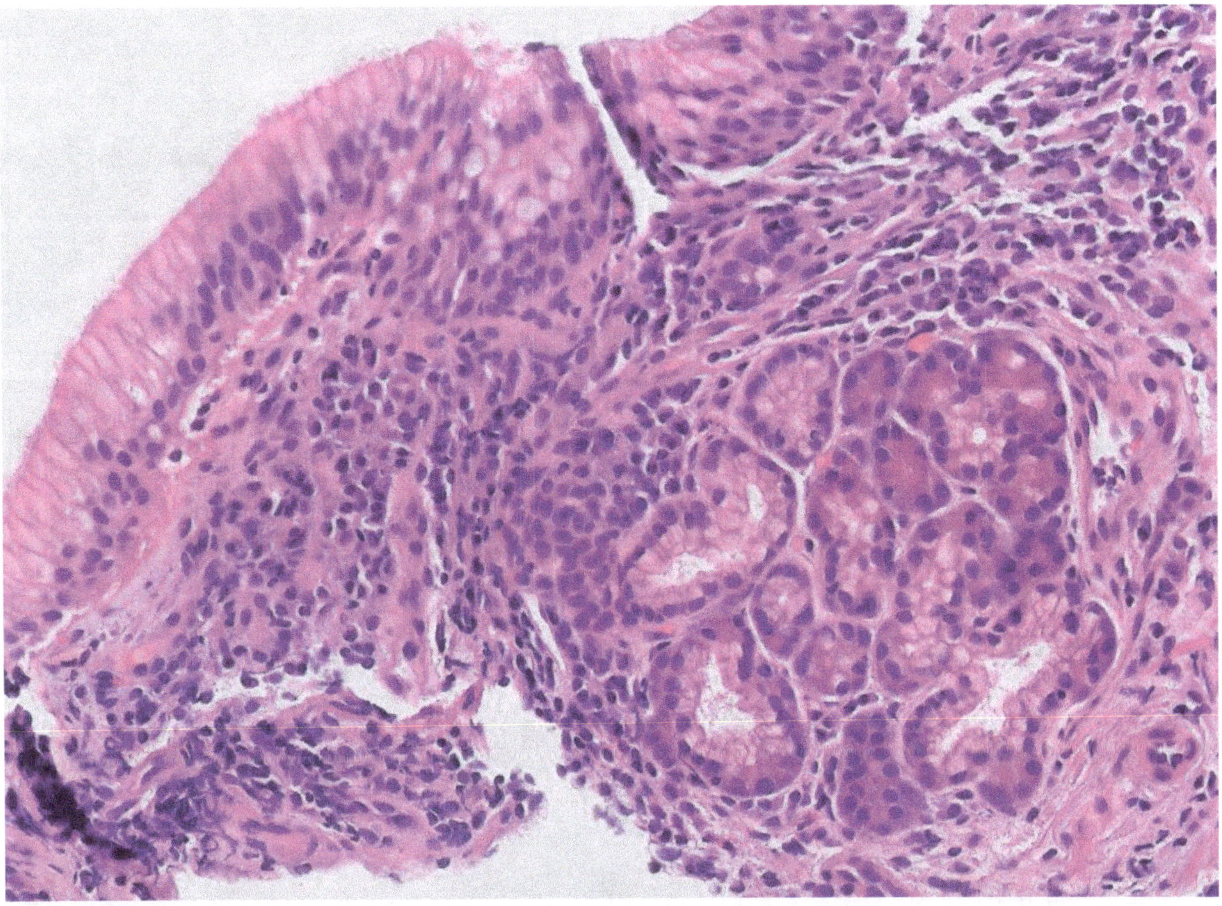

FIGURE 3: Histopathology of the distal esophageal submucosal lesion showing a well-circumscribed small nodule of pancreatic acinar glands.

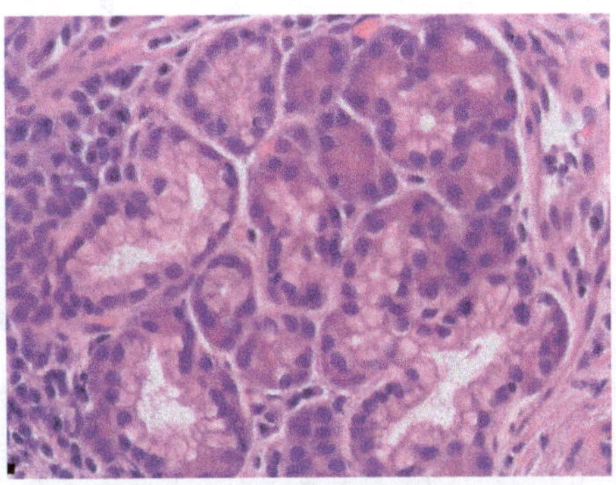

FIGURE 4: Histopathology of the distal esophageal submucosal lesion with higher magnification showing a well-circumscribed small nodule of pancreatic acinar glands.

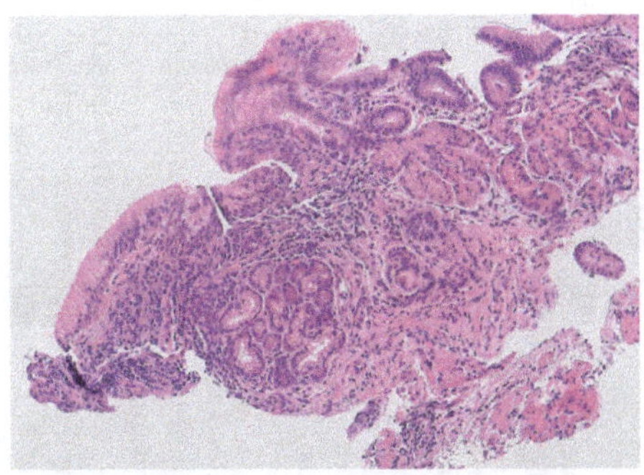

FIGURE 5: Histopathology of the distal esophageal submucosal lesion at low magnification showing a well-circumscribed small nodule of pancreatic acinar glands.

features that may apparel with histologic composition [2]. On MRI, HP is isointense to the orthotopic pancreas with characteristic T1 hyperintensity and early avid enhancement after administration of intravenous gadolinium-based contrast material [2]. Diagnosis occurs usually by EGD, EUS, operation, or autopsy depending on the presentation of symptoms and location of the tissue [4]. When visualized on EGD, a pancreatic rest may appear to be a submucosal bulge covered with normal mucosa with or without a central umbilication [16]. EUS may exhibit an intermediate echogram between the echodense submucosa and hyperechoic muscularis propria (MP) layer; relatively, the lesion appears to be hypoechoic to the submucosa and isoechoic to the MP [2, 16]. Others have suggested, such as Minamoto, that tubular or circular echoless structures may represent pancreatic rest [16, 21]. EUS also allows for sampling via FNA; however, it is not always specific to diagnose HP [2, 16]. Biopsy results are typically nondiagnostic due to the submucosal location of the lesion [10]. Histological evidence is usually achieved after submucosal resection and dissection of the area [10, 22].

Table 1: Reported cases of heterotopic pancreas in the esophagus among adults in the medical literature.

Case	Age	Sex	Location	Presentation	Treatment	Follow-up
Crighton and Botha [15]	58	F	GEJ	Progressive dysphagia due to IPMN	Laparoscopic/thorascopic ILE	Asymptomatic at 3 months
Temes et al. [10]	24	F	4.5 cm mass 3 cm proximal to the GEJ	5 days of nausea, vomiting, fever, chest pain, SOB due to esophageal rupture, and empyema	Esophageal enucleation, esophageal mucosa, and muscle closed	Asymptomatic at 1 year
Lowry et al. [1]	25	M	Mass located in submucosa of distal esophagus	RUQ and epigastric abdominal pain. EGD showed fistulous tracts 3 cm proximal to GEJ and stomach nodule	VATS resection	Asymptomatic at 2 months
Noffsinger et al. [5]	47	F	Distal esophagus	Epigastric abdominal pain, unable to tolerate solid foods, poor appetite, and weight loss for 2 weeks that was found to have 9 cm mass at the GEJ	ILE, pyloroplasty, Witzel jejunostomy	Infections and respiratory distress postoperative
Goto et al. [13]	63	M	~2 cm in diameter submucosal tumor in the middle third of esophagus	Asymptomatic, incidental finding	Conservative management	Asymptomatic for 5 years
Ulrych et al. [17]	34	M	Tumor arising from the lower esophagus	Several years of dyspepsia with 3 months of progressive dysphagia, odynophagia, and regurgitation. Weight loss and weakness.	Left posterolateral thoracotomy, primary anastomosis, and partial fundoplication	Asymptomatic at 3 months
Gananadha and Hunt [12]	26	F	Mass located in the wall of the distal esophagus; caudal portion was involved with GEJ	Episodes of severe epigastric pain, occurring after food intake, and nausea	Diagnostic laparoscopy discovered mass in the wall of distal esophagus. Cephalad portion was cystic which was separated from esophageal mucosa. Caudal portion was excised using endo-GIA stapler. Partial Dor fundoplication performed afterwards.	Asymptomatic at 2 months
Roshe et al. [9]	45	M	Distal esophagus	Dysphagia for 6 weeks	Left thoracoabdominal esophagogastrectomy	Asymptomatic
Razi [7]	43	M	Distal esophagus	Massive upper GI bleeding	Thoracotomy for removal of the pleural over the esophagus; tumor was enucleated from the esophageal wall	Asymptomatic
Salo et al. [6]	25	M	Distal esophagus	Nonspecific upper abdominal discomfort, heartburn, and vomiting for 1 year preoperatively. 3 years postoperatively, EGD showed reflux esophagitis.	Intramural esophageal cyst was enucleated by right thoracotomy. Reflux was treated with metoclopramide and ranitidine.	N/A
Shalaby et al. [16]	52	M	Mass located at GEJ	Episodic dysphagia	Small food boluses	Asymptomatic
Guillou et al. [8]	60	M	Ulcerated mass located at GEJ	Epigastric pain, dysphagia, and weight loss.	Tumor resection by left thoracotomy with proximal stomach resection; esophagogastric anastomosis	Asymptomatic at first but then developed bronchopneumonia and died 3 months postoperatively
Rodriguez et al. [11]	41	F	Submucosal mass found at GEJ extending into lesser curvature of stomach	Dysphagia and epigastric pain	Total gastrectomy with Roux-en-Y esophagojejunostomy	N/A
Garn et al. [14]	38	F	Submucosal tumor of GEJ	GERD	Endoscopically assisted laparoscopic resection	Asymptomatic
Salim et al. [18]	29	M	Irregularity of Z-line in distal esophagus	Epigastric pain radiating to the chest, worsened by hunger. Dysphagia to solids.	N/A	N/A

GEJ: gastroesophageal junction; IPMN: intraductal papillary mucinous neoplasm; SOB: shortness of breath; RUQ: right upper quadrant; VATS: video-assisted thoracoscopic surgery; ILE: Ivor-Lewis esophagectomy; GI: gastrointestinal; GERD: gastroesophageal reflux disease.

Treatment of the condition varies based on symptoms and location. Options include observation, Ivor-Lewis esophagectomy (ILE), and surgical or laparoscopic resection [1]. Although many cases have shown that surgical resection is the primary treatment, conservative treatment when identified by biopsy may be possible as only few cases of malignant transformation have been reported [13]. In our case, this was an incidentally found lesion, and it was unclear whether it was the reason for our symptoms. Therefore, our patient was treated conservatively with one-year surveillance with EGD.

4. Conclusions

We present a 70-year-old male who was diagnosed by histopathology to have a heterotopic pancreas after complaints of heartburn, nausea, and abdominal bloating. This condition is rare with only about 15 adult cases reported. The lesion was resected endoscopically, and PPI was initiated for symptomatic relief as well as gastric inflammation. Patient will be followed with surveillance with biopsy with EUS pending biopsy results.

Disclosure

Between the dates of October 25–30, 2019, our case was presented at the American College of Gastroenterology Annual Scientific Meeting in San Antonio, Texas.

References

[1] D. M. Lowry, T. E. MacK, B. J. Partridge, B. C. Barbick, R. M. Marks, and J. T. Kindelan, "Thorascopic resection of esophageal heterotopic pancreas," *The Annals of Thoracic Surgery*, vol. 96, no. 5, pp. 1850-1851, 2013.

[2] M. Rezvani, C. Menias, K. Sandrasegaran, J. D. Olpin, K. M. Elsayes, and A. M. Shaaban, "Heterotopic pancreas: histopathologic features, imaging findings, and complications," *Radiographics*, vol. 37, no. 2, pp. 484–499, 2017.

[3] T. Mack, D. Lowry, P. Carbone, B. Barbick, J. Kindelan, and R. Marks, "Multimodality imaging evaluation of an uncommon entity: esophageal heterotopic pancreas," *Case Reports in Radiology*, vol. 2014, Article ID 614347, 6 pages, 2014.

[4] V. Yagnik, K. Patel, P. Patel, and F. Mulla, "Ectopic pancreatic tissue in the cecum," *Saudi Journal of Gastroenterology*, vol. 16, no. 3, p. 228, 2010.

[5] A. E. Noffsinger, D. M. Hyams, and C. M. Fenoglio-Preiser, "Esophageal heterotopic pancreas presenting as an inflammatory mass," *Digestive Diseases and Sciences*, vol. 40, no. 11, pp. 2373–2379, 1995.

[6] J. A. Salo, M. Dlouhy, and I. Virtanen, "Congenital cyst and heterotopic pancreatic tissue in the oesophagus," *Annales Chirurgiae et Gynaecologiae*, vol. 82, no. 4, pp. 263–265, 1993.

[7] M. D. Razi, "Ectopic pancreatic tissue of esophagus with massive upper gastrointestinal bleeding," *Archives of Surgery*, vol. 92, no. 1, pp. 101–104, 1966.

[8] L. Guillou, P. Nordback, C. Gerbet, and R. P. Schneider, "Ductal adenocarcinoma arising in a heterotopic pancreas situated in a hiatal hernia," *Archives of Pathology & Laboratory Medicine*, vol. 118, no. 5, pp. 568–571, 1994.

[9] J. Roshe, E. Del Buono, D. Domenico, and T. J. Colturi, "Anaplastic carcinoma arising in ectopic pancreas located in the distal esophagus," *Journal of Clinical Gastroenterology*, vol. 22, no. 3, pp. 242–244, 1996.

[10] R. T. Temes, M. J. Menen, M. S. Davis, S. B. Pett, and J. A. Wernly, "Heterotopic pancreas of the esophagus masquerading as Boerhaave's syndrome," *The Annals of Thoracic Surgery*, vol. 69, no. 1, pp. 259–261, 2000.

[11] F. J. Rodriguez, S. C. Abraham, M. S. Allen, and T. J. Sebo, "Fine-needle aspiration cytology findings from a case of pancreatic heterotopia at the gastroesophageal junction," *Diagnostic Cytopathology*, vol. 31, no. 3, pp. 175–179, 2004.

[12] S. Gananadha and D. R. Hunt, "A unique case of pancreatitis and retention cyst in esophageal heterotopic pancreas," *Surgical Laparoscopy, Endoscopy & Percutaneous Techniques*, vol. 15, no. 6, pp. 345–347, 2005.

[13] J. Goto, S. Ohashi, S. Okamura et al., "Heterotopic pancreas in the esophagus diagnosed by EUS-guided FNA," *Gastrointestinal Endoscopy*, vol. 62, no. 5, pp. 812–814, 2005.

[14] T. Garn, T. Hallenscheidt, B. Schumacher, and H.-J. Krämling, "Tumor des ösophagokardialen Übergangs," *Der Chirurg*, vol. 82, no. 5, pp. 447–450, 2011.

[15] E. Crighton and A. Botha, "Intraductal papillary mucinous neoplasm of the oesophagus: an unusual case of dysphagia," *The Annals of The Royal College of Surgeons of England*, vol. 94, no. 2, pp. e92–e94, 2012.

[16] M. Shalaby, M. L. Kochman, and G. R. Lichtenstein, "Heterotopic pancreas presenting as dysphagia," *The American Journal of Gastroenterology*, vol. 97, no. 4, pp. 1046–1049, 2002.

[17] J. Ulrych, V. Fryba, H. Skalova, Z. Krska, T. Krechler, and D. Zogala, "Premalignant and malignant lesions of the heterotopic pancreas in the esophagus: a case report and review of the literature," *Journal of Gastrointestinal and Liver Diseases*, vol. 24, no. 2, pp. 235–239, 2015.

[18] S. T. Salim, L. Joo, and B. Blair, "Esophageal pancreatic heterotopia and dysphagia in the absence of a mass," *American Journal of Gastroenterology*, vol. 113, no. Supplement, p. S986, 2018.

[19] C. M. Qualia, T. M. Rossi, and A. Ullah, "Heterotopic pancreatic tissue found in the esophagus of a 14-year-old girl," *Gastroenterol Hepatol (N Y)*, vol. 3, no. 12, pp. 939-940, 2007.

[20] B. Papaziogas, I. Koutelidakis, P. Tsiaousis et al., "Carcinoma developing in ectopic pancreatic tissue in the stomach: a case report," *Cases Journal*, vol. 1, no. 1, 2008.

[21] T. Minamoto, H. Ueda, A. Ooi, K. Omote, T. Ogino, and M. Mai, "A limitation of endoscopic ultrasound: an unusual case of early gastric cancer overlying a pancreatic rest," *The American Journal of Gastroenterology*, vol. 86, no. 5, pp. 622–626, 1991.

[22] R. Filip, E. Walczak, J. Huk, R. P. Radzki, and M. Bieńko, "Heterotopic pancreatic tissue in the gastric cardia: a case report and literature review," *World Journal of Gastroenterology*, vol. 20, no. 44, pp. 16779-16781, 2014.

11

A Rare Cause of Ascites-Disseminated TB with Peritonitis in a Middle-Aged Female

Sahathevan Vithoosan,[1] **Ponnudurai Shanjeeban**,[1] **Joseph Philip Anpalahan**,[1] **Paramarajan Piranavan**,[2] **Harindra Karunatilake**,[1] **and Ananda Jayanaga**[1]

[1]*National Hospital, Colombo, Sri Lanka*
[2]*Internal Medicine, Saint Vincent Hospital, Worcester, MA 01608, USA*

Correspondence should be addressed to Sahathevan Vithoosan; vithoosan@gmail.com

Academic Editor: Yoshihiro Moriwaki

Background. Disseminated tuberculosis (TB) has been increasingly recognized in adults in the recent times due to increased prevalence of immune suppression. Here we describe a case of 47-year-old female who presented with disproportionate ascites where the diagnosis of disseminated TB was delayed. *Case Report.* A 47-year-old previously healthy female presented with generalised body swelling with disproportionate ascites and loss of appetite and weight for four-month duration. She denied any contact or past history of TB and reported no respiratory symptoms. Physical examination revealed significant ascites. There was no lymphadenopathy or hepatosplenomegaly. Respiratory system examination was normal. Her Erythrocyte Sedimentation Rate (ESR) was above 100. Tuberculin skin test was positive with 17mm. Contrast Enhanced Computed Tomography (CECT) abdomen revealed chronic liver disease with ascites. Diagnostic laparoscopy was in favour of miliary TB and the peritoneal biopsy revealed granulomatous inflammation with caseous necrosis, suggestive of TB. The patient was started on antituberculosis treatment and subsequently improved. *Conclusion.* TB peritonitis due to disseminated TB should be considered in the differential diagnosis of disproportionate ascites. Even though the diagnosis is difficult, diagnostic laparoscopy and biopsy is very helpful. It is important to have an early diagnosis since delay in treatment can be detrimental in most cases.

1. Introduction

Tuberculosis (TB) is a systemic infectious disease caused by *Mycobacterium tuberculosis* that affects multiple tissues and organs. Because it has diverse presentations, it requires a high index of suspicion. Disseminated TB has been increasingly recognised in adults in recent times. This is due to the increased prevalence of immune suppression due to acquired immunodeficiency syndrome (AIDS) and immunosuppressive therapies for various medical disorders [1]. Tuberculous peritonitis is a rare presentation of disseminated TB [2]. There is usually a delay of about one month from presentation to diagnosis in tuberculous peritonitis [2]. Here, we describe a case of a 47-year-old previously healthy female who presented with disproportionate ascites, where the diagnosis of disseminated TB was delayed. The case highlights the importance of and difficulty in diagnosing disseminated TB.

2. Case Presentation

A 47-year-old previously healthy female presented with generalised body swelling, disproportionate ascites, loss of appetite, and loss of weight for four months' duration. She denied any fever, night sweats, yellowish discolouration of the eyes, hematemesis, melena, chronic cough, and haemoptysis. She reported no history of orthopnoea and paroxysmal nocturnal dyspnoea, and her urine output remained normal.

Her past medical history was not significant for any liver, renal, or cardiac disease. She denied any past or contact history of TB. She reported no use of alcohol or herbal medications and no intravenous drug abuse. She was in a monogamous relationship and she denied any family history of liver or renal disease.

She was afebrile on admission and her vitals included a pulse rate within normal limits. On exam, she was emaciated

TABLE 1: The initial biochemical investigations.

Investigation	Result	Normal range
White cell count(10^9/L)	10.6	4-11
Neutrophil percentage	67%	
Lymphocyte percentage	28%	
Haemoglobin	7.4	11-13
Platelet count(10^9 /L)	511	150-450
C- Reactive Protein (CRP)(mg/L)	128	0-6
ESR(mm/1st hour)	110	<10
Serum creatinine(μmol/L)	52	60-120
Serum sodium (mmol/L)	135	135-148
Serum potassium(mmol/L)	4.2	3.5-5.1
Aspartate Transaminase(AST) (U/L)	56	<40
Alanine Transaminase (ALT) (U/L)	44	<40
Alkaline Phosphatase (ALP) (U/L)	776	30-120
Gamma Glutamyl Transferase (GGT)(U/L)	500	<50
Total bilirubin (mg/dl)	6.6	<1.2
Direct bilirubin (mg/dl)	3.4	<0.3
Serum total proteins(g/L)	58	61-80
Serum Albumin(g/L)	25	36-50
Serum Globulin(g/L)	33	22-40

TABLE 2: Aetiological work-up for CLD.

Investigation	Result
Viral markers	
Hepatitis B surface antigen	Negative
Hepatitis C antibody	Negative
Autoimmune markers	
ANA	Negative
Anti smooth muscle antibody	Negative
Iron studies	
Total binding capacity	252 mcg/dl(240-450)
Serum iron	60μg/dl (50-170)
Serum ferritin	310 ng/ml(12-150)
Serum Ceruloplasmin	28 mg/dl(20-35)

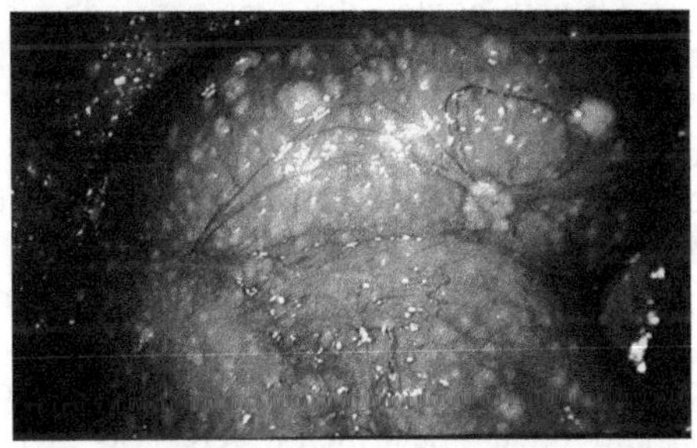

FIGURE 1: Studded miliary tubercles in laparoscopic examination.

with a body mass index of 18, and she had significant ascites with mild ankle oedema. She was anicteric and did not have any lymphadenopathy, hepatosplenomegaly, or the peripheral stigmata of chronic liver disease. Respiratory system and cardiovascular examinations were within normal limits. On eye exam, there was no evidence of choroid tubercles.

The initial laboratory findings are summarised in Table 1.

The anaemia workup, including serum iron studies, vitamin B12, and folate testing, was normal. A blood picture revealed normochromic normocytic anaemia and thrombocytosis, suggestive of anaemia of chronic disease. Thyroid function tests were normal. She did not have any proteinuria, and her international normalised ratio (INR) was normal. Repeated blood cultures, urine culture, and sputum culture were sterile, and a human immunodeficiency virus (HIV) fourth-generation test was negative. CA 125 was mildly elevated to 175 U/ml (<46 U/ml).

The initial chest x-ray (CXR) was normal, and her transthoracic two-dimensional echocardiography showed normal systolic and diastolic functions and no evidence of constrictive pericarditis. A transvaginal ultrasound (US) did not reveal any ovarian pathology. Meanwhile, an abdomen US revealed a mildly hyperechoic liver with moderate ascites. Contrast Enhanced Computed Tomography (CECT) of the abdomen and pelvis revealed a normal-sized liver with evidence of heterogenicity of the liver parenchyma with minimal nodularity of the liver surface and moderate ascites with no portal vein thrombosis or lymphadenopathy. The spleen, gallbladder, biliary tract, and intestines were normal, as were the ovaries. The findings were in favour of possible decompensated chronic liver disease (CLD). However, the CLD workup did not reveal any potential aetiology (Table 2). Upper gastrointestinal endoscopy (UGIE) was normal and did not show any evidence of portal gastropathy or varices.

The initial diagnosis of possible cryptogenic CLD was made, and the patient was started on spironolactone and furosemide. Even though the diagnostic paracentesis was planned on admission, it was delayed due to the patient's refusal, but we were to do initiate after a few days. The analysis of the ascitic fluid revealed an exudative picture. There was no evidence of spontaneous bacterial peritonitis, and the ascitic fluid cytology was negative for malignant cells.

With elevated inflammatory markers and an exudative type of ascites, we decided to proceed with further investigations to rule out possible peritoneal TB. The ascitic fluid acid-fast bacilli (AFB) test was negative. The ascitic fluid bacterial, TB culture, and TB Gene Xpert were negative. The tuberculin sensitivity test (Mantoux) was positive at 17 mm without ulceration. Her repeated sputum for AFB, TB culture, and GeneXpert were negative.

Because the clinical picture did not fit the imaging findings, we decided to proceed with diagnostic laparoscopy and peritoneal biopsy. The laparoscopy was in favour of miliary TB (Figure 1) and the peritoneal biopsy revealed granulomatous inflammation with caseous necrosis favouring TB. She was started on anti-TB treatment (ATT), and on initial follow-up, she showed improvement in her clinical, biochemical, and radiological parameters. Her fever settled with ATT, and her ESR was 15 mm/1st hour and CRP was 12 mg/l at 3 weeks after the initiation of ATT.

3. Discussion

Tuberculous peritonitis is a rare presentation of extra-pulmonary TB. The diagnosis is difficult due to its presentations overlapping with other diseases [2]. The delayed diagnosis leads to a delay in initiating treatment, which worsens outcomes [3]. A high index of suspicion is important for early diagnosis. Abdominal TB can involve the gastrointestinal tract, peritoneum, lymph nodes, or solid organs [4], and it comprises 5% of all cases of TB. Peritoneal TB mostly occurs following the reactivation of latent TB foci in the peritoneum established via the bloodstream and spread from a primary lung focus. Both the visceral and parietal peritonea can be studded with tubercles. Clinical manifestations of peritoneal TB include ascites, abdominal pain, and fever [3]. Three different forms of peritoneal TB have been reported, which include wet TB with ascites, dry type with adhesions, and fibrotic type with omental thickening and loculated ascites [5].

Our patient's ascites were disproportionate to the peripheral oedema. She was investigated for the potential causes for disproportionately predominant ascites, which include cirrhosis with portal hypertension, ovarian carcinoma, constrictive pericarditis, and peritonitis. Other causes of generalised oedema, such as congestive heart failure, nephrotic syndrome, and renal impairment, were also excluded by history, physical examination, and basic investigations. Both the abdominal US and the abdominal CECT revealed CLD with ascites. However, she did not have the peripheral stigmata of CLD and did not have significant risk factors for CLD. Blood investigations revealed an elevated platelet count and a normal INR. The absence of oesophageal varices and portal gastropathy further challenged the diagnosis of CLD. The exudative type of fluid on an ascitic fluid analysis led to the suspicion of any form of peritonitis in our patient. She did not have the typical constitutional symptoms or the risk factors for TB. Her CXR was normal, but her tuberculin sensitivity test (TST) was positive. However, the TST is of limited value in clinical work, especially in countries with a high prevalence of TB and prior Bacillus Calmette-Guerin vaccination. A positive test only indicates the infection but not the presence or extent of tuberculous disease. In our patient, the laparoscopic peritoneal biopsy revealed a peritoneum studded with tubercles, confirming our diagnosis.

It is important to note that the absence of CXR findings does not rule out the possibility of extra-pulmonary TB, as less than 25% of cases with extra-pulmonary TB were found to have an abnormal CXR [5]. The abdominal US can be a useful tool in the investigation for peritoneal TB, which may reveal ascites, lymphadenopathy, bowel wall thickening, and the pseudo kidney sign [5]. Interestingly, our patient's imaging was reported as decompensated CLD.

The ascitic fluid ADA and interferon activity were not checked in our patient due to limited resources. The ascitic fluid ADA is a potentially useful test, which can help when there is a diagnostic dilemma [6]. It was found to be a sensitive test, even in patients with concomitant cirrhosis. However, it must be noted that malignant ascites can give rise to a falsely high ADA [6]. High interferon activity is also noted in TB ascites. Combining ascitic fluid interferon activity with ADA may further increase the sensitivity of TB diagnosis [5]. The ascitic fluid AFB is often negative in cases of peritoneal TB [7]. Even though TB PCR is a useful diagnostic tool, it also has low sensitivity [8].

Our patient's serum CA 125 level was moderately elevated, but further investigations ruled out ovarian pathologies. Although CA 125 is used as a biomarker in the early detection of ovarian carcinoma, there have also been reports of elevated levels of soluble CA 125 in a number of other malignant conditions, such as breast cancer, mesothelioma, non-Hodgkin's lymphoma (NHL), gastric cancer, and leiomyosarcoma of gastrointestinal origin. CA 125 levels have also been found elevated in benign conditions, such as endometriosis, pregnancy, ovulatory cycles, liver diseases, and congestive heart failure, as well as in infectious disease, such as TB peritonitis [9]. There were instances where TB peritonitis has been mistaken as ovarian carcinomatosis based on elevated CA 125 [10]. Localizing CA 125 around tuberculous granuloma using immunohistochemistry was previously reported in literature [11]. Furthermore normalization of CA 125 levels after ATT supports the fact that the raised level could be due to peritoneal TB. So serial measurement of serum CA125 level in TB peritonitis may be of significance in follow-up and monitoring the response of disease to ATT [11].

Reduction in CRP levels after ATT is well described before in several cohorts of tuberculous patients. In one study when CRP levels decrease ≤55% at 2 weeks, it predicted death or hospitalization, with a negative predictive value of 99% [12]. Failure to see a decline after ATT may suggest alternative diagnosis or drug-resistant tuberculosis [13].

In our patient ALP, GGT and bilirubin were significantly elevated compared to other transaminases. The correlation between liver function tests and the site of liver disease in any infiltrative or infective diseases, including TB, was previously reported in the literature. The involvement of the liver parenchyma is usually reflected in elevated transaminases, while the involvement of the biliary tract or porta is usually reflected in elevated ALP and GGT. Bilirubin may be elevated in hepatic TB or miliary TB [14].

The visual appearance during laparoscopy will help in the diagnosis of tuberculous peritonitis [5], and our patient was studded with multiple yellow white tubercles.

Biopsies of the peritoneal lesion, lymph nodes, or other intra-abdominal locations are often necessary for the diagnosis. The laparoscopic biopsy is preferred, as it is minimally invasive and allows for the visualisation of the peritoneum [7]. The biopsy has a diagnostic yield of more than 80% in the diagnosis of tuberculous peritonitis [3]. Our patient's biopsy of the peritoneal lesion revealed granulomatous inflammation with caseous necrosis.

4. Conclusion

Tuberculous peritonitis due to disseminated TB should be considered in the differential diagnosis of disproportionate ascites. Even though the diagnosis is difficult, diagnostic laparoscopy and biopsy are highly helpful. It is important to reach an early diagnosis, as delays in treatment can be detrimental in these cases.

Authors' Contributions

Dr. S. Vithoosan collected data, followed up the patient, did literature review, and drafted the manuscript. Dr. P. Piranavan, Dr. J. P. Anpalahan, and Dr. P. Shanjeeban helped in finding the relevant literature and drafting the manuscript. Dr. A. Jayanaga and Dr. H. Karunatilake were involved in the patient management and corrected the manuscript. All the authors read and approved the final manuscript.

References

[1] M. Aye, C. J. S. F. Cabot, S. Baba, M. C. Thanabalan, and S. F. Chung, "Disseminated tuberculosis - a case study," *Journal of Metabolic Syndrome*, vol. 3, no. 2, pp. 2–5, 2014.

[2] C.-Y. Lee, H.-C. Tsai, S. S.-J. Lee, C. Sy, and Y.-S. Chen, "Disseminated tuberculosis presenting as tuberculous peritonitis and sepsis tuberculosa gravissima in a patient with cirrhosis of the liver: a diagnosis of challenge," *Journal of Microbiology, Immunology and Infection*, vol. 49, no. 4, pp. 608–612, 2016.

[3] K. M. Chow, V. C. Chow, L. C. Hung, S. M. Wong, and C. C. Szeto, "Tuberculous peritonitis-associated mortality is high among patients waiting for the results of mycobacterial cultures of ascitic fluid samples," *Clinical Infectious Diseases*, vol. 35, no. 4, pp. 409–413, 2002.

[4] U. Debi, V. Ravisankar, K. K. Prasad, S. K. Sinha, and A. K. Sharma, "Abdominal tuberculosis of the gastrointestinal tract: revisited," *World Journal of Gastroenterology*, vol. 20, no. 40, pp. 14831–14840, 2014.

[5] M. P. Sharma and V. Bhatia, "Abdominal tuberculosis," *Indian Journal of Medical Research*, vol. 120, no. 4, pp. 305–315, 2004.

[6] Y. J. Liao, C. Y. Wu, S. W. Lee et al., "Adenosine deaminase activity in tuberculous peritonitis among patients with underlying liver cirrhosis," *World Journal of Gastroenterology*, vol. 18, no. 37, pp. 5260–5265, 2012.

[7] M. O. Chaparro, C. A. Reyes-Ortiz, R. Soto, and J. W. Reynolds, "Abdominal tuberculosis presenting as ascites in an older indigenous woman: a case report," *JMM Case Reports*, vol. 2015, pp. 1–5, 2018.

[8] R. Avasthi, S. C. Chaudhary, and P. Jain, "Disseminated tuberculosis manifesting as chronic pancreatitis," *Indian Journal of Tuberculosis*, vol. 3, pp. 19–21, 2008.

[9] E. L. Moss, J. Hollingworth, and T. M. Reynolds, "The role of CA125 in clinical practice," *Journal of Clinical Pathology*, vol. 58, no. 3, pp. 308–312, 2005.

[10] J. D. Boss, C. T. Shah, O. Oluwole, and J. N. Sheagren, "TB peritonitis mistaken for ovarian carcinomatosis based on an elevated CA-125," *Case Reports in Medicine*, vol. 2012, Article ID 215293, 3 pages, 2012.

[11] V. Thakur, U. Mukherjee, and K. Kumar, "Elevated serum cancer antigen 125 levels in advanced abdominal tuberculosis," *Medical Oncology*, vol. 18, no. 4, pp. 289–291, 2001.

[12] D. Wilson, M. S. Moosa, T. Cohen, P. Cudahy, C. Aldous, and G. Maartens, "Evaluation of tuberculosis treatment response with serial C-reactive protein measurements," *Open Forum Infectious Diseases*, vol. 5, no. 11, article ofy253, 2018.

[13] V. Sharma, H. S. Mandavdhare, S. Lamoria, H. Singh, and A. Kumar, "Serial C-reactive protein measurements in patients treated for suspected abdominal tuberculosis," *Digestive and Liver Disease*, vol. 50, no. 6, pp. 559–562, 2018.

[14] A. J. Hickey, L. Gounder, M. S. Moosa, and P. K. Drain, "A systematic review of hepatic tuberculosis with considerations in human immunodeficiency virus co-infection," *BMC Infectious Diseases*, vol. 15, no. 1, article 209, 2015.

12

Acute Liver Failure following a Single Dose of Atezolizumab, as Assessed for Causality using the Updated RUCAM

Roie Tzadok,[1] **Sharon Levy**,[2] **Jessie Aouizerate**,[3] **and Oren Shibolet**[2]

[1]*Department of Internal Medicine C, Tel Aviv Sourasky Medical Center, Tel Aviv, Israel*
[2]*Department of Gastroenterology and Hepatology, Tel Aviv Sourasky Medical Center and the Sackler Faculty of Medicine, Tel Aviv University, Tel Aviv, Israel*
[3]*Institute of Pathology, Tel Aviv Sourasky Medical Center, Tel Aviv, Israel*

Correspondence should be addressed to Roie Tzadok; roie.tzadok@gmail.com

Academic Editor: Marcel Cerqueira Cesar Machado

Immune checkpoint inhibitors have become major therapeutic agents in oncology over the last few years. However, they are associated with a variety of potentially severe autoimmune phenomena. We present a patient with advanced adenocarcinoma of the lung, who presented with acute liver injury two weeks following his first treatment with atezolizumab, rapidly deteriorating to fulminant liver failure. A thorough evaluation of infectious, vascular, metabolic, and autoimmune etiologies did not yield any results. Liver pathology was nonspecific. Using RUCAM as a causality assessment method indicated probable connection between atezolizumab and liver damage. To our knowledge, this is the first documented report of a patient developing acute liver failure shortly after immune checkpoint inhibitor initiation.

1. Introduction

Immune checkpoint inhibitors (ICI) are antineoplastic agents that activate the immune system against tumor cells. Programmed death 1 (PD-1), its ligand-1 (PD-L1), and cytotoxic T-lymphocyte antigen 4 (CTLA-4) are the most common targets of these agents, which operate by relieving tumor-induced T-cell inactivation [1]. Atezolizumab is an Fc-modified IgG1 humanized monoclonal antibody directed against PD-L1 [2]. In the past several years, immunotherapy with ICI has become a leading treatment strategy in oncology, improving response and overall survival rates in a variety of neoplastic diseases [3].

Although ICI are usually well tolerated, their incurred immune activation may lead to autoimmune-like phenomena affecting a variety of organs, including the liver, colon, lungs, pituitary gland, thyroid, and skin. The extent of tissue injury varies but may be severe and even life threatening [4, 5]. All ICI induce autoimmunity, but ipilimumab, a CTLA-4 inhibitor, as well as combinations of ICI are considered more hepatotoxic than other ICI monotherapy regimens [6]. Although the mechanism for this immune-mediated toxicity is still unclear, antigen similarity between tumor cells and native host tissues may play a role [7]. Risk factors contributing to increased risk of ICI-induced liver injury may be the use of higher doses, a preexisting tendency to autoimmunity unmasked by ICI use or a preexisting liver disease [3].

2. Case Presentation

A 46-year-old male was diagnosed with adenocarcinoma of the lung and was treated with neo-adjuvant chemoradiation and lobectomy but was diagnosed with disease recurrence. His disease involved the right lung, cervical and thoracic vertebrae, pleura, mediastinal lymph nodes, and adjacent ribs. He was treated with a single-agent immunotherapy protocol with atezolizumab (without other coadministered drugs).

About two weeks after receiving the first treatment, he presented to our hospital complaining of weakness, vomiting, and epigastric pain in the previous week. He reported sporadic consumption of paracetamol a few days prior to his presentation, well below the considered hepatotoxic range. His physical examination was unremarkable. Laboratory tests demonstrated stable normocytic anemia with a hemoglobin of 8.1 g/dL, 9,400 leukocytes with an absolute lymphocyte count of 300 ($10^3/\mu L$), and 311,000 platelets. The sodium level was 125 mmol/L (normal 135–145 mmol/L), creatinine 1.37 (normal 0.7–1.3 mg/dL), and bilirubin 0.3 (normal 0.1–1.2 mg/dL). A new-onset mixed pattern of liver enzymes elevation was noted, with alanine aminotransferase (ALT) of 485 (normal 8–40 U/L), aspartate aminotransferase (AST) of 253 (normal 7–40 U/L), gamma glutamyltransferase (GGT) of 560 (normal 6–42 U/L), and alkaline phosphatase (ALKP) of 261 (normal 46–116 U/L). The international normalized ratio (INR) was 1.32 (normal 0.97–1.19). Urine tests indicated hypovolemic hyponatremia, most probably due to excessive vomiting. Abdominal and brain imaging ruled out bowel obstruction or intracranial metastases as causes of vomiting.

The patient was hospitalized in stable condition without hypotension and was treated with fluids. Over the next five days, he continued to deteriorate rapidly and progressed from acute liver injury to fulminant liver failure, with new-onset encephalopathy, further prolongation of INR to 2.91, and acute kidney injury with creatinine elevation up to 2.8 mg/dL, with accompanying profound lactic acidosis. His liver test abnormalities progressed with a predominant hepatocellular pattern ($R = 25$) [8], with ALT up to 2124 U/L and AST 1726 U/L. Cholestatic enzymes and bilirubin remained stable, and glucose levels were within the normal range.

The patient was not admitted to an intensive care unit (ICU) but was managed in an internal medicine department. He did not need mechanical ventilation at any stage. During his hospitalization, he underwent a full evaluation to determine the cause of his deterioration. Blood and urine cultures were negative. Liver ultrasonography and Doppler did not demonstrate any focal hepatic or vascular findings (portal vein thrombosis or Budd-Chiari syndrome) (Figure 1). A thorough evaluation for infectious, autoimmune, and metabolic etiologies of acute liver failure yielded no results: viral hepatitis (hepatitis B surface antigen and antibody, hepatitis B core antibody, hepatitis C antibody, and hepatitis A IgG antibody) and HIV serologies were negative. Ethanol levels were not elevated. CMV, EBV, VZV, and HSV serologies indicated past infections. Toxoplasma and celiac serologies were negative. Immunoglobulin levels were normal. Autoantibodies including ANA, ASMA, AMA, and anti-LKM were normal.

He developed large volume ascites and underwent paracentesis, demonstrating high serum-ascites albumin gradient (19 g/L) and ascites protein content of 24 g/L, suggestive of portal hypertension secondary to a hepatic cause. The patient also underwent a percutaneous liver biopsy (Figure 2), which showed zone 3 (centrilobular) necrosis and mild steatosis with bridging necrosis and mild neutrophilic infiltrate. Sinusoidal dilatation was also noted. No fibrosis was seen.

Hepatic sinusoidal dilatation is usually caused by hepatic venous outflow obstruction, whether due to pericardial disease, congestive heart failure, or direct hepatic vascular involvement (as in Budd-Chiari syndrome or sinusoidal obstruction syndrome). It may also happen in extrahepatic inflammatory diseases, without venous outflow obstruction. In these cases, the mechanism is not as clear but may be attributed to hemodynamic changes and overexpression of interleukin-6 (IL-6) [9]. The biopsy was interpreted as nonspecific, but a differential diagnosis of drug-induced liver injury (DILI) was suggested. Because there were no documented hypotensive episodes and blood cultures were sterile, we initiated empirical pulse steroid therapy (1000 mg methylprednisolone daily) and N-acetylcysteine after the biopsy was given. Due to the patient's metastatic disease, liver transplantation was not discussed.

Due to advancing acute liver injury with oliguria and acidosis, which was suspected to be checkpoint inhibitor-induced acute interstitial nephritis, the patient was scheduled to undergo hemodialysis. However, he developed severe shock and died after five days.

3. Discussion

This is a unique case of acute liver failure in a patient with metastatic adenocarcinoma of the lung, which developed shortly after one course of atezolizumab. Rigorous attempts to find other etiologies yielded no results. The pathologic report suggested DILI. The differential diagnosis of ischemic hepatitis seems less relevant as no vascular pathology was noted on Doppler sonography, and no hypotensive events were noted. Right heart failure leading to hepatic congestion and dilated sinusoids, possibly as a result of checkpoint-induced myocarditis, a previously described toxic side effect of ICI [10, 11], was also considered. The patient did not undergo echocardiography, but his physical examination and chest X-ray showed no signs of congestion, and his electrocardiogram demonstrated sinus rhythm without arrhythmias or ischemic changes. Therefore, a cardiac etiology for his condition seems less likely.

The Roussel Uclaf Causality Assessment Method (RUCAM) is a scale based on seven category parameters to assess causality for a liver injury being due to a specific medication. As the patient described in this case presented with a pattern of hepatocellular injury (R value > 5), the relevant RUCAM score was calculated to be +7, indicating atezolizumab to be a probable cause of liver failure. Alternatively, the RUCAM score for causality of acetaminophen-induced injury is +4, indicating only a possible connection, which is not supported by the clinical story [8].

Hepatic side effects have been reported in 3–10% of patients with ICI [12, 13] and most commonly manifest as asymptomatic elevations of liver enzymes, mostly transaminases, and mildly elevated bilirubin [14]. This pattern of liver enzyme abnormality was also present in this case.

Grading the severity of hepatic damage is based on the Common Terminology Criteria for Adverse Events (CTCAE) established by the Cancer Therapy Evaluation Program of the National Cancer Institute and is based on levels of multiples of the upper normal limit of ALT, AST,

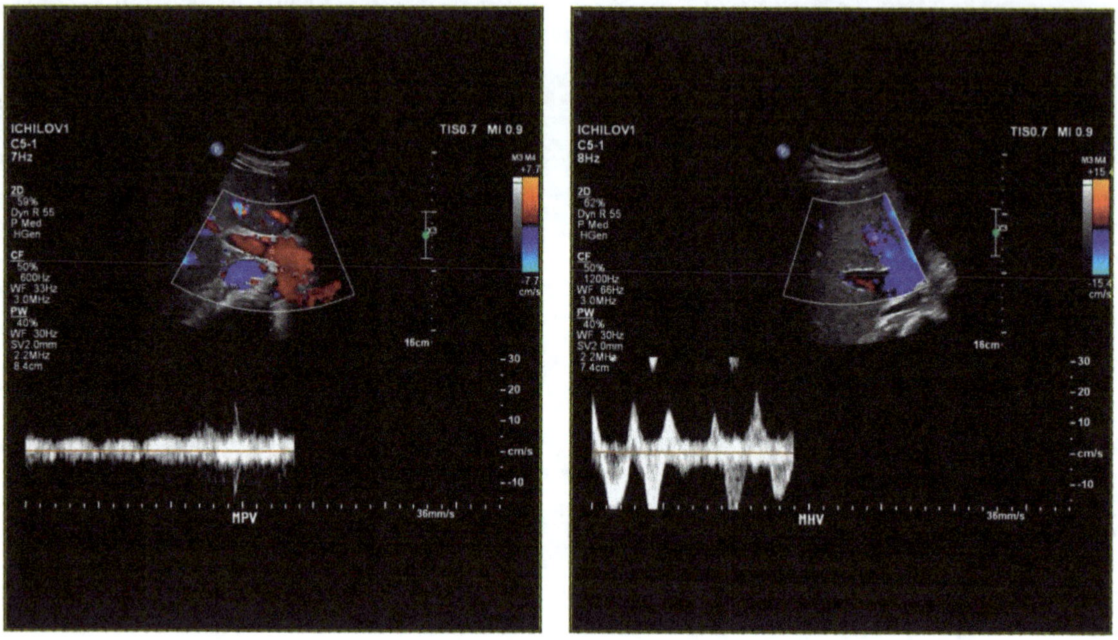

(a) (b)

Figure 1: Liver Doppler sonography showing normal venous flow in the main portal vein (a) and three hepatic veins (b).

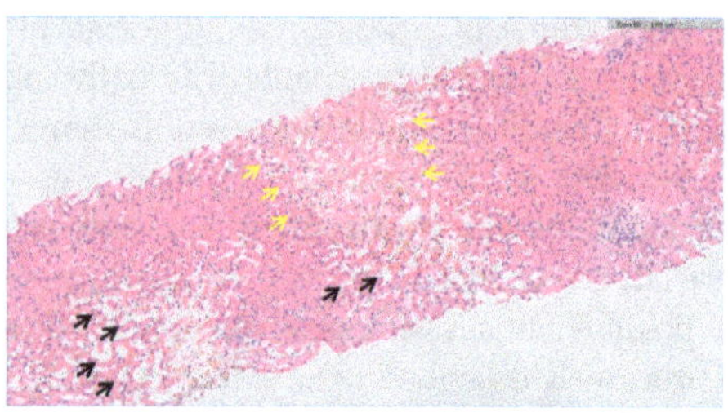

Figure 2: Liver biopsy showing centrilobular coagulative necrosis (yellow arrows) with marked sinusoidal dilatation (black arrows). No significant inflammatory infiltrate is seen.

ALKP, GGT, and bilirubin [15]. Therefore, as in this case, a patient may be classified as grade 4 liver injury without concomitant bilirubin elevation.

The median time of onset of immune-mediated hepatitis is 6–14 weeks from treatment initiation, after a median of 3 doses of immunotherapy. However, it may also occur at a much later phase, or even after therapy cessation [3, 6]. To our knowledge, this is the first documented report of a patient developing acute liver failure shortly after ICI initiation. A single case of nivolumab-induced hepatitis in a patient with renal cell carcinoma which developed within two weeks of therapy initiation was previously reported but was not as clinically severe [16].

In a single-center retrospective analysis of 17 patients with immune ICI-induced hepatotoxicity, Huffman et al. showed that about half of the patients also had concurrent immune-related adverse events in other systems [17]. Our patient also suffered from acute renal failure, which was suspected to be therapy-induced acute interstitial nephritis, a well-documented renal adverse effect of ICI [18].

Pathological reports of anti-PD-1-related hepatic injury described a heterogeneous histological picture, with lobular hepatitis, scattered foci of necrosis, and sometimes lobular fibrosis [14, 19]. These histologic findings are not specific and may also be found in other conditions, such as autoimmune hepatitis (AIH), viral hepatitis, and DILI secondary to various agents. The differentiation from AIH may be particularly difficult: elevated IgG levels and typical autoantibodies, as well as an inflammatory infiltrate of B cells and CD4+ T cells on biopsy, may be suggestive of AIH, whereas temporal association with administration of the ICI and a sinusoidal distribution of histiocytic and CD8+ T-cell infiltration may imply ICI-induced hepatitis. A mixed inflammatory infiltrate containing neutrophils, as described here, is also a common finding [2, 14, 20].

Apart from stopping the offending agent, there is currently no approved therapy for DILI. Corticosteroids are often given, but their benefit is unknown. In a recently published systematic review, the majority of studies suggested a beneficial effect to steroids in moderate to severe DILI, while some showed no effect. Steroids have not shown improvement in survival in drug-induced fulminant hepatic failure. In ICI-induced DILI, they have shown a beneficial effect. Thus, although the data are inconclusive, steroids are routinely given in DILI and in some cases may be beneficial [21].

In conclusion, we report a rare case of acute liver failure after only one infusion of atezolizumab. An extensive work-up for other etiologies was negative.

Although exceptional, the increasing use of ICI for a widening spectrum of neoplastic diseases warrants physicians' awareness of the wide variety of hepatic manifestations, ranging from mild transient enzyme elevation to autoimmune hepatitis and, as shown in this case, to fulminant hepatic failure leading to rapid deterioration and fatal consequences.

References

[1] I. Iranzo, J. M. Huguet, P. Suárez, L. Ferrer-Barceló, V. Iranzo, and J. Sempere, "Endoscopic evaluation of immunotherapy-induced gastrointestinal toxicity," *World Journal of Gastrointestinal Endoscopy*, vol. 10, no. 12, pp. 392–399, 2018.

[2] G. Vitale, G. Lamberti, F. Comito et al., "Anti-programmed cell death-1 and anti-programmed cell death ligand-1 immune-related liver diseases: from clinical pivotal studies to real-life experience," *Expert Opinion on Biological Therapy*, vol. 20, no. 9, pp. 1047–1059, 2020.

[3] EASL Clinical Practice Guidelines, "Drug-induced liver injury," *Journal of Hepatology*, vol. 70, no. 6, pp. 1222–1261, 2019.

[4] D. Y. Wang, J.-E. Salem, J. V. Cohen et al., "Fatal toxic effects associated with immune checkpoint inhibitors," *JAMA Oncology*, vol. 4, no. 12, pp. 1721–1728, 2018.

[5] Y. Wang, S. Zhou, F. Yang et al., "Treatment-related adverse events of PD-1 and PD-L1 inhibitors in clinical trials," *JAMA Oncology*, vol. 5, no. 7, pp. 1008–1019, 2019.

[6] W. Wang, P. Lie, M. Guo, and J. He, "Risk of hepatotoxicity in cancer patients treated with immune checkpoint inhibitors: a systematic review and meta-analysis of published data," *International Journal of Cancer*, vol. 141, no. 5, pp. 1018–1028, 2017.

[7] F. Berner, D. Bomze, S. Diem et al., "Association of checkpoint inhibitor-induced toxic effects with shared cancer and tissue antigens in non-small cell lung cancer," *JAMA Oncology*, vol. 5, no. 7, pp. 1043–1047, 2019.

[8] G Danan and R Teschke, "RUCAM in drug and herb induced liver injury: the update," *International Journal of Molecular Sciences*, vol. 17, no. 1, 2015.

[9] G. Brancatelli, A. Furlan, A. Calandra, and M. Dioguardi Burgio, "Hepatic sinusoidal dilatation," *Abdominal Radiology*, vol. 43, no. 8, pp. 2011–2022, 2018.

[10] S. S. Mahmood, M. G. Fradley, J. V. Cohen et al., "Myocarditis in patients treated with immune checkpoint inhibitors," *Journal of the American College of Cardiology*, vol. 71, no. 16, pp. 1755–1764, 2018.

[11] G. Varricchi, M. R. Galdiero, G. Marone et al., "Cardiotoxicity of immune checkpoint inhibitors," *ESMO open*, vol. 2, no. 4, Article ID e000247, 2017.

[12] P. Cramer and R. S. Bresalier, "Gastrointestinal and hepatic complications of immune checkpoint inhibitors," *Current Gastroenterology Reports*, vol. 19, no. 1, p. 3, 2017.

[13] J. S. Weber, K. C. Kähler, and A. Hauschild, "Management of immune-related adverse events and kinetics of response with ipilimumab," *Journal of Clinical Oncology*, vol. 30, no. 21, pp. 2691–2697, 2012.

[14] D. M. Karamchandani and R. Chetty, "Immune checkpoint inhibitor-induced gastrointestinal and hepatic injury: pathologists' perspective," *Journal of Clinical Pathology*, vol. 71, no. 8, pp. 665–671, 2018.

[15] Services Usdohah, "Common terminology criteria for adverse events (CTCAE)," https://ctep.cancer.gov/protocoldevelopment/electronic_applications/docs/ctcae_v5_quick_reference_5x7.pdf.

[16] V. Mathew Thomas, P. Bindal, S. Ann Alexander, and K. McDonald, "Nivolumab-induced hepatitis: a rare side effect of an immune check point inhibitor," *Journal of Oncology Pharmacy Practice*, vol. 26, no. 2, pp. 459–461, 2020.

[17] B. M. Huffman, L. A. Kottschade, P. S. Kamath, and S. N. Markovic, "Hepatotoxicity after immune checkpoint inhibitor therapy in melanoma," *American Journal of Clinical Oncology*, vol. 41, no. 8, pp. 760–765, 2018.

[18] R. Wanchoo, S. Karam, N. N. Uppal et al., "Adverse renal effects of immune checkpoint inhibitors: a narrative review," *American Journal of Nephrology*, vol. 45, no. 2, pp. 160–169, 2017.

[19] E. De Martin, J.-M. Michot, B. Papouin et al., "Characterization of liver injury induced by cancer immunotherapy using immune checkpoint inhibitors," *Journal of Hepatology*, vol. 68, no. 6, pp. 1181–1190, 2018.

[20] Y. Zen and M. M. Yeh, "Checkpoint inhibitor-induced liver injury: a novel form of liver disease emerging in the era of cancer immunotherapy," *Seminars in Diagnostic Pathology*, vol. 36, no. 6, pp. 434–440, 2019.

[21] E. S. Björnsson, V. Vucic, G. Stirnimann, and M. Robles-Díaz, "Role of corticosteroids in drug-induced liver injury. A systematic review," *Frontiers in Pharmacology*, vol. 13, Article ID 820724, 2022.

13

The Impact of Repeating Endosonography with Confocal Endomicroscopy for the Diagnosis of Cystic Neuroendocrine Tumor

Iqra Haq,[1] Somashekar G. Krishna,[2] Bhaveshkumar Patel,[3] Thavam Thambi-Pillai,[4] Chencheng Xie,[1] Karah Odegaard,[5] Kimberlee Buohy,[5] and Muslim Atiq[3]

[1]*Department of Internal Medicine, University of South Dakota Sanford School of Medicine, Sioux Falls, South Dakota, USA*
[2]*Division of Gastroenterology, Hepatology and Nutrition, The Ohio State University Wexner Medical Center, Columbus, Ohio, USA*
[3]*Department of Gastroenterology, University of South Dakota Sanford School of Medicine, Sioux Falls, South Dakota, USA*
[4]*Department of Surgery, University of South Dakota Sanford School of Medicine, Sioux Falls, South Dakota, USA*
[5]*Department of Pathology, University of South Dakota Sanford School of Medicine, Sioux Falls, South Dakota, USA*

Correspondence should be addressed to Iqra Haq; iqra.haq@usd.edu

Academic Editor: Daniel C. Damin

Cystic pancreatic neuroendocrine tumors represent around 13% of all neuroendocrine tumors (Hurtado-Pardo 2017). There has been an increase in the incidence of cases due to improvement in imaging modalities. This is a case of a 68-year-old male with the incidental finding of a pancreatic cyst on CT. Initial Endoscopic Ultrasound with Fine Needle Aspiration (EUS-FNA) showed sonographic and cytology features suggestive of a pancreatic pseudocyst. However the cyst persisted with no change in size after aspiration leading to a follow-up EUS- FNA, which was combined with needle based confocal laser endomicroscopy (nCLE). The nCLE features were consistent with a cystic pancreatic neuroendocrine tumor, which was later confirmed on histology after surgical resection.

1. Introduction

Cystic tumors of the pancreas are being increasingly recognized as incidental findings with the advancement of imaging modalities. With reported prevalence being up to 13.5% in some studies [1, 2]. Management of indeterminate cystic lesions of the pancreas can be challenging, particularly with concern for early malignant cystic lesions of the pancreas. We are presenting a case in which nCLE was effectively utilized to make a definitive diagnosis.

2. Case Report

Our patient is a 68-year-old male with a past medical history of hyperlipidemia, hypertension, and smoking, who presented with an incidental pancreatic cyst on lung cancer screening helical CT. His CT had shown a 23 × 18 mm fluid density lesion in the distal pancreatic body, without pancreatic ductal dilation. He underwent an EUS-FNA which revealed an anechoic and septated cyst. Needle aspiration with a 19 G Boston Sci. needle was performed for amylase, tumor marker (CEA), and cytology. Cyst fluid analysis showed amylase of 1532 and a CEA of less than 200. FNA cytology revealed a moderately cellular aspirate with no identifiable malignant cells (Figure 1). These findings were consistent with a pseudocyst or a benign cyst.

On follow-up CT abdomen and pelvis with IV contrast in six months, the cyst persisted and the size was unchanged (Figure 2).

This prompted a repeat EUS-FNA using 19G Boston Scientific needle combined with nCLE (using AQ-Flex 19; Mauna Kea Technologies). The tip of the AQ-Flex probe was advanced with the needle under EUS guidance until there was contact with the cyst wall without putting pressure. Fluorescein (2.5 to 5 mL of 10% Fluorescein) was injected intravenously immediately prior to CLE imaging.

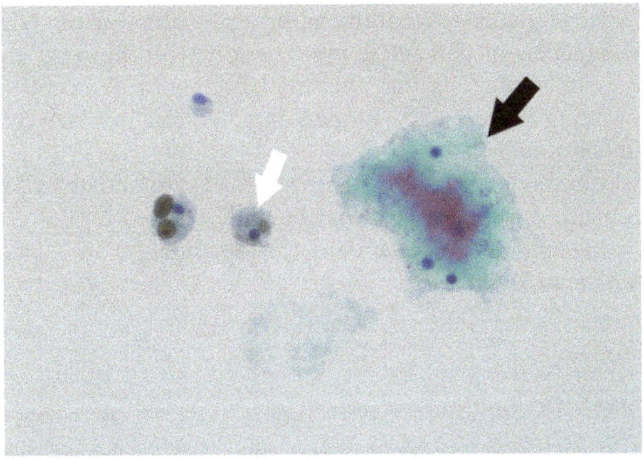

FIGURE 1: FNA cytology showing benign mesothelial cells (white arrow) and hemosiderin-laden macrophages (black arrow).

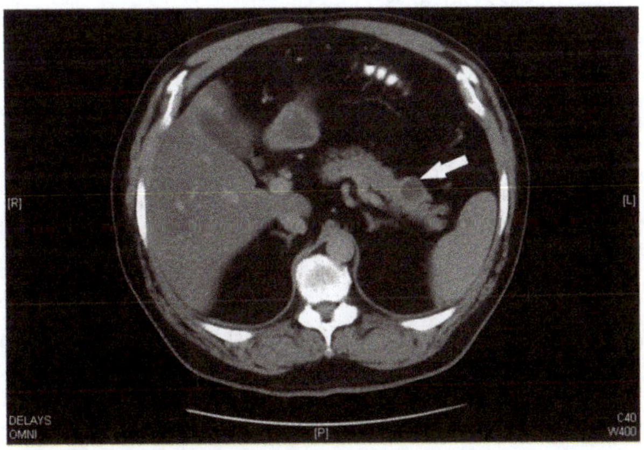

FIGURE 2: CT abdomen pelvis performed after EUS-FNA aspiration showing persistence of the cyst (arrow).

Around-3-minute-long video was acquired with permissible needle angulation. nCLE revealed thick cord like and dark nest like structures (Figures 3 and 4).

There was no evidence for dark rings, vasculature network, or papillary projections to suggest intraductal papillary mucinous neoplasm. These findings were consistent with cystic neuroendocrine tumor of the pancreas [3]. These findings prompted us to send the patient for surgical evaluation. Final histopathology (Figures 4 and 5) confirmed the preoperative nCLE based diagnosis of the cystic neuroendocrine tumor of the pancreas.

3. Discussion

The differential diagnosis of cystic lesions of the pancreas includes pseudocysts, intraductal papillary mucinous neoplasms, mucinous cyst neoplasms, and serous cystadenoma.

These cystic tumors have a wide range of presentations on nCLE: intraductal papillary mucinous neoplasm, in which papillae can be visualized. Serous cystadenomas found to have a branching and tortuous network of multiple blood vessels in a "fern like" pattern, which has been termed as

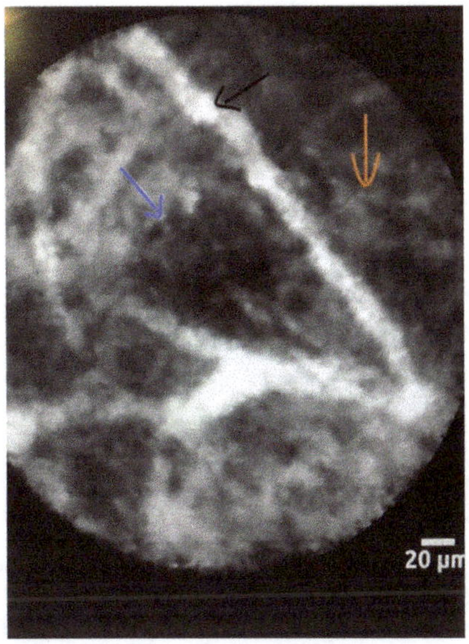

FIGURE 3: EUS guided needle based confocal laser endomicroscopy reveals clusters of cells (blue arrow) with surrounding areas of fibrosis (orange arrow) and vascularity (black arrow).

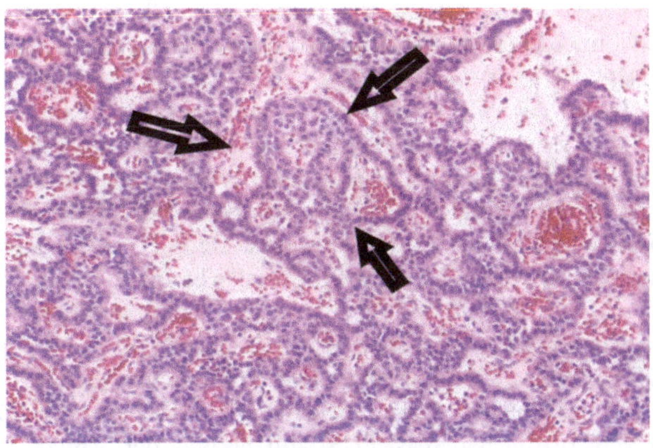

FIGURE 4: Histology showed a mass composed of trabeculae and solid nests of round, monotonous cells with crowded nuclei and stippled, open chromatin consistent with a cystic well-differentiated neuroendocrine tumor. Few mitotic figures were identified within the tumor.

"superficial vascular network"; pseudocyst in which "clusters of bright, floating particles are found in a background of nondescript appearance lacking blood vessels"; finally, mucinous cystic neoplasms which present as solitary epithelial bands without papillae [2]. The nCLE findings in our case reveal nests and clusters of cells separated by stroma of the cyst. This pattern is diagnostic of a neuroendocrine tumor.

Incidences of pancreatic neuroendocrine tumors are rare and account for 1 to 2% of all pancreatic tumors [4]. Cystic neuroendocrine tumors of the pancreas are even rarer, comprising up to 3-17% of all the pancreatic neuroendocrine tumors [5]. Conventional imaging (CT scan and/or MRI with pancreatic protocol) has limited value in definitive diagnosis of cystic neuroendocrine tumors of the pancreas. EUS with FNA is a helpful tool in making the diagnosis. However, it

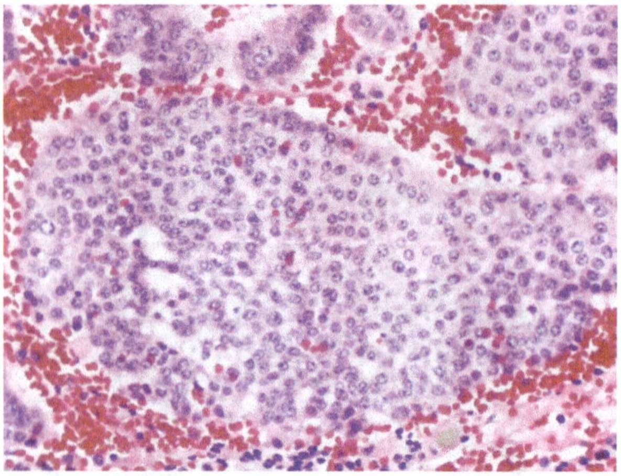

FIGURE 5: Histology showed a mass composed of trabeculae and solid nests of round, monotonous cells with crowded nuclei and stippled, open chromatin consistent with a cystic well-differentiated neuroendocrine tumor. Few mitotic figures were identified within the tumor.

does have its limitations which include small sample sizes and limited cells in the aspirated fluid which can decrease sensitivity.

In our case, EUS-FNA did not yield a correct diagnosis and the cyst persisted on repeat imaging at six-month follow-up. Therefore a nCLE was performed with repeat EUS-FNA, which revealed findings consistent with cystic neuroendocrine tumor of the pancreas. Recent studies have suggested that nCLE has shown promise in aiding diagnosis of solid tumors with good accuracy when compared to post-op diagnoses [6, 7]. There is evidence suggesting the use of nCLE in the work-up of cystic lesions of pancreas [3, 8–10].

Typically when evaluating cystic lesions greater than 2 to 3 cm of the pancreas, EUS with FNA is performed [11, 12]. This has proven to be superior to conventional imaging by most literature, but it can be very operator dependant. EUS with FNA has sensitivity and specificity at 91 and 94%, respectively. However, meta-analyses have shown that EUS-FNA has positive predictive value of 98% but a negative predictive value of 72% [13].

There are several studies on using nCLE for diagnosis of pancreatic masses, solid or cystic, which have shown promising results with an accuracy of ≥90% with low to no interobserver variability [6, 7, 14]. Krishna et al. concluded that nCLE is a good adjunct to use in an inconclusive EUS-FNA as in our case to differentiate mucinous versus nonmucinous primary cystic lesions (PCLs) as nCLE provides virtual histology of PCLs with a higher degree of accuracy, positive predictive value, and negative predictive value [15, 16].

The current IAP, AGA, and ACG guidelines indicate the use of EUS-FNA for evaluation of cysts >3 cm with no high-risk features or any size cyst with high-risk features; however the guidelines are not specific on indication and utility of nCLE in preoperative diagnoses as evidence is limited when compared to the gold standard of histopathology [12, 17, 18]. Currently recent European guidelines state that there is grade 1C level of evidence recommending against the use of nCLE for diagnosis of pancreatic cystic lesions [19]; however the same study suggests that this modality could be useful in preventing unnecessary surgical intervention in a selected number of patients.

Even though there are many studies to substantiate nCLE, it remains a modality that may be underutilized until it can be compared to gold standard (histopathology) in a large multicenter study.

References

[1] K. de Jong, C. Y. Nio, J. J. Hermans, M. G. Dijkgraaf, D. J. Gouma et al., "High prevalence of pancreatic cysts detected by screening magnetic resonance imaging examinations," *Clinical Gastroenterology and Hepatology: the official clinical practice journal of the American Gastroenterological Association*, vol. 8, no. 9, pp. 806–811, 2010.

[2] K. S. Lee, A. Sekhar, N. M. Rofsky, and I. Pedrosa, "Prevalence of incidental pancreatic cysts in the adult population on MR imaging," *American Journal of Gastroenterology*, vol. 105, no. 9, pp. 2079–2084, 2010.

[3] T. Tsujino, J. Y. Huang, J. B. Samarasena, A. Lemaistre, B. Napoleon, and K. J. Chang, "EUS-Guided Needle-Based Confocal Laser Endomicroscopy in the Diagnosis of Cystic Pancreatic Neuroendocrine Tumor: Surgical Pathologic Correlation in Six Cases," *Gastrointestinal Endoscopy*, vol. 83, no. 5, p. AB353, 2016.

[4] J. Hallet, C. H. L. Law, M. Cukier, R. Saskin, N. Liu, and S. Singh, "Exploring the rising incidence of neuroendocrine tumors: a population-based analysis of epidemiology, metastatic presentation, and outcomes," *Cancer*, vol. 121, no. 4, pp. 589–597, 2015.

[5] L. Bordeianou, P. A. Vagefi, D. Sahani et al., "Cystic Pancreatic Endocrine Neoplasms: A Distinct Tumor Type?" *Journal of the American College of Surgeons*, vol. 206, no. 6, pp. 1154–1158, 2008.

[6] P. Kongkam, R. Pittayanon, P. Sampatanukul et al., "Endoscopic ultrasound-guided needle-based confocal laser endomicroscopy for diagnosis of solid pancreatic lesions (ENES): a pilot study," *Endoscopy International Open*, vol. 4, no. 1, pp. E17–E23, 2016.

[7] S. G. Krishna, W. R. Brugge, J. M. Dewitt et al., "Needle-based confocal laser endomicroscopy for the diagnosis of pancreatic cystic lesions: an international external interobserver and intraobserver study (with videos)," *Gastrointestinal Endoscopy*, vol. 86, no. 4, pp. 644–654.e2, 2017.

[8] F. Otaki, P. Kedia, N. A. Kumta, and M. Kahaleh, "Needle confocal microendoscopy of a pancreatic neuroendocrine tumor," *Gastrointestinal Endoscopy*, vol. 81, no. 4, pp. 1009-1010, 2015.

[9] A. K. Kamboj, B. Swanson, M. E. Dillhoff, D. L. Conwell, and S. G. Krishna, "Cystic pancreatic neuroendocrine tumors: correlation of in vivo needle-based confocal endomicroscopic findings by ex vivo analysis," *Gastrointestinal Endoscopy*, vol. 85, no. 1, pp. 259-260, 2017.

[10] S. G. Krishna and J. H. Lee, "Appraisal of needle-based confocal laser endomicroscopy in the diagnosis of pancreatic cysts," *World Journal of Gastroenterology*, vol. 22, no. 4, pp. 1701–1710, 2016.

[11] B. K. P. Goh, L. L. P. J. Ooi, Y. M. Tan et al., "Clinico-pathological features of cystic pancreatic endocrine neoplasms and a

comparison with their solid counterparts," *European Journal of Surgical Oncology*, vol. 32, no. 5, pp. 553–556, 2006.

[12] G. H. Elta, B. K. Enestvedt, and B. G. Sauer, "Diagnosis and Management of Pancreas cysts," *American Journal of Gastroenterology*, 2018.

[13] M. J. Hewitt, M. J. W. McPhail, L. Possamai, A. Dhar, P. Vlavianos, and K. J. Monahan, "EUS-guided FNA for diagnosis of solid pancreatic neoplasms: a meta-analysis," *Gastrointestinal Endoscopy*, vol. 75, no. 2, pp. 319–331, 2012.

[14] B. Napoleon, A.-I. Lemaistre, B. Pujol et al., "In vivo characterization of pancreatic cystic lesions by needle-based confocal laser endomicroscopy (nCLE): proposition of a comprehensive nCLE classification confirmed by an external retrospective evaluation," *Surgical Endoscopy*, vol. 30, no. 6, pp. 2603–2612, 2016.

[15] M. Giovannini, F. Caillol, G. Monges et al., "Endoscopic ultrasound-guided needle-based confocal laser endomicroscopy in solid pancreatic masses," *Endoscopy*, vol. 48, no. 10, pp. 892–898, 2016.

[16] V. J. A. Konda, A. Meining, L. H. Jamil et al., "A pilot study of in vivo identification of pancreatic cystic neoplasms with needle-based confocal laser endomicroscopy under endosonographic guidance," *Endoscopy*, vol. 45, no. 12, pp. 1006–1013, 2013.

[17] M. Tanaka, C. Fernández-del Castillo, V. Adsay et al., "International consensus guidelines 2012 for the management of IPMN and MCN of the pancreas," *Pancreatology*, vol. 12, no. 3, pp. 183–197, 2012.

[18] S. S. Vege, B. Ziring, R. Jain, P. Moayyedi, and Clinical Guidelines Committee, "American gastroenterological association institute guideline on the diagnosis and management of asymptomatic neoplastic pancreatic cysts," *Gastroenterology*, vol. 148, no. 4, pp. 819–822, 2015.

[19] European Study Group on Cystic Tumours of the Pancreas, "European evidence-based guidelines on pancreatic cystic neoplasms," *Gut*, vol. 67, no. 5, pp. 789–804, 2018.

14

A Patient with Eosinophilic Esophagitis and Herpes Simplex Esophagitis: A Case Report and Literature Review

Hemnishil K. Marella[1] **Jiten P. Kothadia,**[1] **Nasir Saleem,**[1] **Bilal Ali,**[1] **Yousef Abdel-Aziz,**[1] **Vamsee Mupparaju,**[2] **Twisha Oza,**[3] **Abdallah Azouz,**[3] **and Colin W. Howden**[1]

[1]*Division of Gastroenterology and Hepatology, University of Tennessee Health Science Center, Memphis, TN 38104, USA*
[2]*Methodist University Hospital, Memphis, TN 38104, USA*
[3]*Department of Pathology, University of Tennessee Health Science Center, Memphis, TN 38104, USA*

Correspondence should be addressed to Hemnishil K. Marella; hkmarella@gmail.com

Academic Editor: Ken Haruma

Acute herpes simplex esophagitis (HSE) is common in immunocompromised patients. Eosinophilic esophagitis (EoE) is characterized by immune-mediated eosinophil-predominant esophageal inflammation. We report a patient with human immunodeficiency virus infection who presented with dysphagia and odynophagia and was found to have HSE and EoE. The combination of these two relatively rare conditions suggests possible predisposition.

1. Introduction

Eosinophilic esophagitis (EoE) is a chronic immune and antigen-mediated disorder characterized by an eosinophil-predominant inflammation of the esophagus resulting in esophageal dysfunction symptoms [1]. Although once considered rare, its reported incidence is increasing partly due to better recognition and improved understanding of the disease process [2–4]. Its most frequent symptoms in adults are dysphagia and food impaction [1]. The diagnosis of EoE is established on clinical, endoscopic, and histologic grounds after other etiologies of symptoms and esophageal eosinophilia are excluded. Histological diagnosis is based on the presence of at least 15 eosinophils per high-power field (hpf) on esophageal mucosal biopsies [1]. Environmental factors, atopy, genetics, and impaired esophageal epithelial barrier function are possible predisposing factors for EoE [1].

Herpes simplex esophagitis (HSE) is an acute viral infection of the esophagus that may cause odynophagia and/or dysphagia, chest pain, and fever [5]. Herpes simplex virus (HSV) lesions are typically found in the mid-to-distal esophagus and can be confirmed histologically by immunohistochemistry, viral culture, or polymerase chain reaction [6]. The occurrence of concomitant HSE and EoE is rare [7–10]. We report a case of concomitant HSE and EoE in an immunocompromised patient and have described a well-referenced review on the subject.

2. Case Report

A 51-year-old African American woman with a past medical history significant for a history of gastroesophageal reflux disease and HIV presented with a one-year history of dysphagia and odynophagia. She was receiving elvitegravir, cobicistat, emtricitabine, and tenofovir alafenamide for HIV infection. Her most recent CD4 count was 207 cells/mm^3, and her viral load was 84,700 copies/mL. She complained of odynophagia and dysphagia at the level of her neck, as well as some epigastric discomfort. She reported weight loss of 5 pounds over six months. She denied any history of atopic disorders. She noticed painful lesions at the edge of her tongue. She had been taking omeprazole 40 mg daily for the preceding six months without symptom improvement. Over the preceding 2-3 years, her CD4 count had been ≤200 with high viral loads. Despite previous poor compliance, she had recently been compliant with all her HIV medications.

On examination, there were several 2 mm shallow ulcers at the edge of her tongue but no evidence of oral *Candida* infection. Her blood count, biochemistry, and liver function tests were within normal limits. Before EGD, she was started on empiric fluconazole because of suspicion for esophageal candidiasis. At EGD, there were multiple, discrete, 1-2 mm shallow ulcers with heaped-up edges in the distal esophagus (Figure 1). The stomach and duodenum were unremarkable. Proximal, mid, and distal esophageal biopsies revealed margination, multinucleation, and moulding consistent with HSE (Figure 2). Additionally, there were 20 eosinophils/hpf (Figure 3) along with eosinophil microabscesses, extracellular eosinophil granules, and Bazel zone hypertrophy. Immunohistochemical staining was positive for HSV. Grocott methenamine silver and periodic acid-Schiff stains did not show fungal microorganisms. The PCR test for cytomegalovirus (CMV) and Epstein–Barr virus (EBV) was negative. The patient was treated with acyclovir 400 mg five times daily for 14 days and was continued omeprazole 40 mg daily. Following treatment, the patient reported significant improvement in her dysphagia and odynophagia.

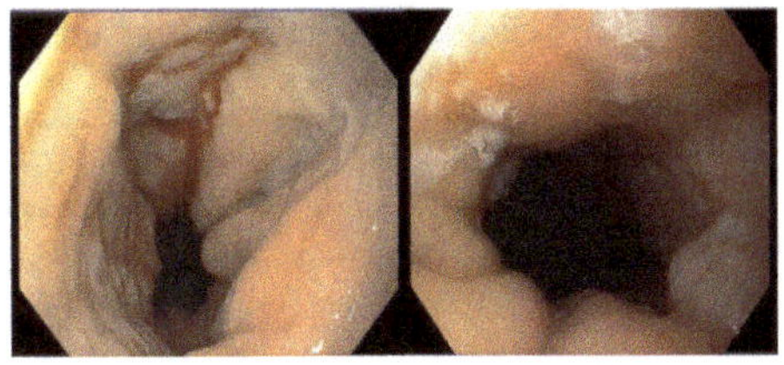

Figure 1: Multiple, discrete, 1-2 mm shallow ulcers with heaped-up edges in the distal esophagus.

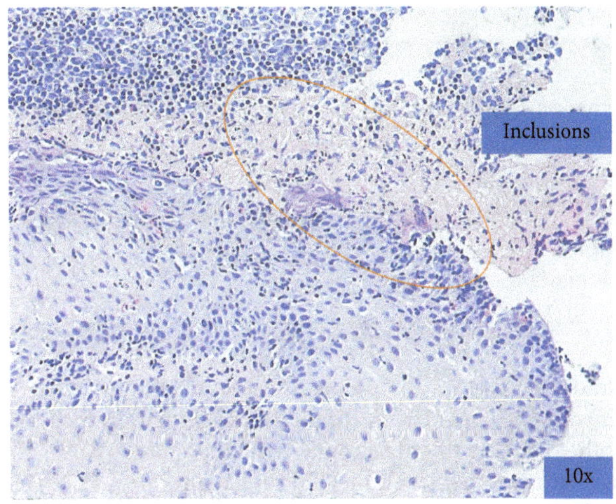

Figure 2: Margination, multinucleation, and moulding consistent with HSV infection.

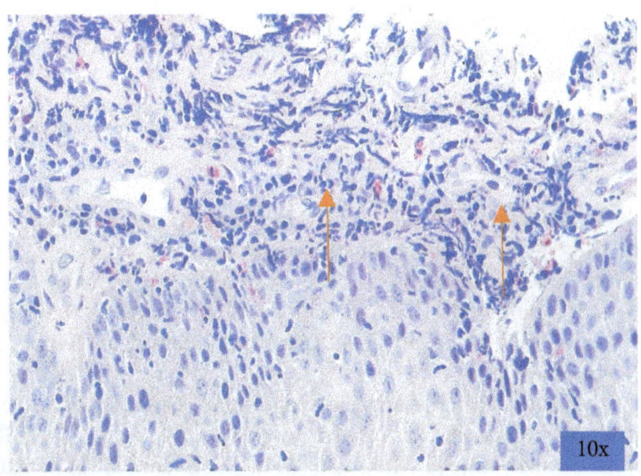

Figure 3: Presence of eosinophils (20/hpf), eosinophilic microabscesses, and eosinophil degranulation and Bazel zone hypertrophy.

3. Discussion

The clinical separation between EoE and GERD is challenging, and an overlap in symptom presentation is recognized. In our case, the major clinical symptom of dysphagia, the histological findings (20 eosinophils/hpf), and the lack of resolution of the symptoms despite the patient taking omeprazole in the preceding months are the main distinguished factors that point towards EoE rather than GERD. The occurrence of concomitant HSE and EoE is rare [7–10]. Our patient's case further adds to the evidence base for a possible relationship between EoE and HSE. It is unknown whether our patient had EoE or HSE first. It is unlikely that these two conditions would coexist by chance alone. With these observations in mind, it is essential to consider possible mechanisms for the coexistence.

First, HSE could predispose to EoE. HSE damages the esophageal mucosa resulting in immune hyperactivity and initiation of the inflammatory cycle [11]. Increased esophageal permeability from mucosal damage may allow access to antigenic stimuli from ingested food and environmental antigens. Antigen-presenting cells can induce T helper 2 (Th2) cells leading to eosinophilic infiltration/inflammation of the esophageal lamina propria and submucosa [11]. Also, acute inflammation resulting from HSE can induce predominantly neutrophilic infiltrate, and EoE may be masked if there is an underlying disease [12].

Alternatively, EoE might predispose patients to HSE. Interleukin 13 (IL-13) has been implicated in the pathogenesis of EoE [11]. IL-13 leads to downregulation of the desmosomal protein, desmoglein-1 [11, 13]. Downregulation of intracellular junction proteins can lead to exacerbation of inflammation and may also lead to impairment of the mucosal barrier, thereby facilitating candidiasis, HSV, and other viral infections [11, 13].

On review of the literature, we found eight adult cases related to EoE and HSE reported (Table 1). The average age was 24.8 years, and three had a definite history of atopy. HSE preceded EoE in three out of eight cases. EoE preceded HSE in three out of the eight cases. Concomitant HSE and EoE were detected in three cases, including our case. Patients with atopy were diagnosed with HSE before EoE. However, it is imperative to ask all patients with EoE about atopic disorders and food and environmental allergies. In most of the previously reported cases, treatment comprised a proton-pump inhibitor and acyclovir/valacyclovir (Table 1).

Additionally, the association between EoE and HIV is not well established. There is only one case report in the literature about the occurrence of EoE in HIV patients [14]. A recently published cross-sectional study showed that HIV patients are twice as likely to have EoE compared to those

Table 1: Summary of clinical characteristics of published cases associated with eosinophilic esophagitis and herpes simplex virus esophagitis.

Author (year)	Country	Age of the patient (yr)	Sex	Immunocompromised (yes/no)	Atopy	HSV or EoE diagnosed first (or concurrently)	Reported treatment
Monsanto et al. [9]	Portugal	20	M	No	Asthma	HSV 6 weeks before	Acyclovir + PPI followed by fluticasone
Machicado et al. [8]	USA	18	M	No	Allergic rhinitis and wheat allergy	Concurrently	Acyclovir (3 days) + valacyclovir (11 days) + PPI
Zimmermann et al. [10]	Switzerland	27	F	No	Unknown	EoE 5 years before	Acyclovir + PPI followed by fluticasone
		25	F	No	Unknown	EoE	Acyclovir
		30	M	No	Unknown	EoE 6 years before	Acyclovir
		28	M	No	Asthma and allergic rhinitis	HSV 9 weeks before	None (asymptomatic and lost to follow-up)
		29	M	No	Unknown	Concurrently	Acyclovir + PPI
Iriarte Rodríguez et al. [7]	Spain	21	M	No	None	HSV 12 weeks before	Acyclovir + lidocaine

without HIV [15]. The proposed mechanism of association between EoE and HIV is due to Th2 inflammation mediated by the cytokine thymic stromal lymphopoietin (TSLP), and there are elevated levels of TSLP in patients with HIV [15].

In conclusion, regardless of a patient's immune status, HSE and EoE can occur simultaneously or successively. However, it is challenging to identify the causal relationship between EoE and HSE, and one disease may predispose to the other. Future studies are needed to evaluate the pathogenicity and coexistence of these two disease processes.

References

[1] G. T. Furuta and D. A. Katzka, "Eosinophilic esophagitis," *New England Journal of Medicine*, vol. 373, no. 17, pp. 1640–1648, 2015.

[2] E. S. Dellon and I. Hirano, "Epidemiology and natural history of eosinophilic esophagitis," *Gastroenterology*, vol. 154, no. 2, pp. 319–332, 2018.

[3] F. J. Moawad, "Eosinophilic esophagitis," *Gastrointestinal Endoscopy Clinics of North America*, vol. 28, no. 1, pp. 15–25, 2018.

[4] N. J. Shaheen, V. Mukkada, C. S. Eichinger, H. Schofield, L. Todorova, and G. W. Falk, "Natural history of eosinophilic esophagitis: a systematic review of epidemiology and disease course," *Diseases of the Esophagus*, vol. 31, 2018.

[5] E. Canalejo, F. García Durán, N. Cabello, and J. García Martínez, "Herpes esophagitis in healthy adults and adolescents," *Medicine*, vol. 89, no. 4, pp. 204–210, 2010.

[6] J. Ramanathan, M. Rammouni, J. Baran Jr., and R. Khatib, "Herpes simplex virus esophagitis in the immunocompetent host: an overview," *The American Journal of Gastroenterology*, vol. 95, no. 9, pp. 2171–2176, 2000.

[7] A. Iriarte Rodríguez, I. Frago Marquínez, and G. P. De Lima Piña, "A case report: asymptomatic esophageal eosinophilia after herpes simplex esophagitis. Controversies in the therapeutic approach," *Revista Española de Enfermedades Digestivas*, vol. 110, pp. 471-472, 2018.

[8] J. D. Machicado, M. Younes, and D. S. Wolf, "An unusual cause of odynophagia in a patient with eosinophilic esophagitis," *Gastroenterology*, vol. 147, no. 1, pp. 37-38, 2014.

[9] P. Monsanto, N. Almeida, M. A. Cipriano, H. Gouveia, and C. Sofia, "Concomitant herpetic and eosinophilic esophagitis--a causality dilemma," *Acta Gastro-Enterologica Belgica*, vol. 75, pp. 361–363, 2012.

[10] D. Zimmermann, D. H. Criblez, E. S. Dellon et al., "Acute herpes simplex viral esophagitis occurring in 5 immunocompetent individuals with eosinophilic esophagitis," *ACG Case Reports Journal*, vol. 3, no. 1, pp. 165–168, 2016.

[11] K. M. O'Shea, S. S. Aceves, E. S Dellon et al., "Pathophysiology of eosinophilic esophagitis," *Gastroenterology*, vol. 154, no. 2, pp. 333–345, 2018.

[12] J. Kim, K. Lee, and W. Lee, "A case of eosinophilic esophagitis associated with herpes esophagitis in a pediatric patient," *Clinical Endoscopy*, vol. 52, no. 6, pp. 606–611, 2019.

[13] J. D. Sherrill, K. Kc, D. Wu et al., "Desmoglein-1 regulates esophageal epithelial barrier function and immune responses in eosinophilic esophagitis," *Mucosal Immunology*, vol. 7, no. 3, pp. 718–729, 2014.

[14] C. Batog, G. Psevdos Jr., A. Paniz-Mondolfi, S. Srivastava, and V. L. Sharp, "Eosinophilic oesophagitis: an unsuspected aetiology for dysphagia in an HIV-positive patient," *International Journal of STD & AIDS*, vol. 21, no. 12, pp. 842–844, 2010.

[15] M. M. Asfari, K. Kendrick, M. T. Sarmini, P. Uy, and K. J. Vega, "Association of eosinophilic esophagitis and human immunodeficiency virus," *Digestive Diseases and Sciences*, vol. 2020, 2020.

15

Colocolic Intussusception in an Adult Patient Secondary to Caecal Adenocarcinoma

Hicham Elmajdoubi, Marouane Baiss, Mohamed El Absi, El Hassan El Faricha El Alami, Mohamed El Ouanani, El Mahjoub Echarrab, Mohamed El Amraoui, and Abdelkader Errougani

Surgical Emergency Department, Avicenna Hospital, Mohammed V University, Rabat, Morocco

Correspondence should be addressed to Hicham Elmajdoubi; el.hicham87@gmail.com

Academic Editor: Haruhiko Sugimura

Acute intestinal invagination is the pathology of infants and small children. Its occurrence in adults is rare, and it represents 1 to 5% of intestinal occlusions often leading to the discovery of an organic cause that may be tumor. We report the case of a 72-year-old patient admitted to the emergency room of Ibn Sina Rabat, Morocco, for intestinal occlusion. The abdominal CT scan showed a voluminous intestinal invagination on a very probable heterogeneous digestive mass. The treatment was an open right hemicolectomy. The histopathological examination of the surgical specimen concluded a colonic well-differentiated adenocarcinoma with a 30% mucinous component. By review of literature, we discuss diagnostic and therapeutic procedures in emergency.

1. Introduction

Intestinal invaginations are rare in adults, and they represent 1 to 5% of intestinal occlusions often leading to the discovery of an organic cause that may or may not be tumoral, unlike in children, where the majority of cases are primitive.

It is defined by the incorporation of an intestinal segment into the one immediately downstream.

Abdominal CT scan can diagnose easily the invagination, but the characterization on the underlying lesion is much more difficult, if not impossible.

Treatment is always surgical. We report the case of an elderly woman being treated in the emergency room of the IBN SINA Rabat hospital.

2. Case Report

A 72-year-old female with no significant past medical history presented with diffuse abdominal pain, vomiting, and subocclusive syndrome for 10 days without any notion of rectorrhagia, in a context of deterioration of the general state and apyrexia.

At the time of presentation to the emergency room, her temperature was 37 C, blood pressure was 110/60 mm Hg, pulse was 60 beats per minute, respiratory rate was 16 breaths per minute, and oxygen saturation was 99% while breathing ambient air.

The abdominal examination showed a slightly distended abdomen with the perception of a mass on the left flank extended to the left iliac fossa without adhesion to the abdominal wall. In addition, there was no hepatomegaly or splenomegaly; digital rectal examination does not revealed a palpable masse and rectum was empty; the rest of the clinical examination was without particularities; the biological assessment was normal; an abdominal X-ray radiography was performed showing some air fluid levels, Ultrasound revealed a mass on the left flank (Figure 1), and abdominal CT scan was performed for a better characterization, which showed a large intestinal invagination on a very probable heterogeneous digestive

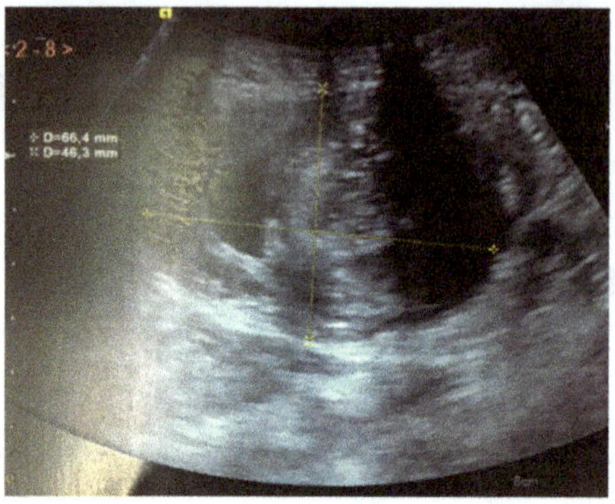

FIGURE 1: Abdominal ultrasound showing a left flank mass.

mass measuring 40 × 37 mm with invagination of the mesentery and signs of parietal pain on a digestive tumor mass (Figures 2 and 3).

We performed an exploratory laparotomy that revealed colocolic intussusception caused by colonic tumor (Figure 4 and 5), an ascending 4.0 × 3.0 × 3.0 cm tumor as the lead point of intussusception into the proximal transverse colon with palpable mesentery lymph nodes Moreover, macroscopically, the tumor was ball-like with a regular surface and firm consistency. The cut surface was white. The appendix was aspirated by tumor; the exploration did not objectively reveal liver metastases or carcinoid nodules.

The patient underwent a right hemicolectomy with terminolateral ileotransverse anastomosis in a single step (Figure 6). The postoperative course was uneventful, and she was discharged home after 6 days in good general condition.

Histopathological examination of the surgical specimen revealed a well-differentiated adenocarcinoma infiltrating the colonic musculosa with mucinous component estimated at 30%, tumor-classified PT2N0Mx.

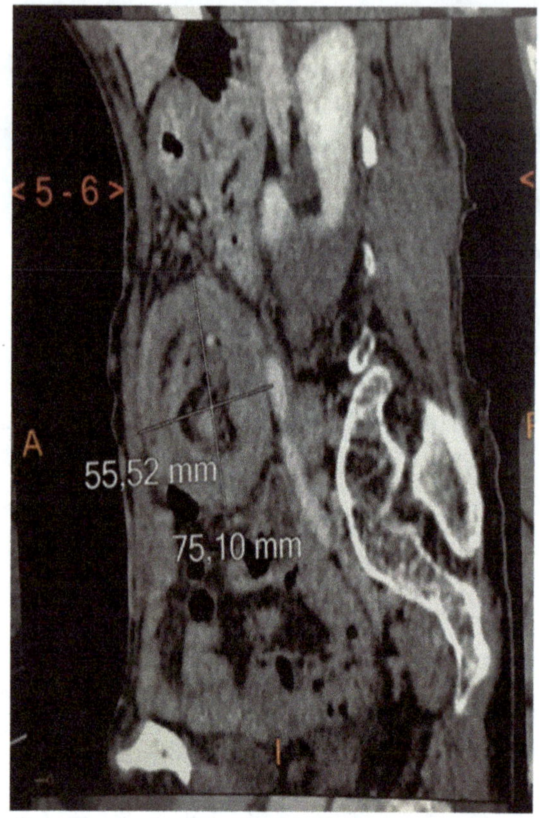

FIGURE 2: Abdominal CT scan showing large intestinal invagination (heterogeneous digestive mass).

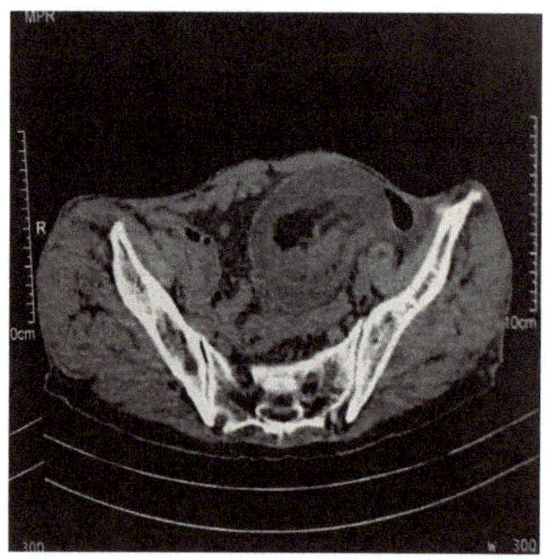

FIGURE 3: Abdominal CT scan showing large intestinal invagination (heterogeneous digestive mass).

3. Discussion

Intestinal invaginations are relatively rare in adults; they represent 2 to 4% of intestinal occlusions in adults [1], where an organic cause is found in 70 to 90% of cases and an idiopathic cause in 8 to 20%, whereas in children, intestinal invagination is primitive in 90% of cases [2, 3]. Adult intussusception of the small intestine is usually attributed to benign neoplasms, contrary to the large intestine, where malignancies constitute the majority [4].

The clinical presentation is polymorphic and often nonspecific: progressive installation of subocclusive syndrome over several days, acute intestinal occlusion, and nonspecific abdominal syndromes (altered transit, diffuse abdominal pain, and digestive bleeding), sometimes evolving over several months, with or without deterioration of the general state [5, 6].

Classically, in adults, the evolution is chronic with intermittent abdominal pain associated with subocclusive seizures. The acute form is mainly the prerogative of the ileoileal forms. For Mondor, the acute form would be the final stage of a chronic invagination for which an early diagnosis would not have been made [7]. This is the case of our patient who reported intermittent abdominal pain with a subocclusive syndrome before the installation of the acute picture.

The clinical presence of a palpable mass is a sign of great value in particular, if it appears to be of different location and consistency during repeated examinations it corresponds to the invagination coil, which should be carefully sought in the right and left lateral decubitus, in the dorsal decubitus, and Trendelenburg position [8].

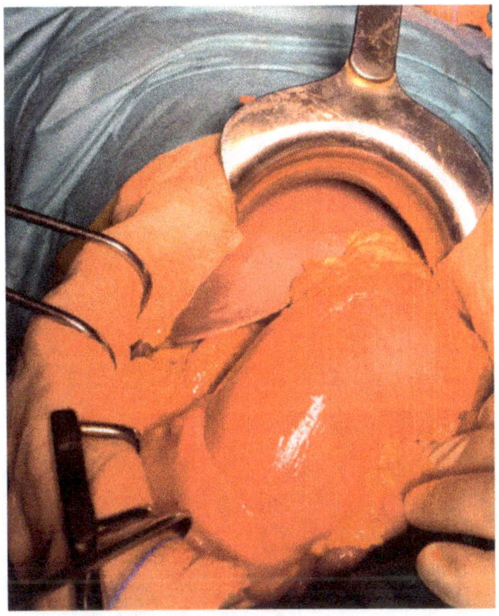

Figure 4: Operative image showing colocolic intussusception.

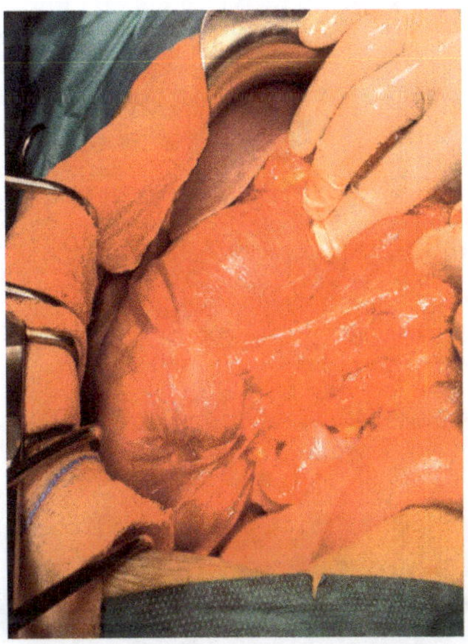

Figure 5: Operative image showing colocolic intussusception.

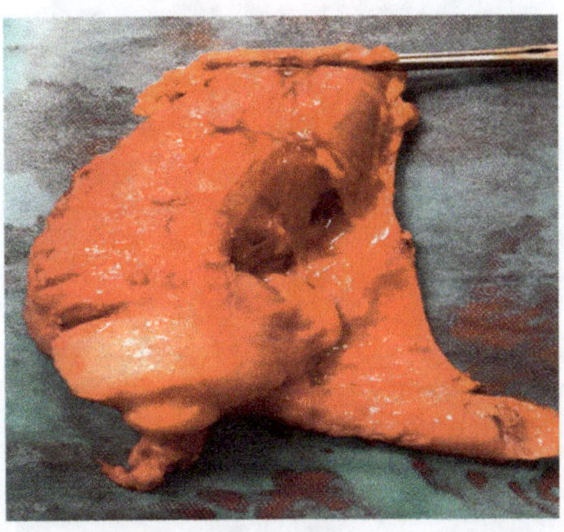

Figure 6: Right hemicolectomy for caecal mass.

Abdominal X-ray shows air fluid levels related to the occlusive syndrome, which is the case of our patient. Abdominal ultrasound can be useful to visualize the classical target sign with a thick peripheral hypoechoic band with central echogenicity zone. These correspond to the bowel wall surrounding hyperecohoic mesenteric fat contained within the intussusception, and it often remains hindered by the presence of air.

Abdominal CT scan confirms the diagnosis of the occlusive syndrome and shows the invagination, its precise location, and etiology. It can detect an organic cause in 71% of cases [9]. In CT, the typical target-like image consists of a thickened hyperdense external segment circumscribing a hypo- or hyperdense eccentric ring depending on the underlying cause and a stratified tissue ring with hypodense or discreetly hyperdense serous edema corresponding to the oedematous walls of the invaginated loop [10].

Treatment modalities for intussusception are variable. Because ileocolic is the most common type seen in children, reduction is often successful by using pneumatic or hydrostatic edema. Moreover, enteroenteric intussusceptions usually reduce spontaneously. This approach should be employed with great caution to avoid missing potentially serious underlying conditions such as malignancy. The operative approach is necessary in patients who present with bowel obstruction, those with mass seen on imaging, those with constitutional symptoms of malignancy (such as weight loss, anorexia and night sweats), and those with colocolic and ileocolic intussusception (given their higher association with malignancy) [11].

When surgical intervention is performed, if underlying malignancy is suspected, oncologic en bloc resection of the involved intestine and the associated mesentery should be sought [12]. This is recommended to avoid perforations and possible dissemination of cancerous cells.

Laparoscopy is currently a real means of diagnosis and sometimes treatment of intestinal intussusception [13]. In the case of intestinal obstruction, it requires expertise in laparoscopic surgery due to the distension of the small intestines, which hinders vision and makes it difficult to mobilise them, with a high risk of iatrogenic wounds. The anastomosis is realized immediately either by mechanical sutures or manual anastomosis after right hemicolectomy for carcinoma.

The prognosis is related to the duration of evolution, the extent of the lesions, and the nature of the cause [14].

4. Conclusion

Colocolic invagination in adults remains a rare condition. The abdominal CT scan is essential for the diagnosis of the invagination and its etiology. Concerning the treatment, a carcinological resection is necessary when a tumor with evidence of malignancy is discovered.

References

[1] R. Lebeau, E. Koffi, B. Diané, A. Amani, and J.-C. Kouassi, "Invaginations intestinales aiguës de l'adulte: analyse d'une série de 20 cas," *Annales de Chirurgie*, vol. 131, no. 8, pp. 447–450, 2006.

[2] C. Toso and P. M. Erne, "Lenz linger Intussusception as a cause of bowel obstruction in adults," *Swiss Med WKLY*, vol. 135, pp. 87–99, 2005.

[3] B. Y. Huang and D. M. Warshauer, "Adult intussusception," *Radiologic Clinics of North America*, vol. 41, no. 6, pp. 1137–1151, 2003.

[4] M. Adloff, "Occlusion intestinale aiguë de l'adulte," *Encyclo Med Chir*, vol. 24059 A, p. 10, 1984.

[5] F. Abou-Nukta, J. Gutweiler, J. Khaw, and G. Yavorek, "Giant lipoma causing a colo-colonic intussusception," *American Surgeon*, vol. 73, no. 4, p. 417, 2007.

[6] K. Y. Tan, S.-M. Tan, A. G. S. Tan, C. Y. Y. Chen, H.-C. Chng, and M. N. Y. Hoe, "Adult intussusception: experience in Singapore," *ANZ Journal of Surgery*, vol. 73, no. 12, pp. 1044–1047, 2003 Dec.

[7] D. Sirinelli, C. Guilley, and M. Boscq, "Invagination intestinale aiguë la désinvagination, quand et comment?" *Journal Radiology*, vol. 84, pp. 269–274, 2003.

[8] P. Tabrizian, S. Q. Nguyen, A. Greenstein et al., "Significant parameters for surgery in adult intussusception," *Surgery*.

[9] G. Bierry, M.-N. Roedlich, A. Neuville, F. Reche, F. Veillon, and J.-L. Dietemann, "Invagination intestinale iléo-iléale secondaire à une tumeur stromale gastro-intestinale (GIST)," *Feuillets de Radiologie*, vol. 46, no. 2, pp. 148–154, 2006.

[10] N. Lvoff, R. S. Breiman, F. V. Coakley, Y. Lu, and R. S. Warren, "Distinguishing features of self-limiting adult small-bowel intussusception identified at CT," *Radiology*, vol. 227, no. 1, pp. 68–72, 2003.

[11] J. D. Rea, M. E. Lockhart, D. E. Yarbrough, R. R. Leeth, S. E. Bledsoe, and R. H. Clements, "Approach to management of intussusception in adults: a new paradigm in the computed tomography era," *The American Surgeon*, vol. 73, no. 11, pp. 1098–1105, 2007 Nov.

[12] T. Hadid, Z. Elazzamy Kafri, H. Elazzamy, and Z. Kafri, "Bowel intussusception in adults: think cancer!" *Case Reports in Gastroenterology*, vol. 14, no. 1, pp. 27–33, 2020.

[13] Y. Ishibashi, S. Yamamoto, Y. Yamada, S. Fujita, T. Akasu, and Y. Moriya, "Laparoscopic resection for malignant lymphoma of the ileum causing ileocecal intussusception," *Surgical Laparoscopy, Endoscopy & Percutaneous Techniques*, vol. 17, no. 5, pp. 444–446, 2007.

[14] C. J. Zeebregts, R. L. Prevo, and J. M. Klaase, "Jejunojejunal intussusception secondary to adenocarcinoma," *The American Journal of Surgery*, vol. 187, no. 3, pp. 450-451, 2004.

16

Recurrent Aphthous Stomatitis Improved after Eradication Therapy for *Helicobacter pylori*

Yinglin Gao,[1] **Nikhil Gupta**,[2] **and Maisa Abdalla**[2]

[1]*Internal Medicine, Loma Linda University Medical Center, Loma Linda, CA, USA*
[2]*Gastroenterology Department, Loma Linda University Medical Center, Loma Linda, CA, USA*

Correspondence should be addressed to Yinglin Gao; ygao@llu.edu

Academic Editor: Ken Haruma

Helicobacter pylori (*H. pylori*) is a Gram-negative bacterium that colonizes gastric mucosa and is often transmitted through direct contact with saliva, contaminated food or water, and vomit. The majority of the infected individuals remain asymptomatic for a long period. Infection with *H. Pylori* often presents with dyspepsia, nausea, frequent belching, bloating, abdominal discomfort, burning abdominal pain, and peptic ulcer. A potential association between *H. Pylori* and recurrent aphthous stomatitis was previously reported; however, the presence of causative relationship between the two remained controversial. We are presenting a case of recurrent aphthous stomatitis of twenty-four-year history resolved after *H. pylori* treatment.

1. Introduction

Recurrent aphthous stomatitis (RAS) is a recurrent painful ulcerative disorder that commonly affects the oral mucosa. The diagnosis of RAS is clinical, and the etiology remains unclear. Some predisposing factors include trauma, hormonal changes, diet, nutritional deficiency, celiac disease, and immunological disorders. Nutritional deficiency that could potentially lead to RAS includes decreased level of iron, vitamins B3 and B12, vitamin C, and folic acid [1].

Helicobacter pylori (*H. pylori*) is a Gram-negative bacterium that colonizes gastric mucosa and is often transmitted through direct contact with saliva, contaminated food or water, and vomit. The majority of infected individuals remain asymptomatic for a long period. Consequently, it can lead to various gastrointestinal disorders such as gastritis, peptic ulcers, and even malignancy. In fact, *H* pylori leads to roughly 89% of all gastric cancers [2]; therefore, early recognition and eradication is of great importance. Although *H. pylori* infection has been suggested to be involved in the pathogenesis of RAS, this association is debatable. We present a case in which RAS resolved with *H. pylori* eradication therapy suggesting possible association between RAS and *H. pylori*.

2. Case Presentation

Our patient is a 49-year-old Hispanic immigrant female with a 24-year history of painful RAS in the oral cavity (Figure 1). Her symptoms were associated with nausea and odynophagia. She reports that the sores last approximately one week at a time and can present with as many as thirteen at a single time. There was never a period of time when she had not had an oral ulcer present for the past 20 years and often she would have an average of 5–6 oral ulcers at any given time. Within the past 20 years, she has seen many doctors before immigrating to the US, but it is unclear what kind of treatment she tried in the past and she never got a formal diagnosis of her problem as well. She has only been controlled with pain medication for symptom relief. She also reports a longstanding history of intermittent postprandial bloating and a history of constipation. She denies diarrhea, hematochezia, and personal or family history of colon cancer or gastric cancer. Other past medical history includes anxiety, history of stroke, and hypertension. Her anxiety is very well controlled. She denies drinking or smoking. Differentials such as lupus, Crohn's, ulcerative colitis, Behcet syndrome, HIV, deep mycosis, tuberculosis, syphilis, celiac disease, vasculitis, drug-induced injury (NSAIDs or

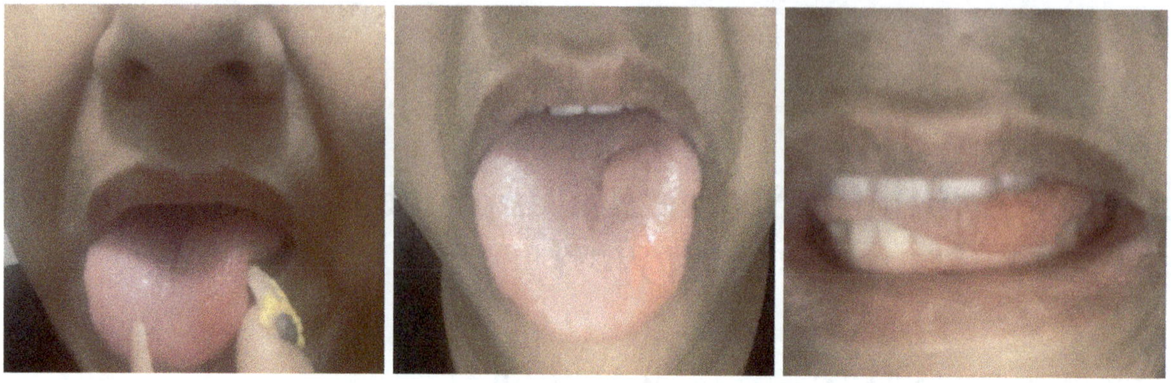

Figure 1: Aphthous stomatitis noted over the left anterolateral tongue (pictures were provided by the patient).

alendronate), and genital ulcers were all considered. The patient had an extensive lab workup for her aphthous ulcers by her PCP (Table 1) including antinuclear antibody, tissue transglutaminase IgA, HIV 1&2 Ab, and HSV-1 IgM, which were all negative. HSV-1 IgG was positive, but the patient had received multiple courses of acyclovir without resolution of her symptoms. The nutrition panel revealed vitamin B and zinc deficiencies for which a three-month supplementation was given without improvement in her symptoms. Repeat vitamin levels were ordered, but the patient did not follow up. She was seen by a dermatologist who recommended triamcinolone paste to affected areas in her mouth without help. She was then referred to gastroenterology for further workup.

For her physical exam, oral cavity revealed normal lips, normal dentition, and occlusion; two aphthous ulcers on the right buccal mucosa, approximately 0.5 cm in size were seen. No drainage or purulent discharge was noted so the ulcer was not swabbed for examination. Other reviews of systems including skin, eye, lymphatics, cardiovascular, abdomen, thyroid, neurologic, and respiratory systems were all normal. Esophagogastroduodenoscopy was done and revealed erythematous gastric mucosa (Figure 2). The biopsy of this area was positive for *H. Pylori* infection and mild active chronic gastritis. She was then prescribed quadruple therapy consisting of a proton pump inhibitor, tetracycline, metronidazole, and bismuth subsalicylate. After completion of the therapy, she reported simultaneous resolution of RAS. *H. pylori* stool antigen was performed after completion of quadruple therapy and confirmed eradication. She was seen in follow-up five months later and denies the presence of RAS which has not happened for the last 20 years.

3. Discussion

It was estimated that the prevalence of *H. Pylori* infection is approximately 20 percent for people less than 30 years and 50 percent for those greater than 60 years in the United States [3]. The exact etiologies for RAS is unclear and could be multifactorial; risk factors could be categorized into local, systemic, immunologic, positive family history with genetic predisposition, allergic, nutritional problems such as B12 deficiency, microbial factors, and anxiety or immunosuppressive drugs [4, 5]. A potential association between *H. Pylori* and recurrent aphthous stomatitis was previously reported; however, the presence of causative relationship between the two remained controversial. It was previously hypothesized *H. pylori* could modify the immune response directly and release proinflammatory mediators, leading to the irritation of surface epithelial cells. [6] In addition, *H. pylori* could potentially multiply in macrophages, dendritic cells, and epithelial cells and then indirectly lead to vitamin B deficiency, which would then cause changes in the epithelium of the tongue and buccal mucosa that would lead to mucosal bleeding and glossitis, given its important role in DNA synthesis [6].

As mentioned previously, the association between *H. pylori* and RAS is unclear. Multiple studies in the past have shown conflicting results regarding the association between RAS and *H. pylori*. In our case, the inability to identify other causes for the patient's 20+ year history of recurrent aphthous ulcers, the lack of response to other commonly used therapies (acyclovir, topical corticosteroids, and vitamin supplementations), and the rapid and sustained resolution of all oral ulcers after completing *H. pylori* treatment support the degree of clinical correlation between recurrent aphthous stomatitis and *H. pylori*. In a prospective study by Karaca et al., a total of 23 patients with RAS were assessed for the association with *H. pylori* and the effect of eradication therapy on the recurrence. All patients underwent endoscopy and had gastric biopsies evaluated for *H. pylori*. The ones with confirmed *H. pylori* were followed up for up to a year after treatment. The result revealed a statistically significant decrease in recurrence rate of RAS with eradication therapy [7]. Similarly, Tas et al. also evaluated 46 patients with aphthous lesions, and they also underwent endoscopic biopsy to evaluate *H pylori*. It was found *H. pylori* positive in 30 patients and negative in 16 patients. The 30 patients with positive results received treatment and were followed up. The result revealed that vitamin B12 levels were significantly increased in the *H. pylori*-eradicated group ($P = 0.001$); however, no significant change was found in the control group ($P = 0.638$). In addition, the average number of aphthous lesions (per 6 months) of *H. pylori*-eradicated group was significantly decreased after eradication ($P = 0.0001$) as compared to the control group ($P = 0.677$) [8]. Furthermore, in a meta-analysis study in 2014, Li et al. assessed seven case-control

TABLE 1: Lab work in diagnosis of the etiology of the recurrent aphthous stomatitis.

CBC	WBC	9.5 th/μL	3.8–10.8 th/μL
	Hgb	13.5 g/dL	11.7–15.5 g/dL
	Hct	42.1%	35–45.0%
	MCV	86.1 fL	80–100 fL
	Platelet	301 th/uL	7.5–12.5 th/uL
	Absolute lymphocyte	3891 cells/uL	200–950 cells/uL
CMP	Na	143 MEQ/L	135–146 MEQ/L
	K	5.0 MEQ/L	3.5–5.3 MEQ/L
	Cl	106 MEQ/L	98–110 MEQ/L
	CO2	32 MEQ/L	20–32 MEQ/L
	Albumin	4.4 g/dL	3.6–5.1 g/dL
	Bilirubin	0.3 g/dL	0.2–1.2 g/dL
	AST	27 IU/L	10–35 IU/L
	ALT	37 IU/L	6-29 IU/L
	BUN	17 mg/dL	7–25 mg/dL
	Creatinine	0.83 mg/dL	0.5–1.10 mg/dL
	Calcium	12.1 mg/dL	8.6–10.2 mg/dL
Micronutrients/vitamins	B12	484 pg/mL	254–1320 pg/mL
	B1	<7 nmol/L	8–30 nmol/L
	B6	<2 ng/μL	2.1–21.7 ng/μL
	B2	43.5 nmol/L	6.2–39 nmol/L
	B3	<20 ng/mL	<20–30000 ng/mL
	Vitamin D 25 (OH)	19 ng/mL	30–100 ng/mL
	Transthyretin	27.7 mg/dL	20–40 mg/dL
	Folate	13.1 ng/mL	3.1–17.5 ng/mL
	TIBC	370 mcg/dL	250–450 mcg/dL
	Ferritin	147.8 ng/mL	8–252.0 ng/mL
	Iron	48 ng/mL	50–170 ng/mL
	Zinc	53 mcg/dL	60–130 mcg/dL
Serologies/autoimmune work up	ANCA	Negative	Negative
	ANA	Negative	Negative
	Rheumatoid factor	Negative	Negative
	TTG-IGA	Negative	Negative
	Lupus panel	Negative	Negative
	SSA/SSB	Negative	Negative
	T4	1.02 ng/dL	0.76–1.46 ng/dLf
	TSH	1.12 mIU/L	0.358–3.740 mIU/L
	A1c	6.2%	<5.5%
Infectious work up	HIV	Negative	Negative
	HSV 1	Positive abs	Negative
	Hepatitis C ab	Negative	Negative
	H pylori (stool antigen)	Negative (after eradication)	Negative
Lipid Panel	Total cholesterol	217 mg/dL	<200 mg/dL
	HDL	67 mg/dL	>50 mg/dL
	Triglyceride	263 mg/dL	<150 mg/dL

CBC: complete blood count, WBC: white blood cell, Hgb: hemoglobin, Hct: hematocrit, MCV: mean corpuscular volume. CMP: comprehensive metabolic panel. AST: aspartate aminotransferase. ALT: alanine transaminase. TIBC: total iron-binding capacity. ANCA: antineutrophil cytoplasmic antibodies. ANA: antinuclear antibodies. TTG-IGA: tissue transglutaminase-immunoglobulin A. SSA/SSB: Sjögren's-syndrome-related antigen A/Sjögren's-syndrome-related antigen B. TSH: thyroid stimulating hormone. HIV: human immunodeficiency virus.

studies containing 339 cases and 271 controls. The result revealed that patients with RAS had significantly higher rates of *H. pylori* infection than non-RAS controls. They concluded that *H. Pylori* is associated with an increased risk of RAS [9].

On the contrary, few studies were found to have no association between *H pylori* infection and RAS. In a study by Mansour-Ghanaei et al., toothbrush was used to obtain the oral aphthous ulcer from 50 patients that aged from 18 to 60 years old, and samples were sent for both DNA PCR and ELISA tests to evaluate for *H. Pylori*. The result revealed 26 patients (52%) had positive ELISA tests, and only one patient (2%) was positive for DNR PCR [10]. Similarly, Fritscher et al. also evaluated 105 children and adolescents, where 53 patients were found to have RAS and 52 without it. They analyzed samples obtained by swabbing aphthous lesions, oral mucosa, and dental plaque. These samples were then sent for nested PCR to be evaluated for *H. pylori*, and results were similar to the study conducted by Fritscher et al. [11]. Moreover, Iamaroon et al. evaluated the association of *H. pylori* and RAS by nested PCR, the oral samples were also obtained by using toothpicks to brush the ulcer surfaces and/

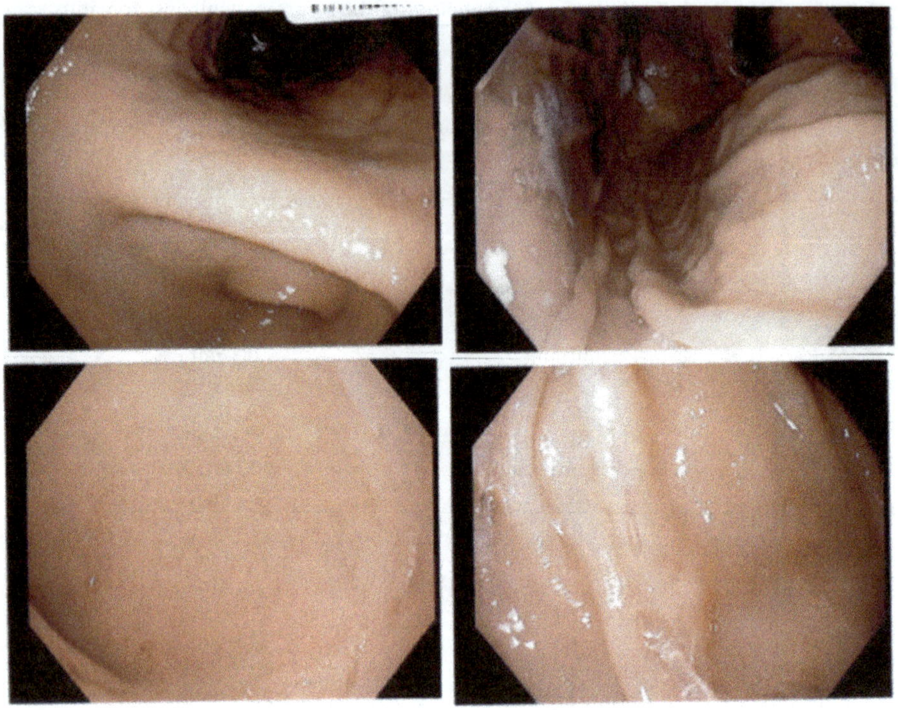

Figure 2: Endoscopic appearance of stomach.

or the dorsum of the tongue in 22 patients with RAS that ages ranging from 12–36 years. The results revealed *H. pylori* does not play a role in the pathogenesis of RAS [12]. The negative associations found in the above studies could be due to the level of bacteria in the oral cavity under undetectable level by one round of PCR (Kignel et al. 2005), the location in the mouth for collection, or sensitivity of PCR difference with saliva vs gastric biopsies [13]. Kignel pointed out that the location mouth used for the collection of the samples can influence the prevalence of the microorganism [13]. This statement was further supported by Song et al. (2000), who found 82% prevalence in the molar region, 64% in premolar region, and 59% in the incisor region [14]. Besides the location, the PCR sensitivity difference in gastric biopsy sample and saliva sample remained unclear, and the evidence is limited. Sekhar et al. found sensitivity and specificity of PCR for saliva were found to be 80% and 70% [15] which is lower compared to gastric biopsy in detecting *H. pylori* which might explain the potential variance in result [16].

4. Conclusion

The debate on the association between RAS and *H. pylori* remains. The variable results could stem from the broad inclusion and exclusion criteria each study had, small sample sizes, demographics, and the various detection methods that differ among studies. This association requires further investigation. Despite the ongoing debate between association between *H. pylori* and RAS, *H. pylori* should still always be considered as one of the potential factors contributing to recurrent aphthous stomatitis. Eradication of *H. Pylori* could potentially make a drastic impact on a patient's quality of life and help prevent potential detrimental consequences of untreated *H. pylori* infection such as lymphoma or other gastric malignancies.

Disclosure

The authors certify that they have no affiliations with or involvement with any organization with any financial interest in the subject matter discussed.

References

[1] C. C. Gomes, R. S. Gomez, L. G. Zina, and F. R. Amaral, "Recurrent aphthous stomatitis and *Helicobacter pylori*," *Medicina Oral, Patologia Oral y Cirugia Bucal*, vol. 21, no. 2, pp. e187–e191, 2016.

[2] J. K. Y. Hooi, W. Y. Lai, W. K. Ng et al., "Global prevalence of *Helicobacter pylori* infection: systematic review and meta-analysis," *Gastroenterology*, vol. 153, no. 2, pp. 420–429, 2017.

[3] J. E. Everhart, D. Kruszon-Moran, G. I. Perez-Perez, T. S. Tralka, and G. McQuillan, "Seroprevalence and ethnic differences inHelicobacter pyloriInfection among adults in the United States," *The Journal of Infectious Diseases*, vol. 181, no. 4, pp. 1359–1363, 2000.

[4] S. O. Akintoye and M. S. Greenberg, "Recurrent aphthous stomatitis," *Dental Clinics of North America*, vol. 58, no. 2, pp. 281–297, 2014.

[5] S. Koybasi, A. H. Parlak, E. Serin, F. Yilmaz, and D. Serin, "Recurrent aphthous stomatitis: investigation of possible etiologic factors," *American Journal of Otolaryngology*, vol. 27, no. 4, pp. 229–232, 2006.

[6] B. Tarakji, G. Gazal, S. A. Al-Maweri, S. N. Azzeghaiby, and N. Alaizari, "Guideline for the diagnosis and treatment of

recurrent aphthous stomatitis for dental practitioners," *Indian Journal of Forensic Medicine & Toxicology*, vol. 14, no. 4, 2020.

[7] S. Karaca, M. Seyhan, M. Senol, M. M. Harputluoglu, and A. Ozcan, "The effect of gastric *Helicobacter pylori* eradication on recurrent aphthous stomatitis," *International Journal of Dermatology*, vol. 47, no. 6, pp. 615–617, 2008.

[8] D. A. Tas, T. Yakar, H. Sakalli, and E. Serin, "Impact of *Helicobacter pylori* on the clinical course of recurrent aphthous stomatitis," *Journal of Oral Pathology & Medicine*, vol. 42, pp. 89–94, 2013.

[9] L. Li, H. Gu, and G. Zhang, "Association between recurrent aphthous stomatitis and *Helicobacter pylori* infection: a meta-analysis," *Clinical Oral Investigations*, vol. 18, no. 6, pp. 1553–1560, 2014.

[10] F. Mansour-Ghanaei, M. Asmar, A. H. Bagherzadeh, and S. Ekbataninezhad, "*Helicobacter pylori* infection in oral lesions of patients with recurrent aphthous stomatitis," *Medical Science Monitor*, vol. 11, no. 12, 2005.

[11] A. M. G. Fritscher, K. Cherubini, J. Chies, and A. C. O. Dias, "Association between *Helicobacter pylori* and recurrent aphthous stomatitis in children and adolescents," *Journal of Oral Pathology and Medicine*, vol. 33, no. 3, pp. 129–132, 2004.

[12] A. Iamaroon, S. Chaimano, S. Linpisarn, S. Pongsiriwet, and K. Phornphutkul, "Detection of *Helicobacter pylori* in recurrent aphthous ulceration by nested PCR," *Journal of Oral Science*, vol. 45, no. 2, pp. 107–110, 2003.

[13] S. Kignel, F. Almeida Pina, E. André, M. Alves Mayer, and E. Birman, "Occurrence of *Helicobacter pylori* in dental plaque and saliva of dyspeptic patients," *Oral Diseases*, vol. 11, no. 1, pp. 17–21, 2005.

[14] Q. Song, T. Lange, A. Spahr, G. Adler, and G. Bode, "Characteristic distribution pattern of *Helicobacter pylori* in dental plaque and saliva detected with nested PCR," *Journal of Medical Microbiology*, vol. 49, no. 4, pp. 349–353, 2000.

[15] E. V. S. Goud, R. Kannan, U. Rao, E. Joshua, R. Tavaraja, and Y. Jain, "Identification of *Helicobacter pylori* in saliva of patients with and without gastritis by polymerase chain reaction," *Journal of Pharmacy and Bioallied Sciences*, vol. 11, no. Suppl 3, pp. 523–S529, 2019.

[16] Y.-K. Wang, F. C. Kuo, C. J. Liu et al., "Diagnosis ofHelicobacter pyloriinfection: current options and developments," *World Journal of Gastroenterology*, vol. 21, no. 40, pp. 11221–11235, 2015.

17

Persistent Anemia in the Setting of a Rare Pancreatic Pseudoaneurysm

Olivia Peralta,[1] Christopher Chew,[2] and Matthew Newcomb[3]

[1]*American University of the Caribbean School of Medicine, Cupecoy, Saint Martin*
[2]*Department of Graduate Medical Education, Northeast Georgia Health System, Gainesville, GA, USA*
[3]*Department of Hospital Medicine, Northeast Georgia Health System, Gainesville, GA, USA*

Correspondence should be addressed to Matthew Newcomb; matthew.newcomb@nghs.com

Academic Editor: Hirotada Akiho

Introduction. Pancreatic pseudoaneurysm is a rare but potentially fatal complication that can follow pancreatitis. While early detection is critical to preventing poor long-term outcomes, clinical features vary significantly. Most often, abdominal pain is the presenting complaint, but this can be complicated as classic symptoms of pancreatitis also present with abdominal pain. Herein, we present a patient with an acute on chronic gastrointestinal bleed that was finally attributed to a pancreatic pseudoaneurysm. *Case Presentation.* The patient was a 56-year-old male with a past medical history significant for epilepsy, alcohol abuse, and hypertension who presented as a transfer from an outside facility for a gastrointestinal bleed. Prior to presentation, the patient reported rectal bleeding over the prior 1.5 months but had not sought care until bleeding increased along with increased abdominal pain. The patient's hemoglobin was 6.3 at presentation of the outside facility and received a total of four units of packed red blood cells (PRBCs) prior to arrival. After arrival, persistent bleeding was noted, and an additional 2 units of PRBCs were transfused. A computed tomography angiography (CTA) of the abdomen was obtained to identify the source for embolization. This, however, revealed a $4 \times 4 \times 3.5$ cm intrinsically dense or enhanced mass of the pancreatic head. *Discussion.* Pancreatic pseudoaneurysm is a rare but potentially fatal complication that can follow pancreatitis. In chronic pancreatitis patients who underwent imaging incidence is estimated to be up to 10%. Treatment is difficult, and coil embolization is often used, though this can lead to splenectomy due to splenic ischemia. Stent grafts can be used in the surrounding arteries to maintain the integrity of viscera but carry risk of stent-related thrombosis. Further research is needed on the optimal management of this potentially lethal complication of pancreatitis.

1. Introduction

Pancreatic pseudoaneurysm is a rare but potentially fatal complication that can follow pancreatitis. Thought to be due to an erosion of vessels by pancreatic enzymes, aneurysms most often involve the splenic artery but can affect other branches [1]. Approximately 10% of chronic pancreatitis patients who undergo imaging are found to have developed pseudoaneurysms, with many of these developing within pseudocysts or forming fistulas with surrounding structures [1]. Due to their complexity, it is thought that these pseudoaneurysms can take from weeks to even years to form [2]. While early detection is critical to preventing poor long-term outcomes, clinical features vary significantly. Most often, abdominal pain is the presenting complaint, but this can be complicated as classic symptoms of pancreatitis also present with abdominal pain [3]. Herein, we present a patient with an acute on chronic gastrointestinal bleed that was finally attributed to a pancreatic pseudoaneurysm.

2. Case Report

The patient was a 56-year-old male with a past medical history significant for epilepsy, alcohol abuse, and hypertension who presented as a transfer from an outside facility for a gastrointestinal bleed. Prior to presentation, the patient reported rectal bleeding over the prior 1.5 months but had not sought care until bleeding increased along with increased abdominal pain. The patient's hemoglobin was 6.3 g/dL (normal range: 13.5–17.5 g/dL for men) at presentation of the outside facility and received a total of four units of packed red blood cells (PRBCs) prior to arrival due to continued bleeding. Upon arrival to our facility, the patient was experiencing alcohol withdrawals requiring ongoing management with lorazepam and dexmedetomidine. Upon arrival, there was initial moderate abdominal pain that was diffuse. The patient was started on intravenous (IV) pantoprazole twice daily along with hemoglobin monitoring. Gastroenterology performed an esophagogastroduodenoscopy (EGD) on hospital day one that did not identify a source of bleeding. With continued bleeding, a tagged red blood cell (tRBC) scan was performed which showed an upper gastrointestinal (GI) source of bleeding, likely in the distal stomach or proximal duodenum. With persistent bleeding and having received a total of 9 units of PRBCs at this time, a computed tomography angiography (CTA) of the abdomen was obtained to identify the source for potential embolization. This, however, revealed a $4 \times 4 \times 3.5$ cm intrinsically dense or enhanced mass of the pancreatic head, as shown in Figures 1 and 2. Magnetic resonance cholangiopancreatography (MRCP) was obtained which showed findings suggestive of pseudoaneurysm involving the pancreatic head, as shown in Figures 3 and 4.

Vascular surgery was consulted, and percutaneous embolization of the pseudoaneurysm was attempted as shown in Figures 5 and 6. Specifically, a catheter was inserted into the common femoral artery with ultrasound guidance, and it was then guided into the superior mesenteric artery and celiac axis and trunk. Selective injection of contrast was performed there, and then it was guided further into the gastroduodenal artery where a microcatheter was positioned at the distal end, corresponding to the location noted in the CT scan. Four 3 to 5 mm diameter coils were delivered, as shown in Figure 7, and the procedure ended. Bleeding failed to improve after the procedure, likely due to the sheer size and length of time it had been developing. After discussion with the general surgery team and consultation with an outside hepatobiliary surgeon, the patient was then transferred to a tertiary care center for surgical intervention.

When he arrived at the tertiary care center, he was monitored for seven days to evaluate for resolution since embolization was attempted immediately prior to transfer. After there was no resolution, he was taken to the operating room for an open Whipple procedure, cholecystectomy, and repair of a portal vein. All removed specimens were sent for surgical pathology evaluation. The gall bladder showed chronic cholecystitis, and pancreatic slices for the frozen section showed chronic pancreatitis with a dilated pancreatic duct negative for high-grade dysplasia or malignancy. The Whipple procedure yielded a bile duct, small intestine, and stomach that were all unremarkable and negative for carcinomas, as well as surgical margins and 31 lymph nodes that were also negative for carcinomas. The pancreas removed during the Whipple showed intraductal papillary mucinous neoplasm with focal high-grade dysplasia in the main duct, as well as chronic pancreatitis.

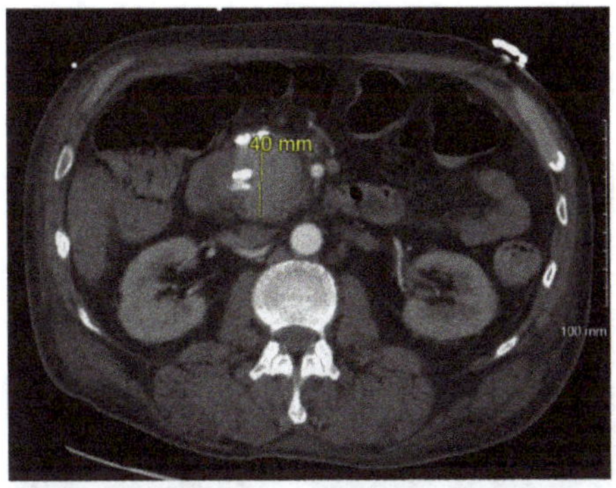

Figure 1: Computed tomography with angiography with measurement of pseudoaneurysm.

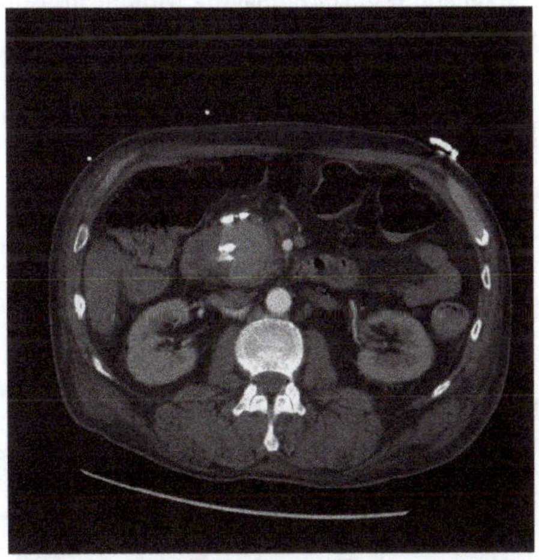

Figure 2: Computer tomography without measurements of pseudoaneurysm.

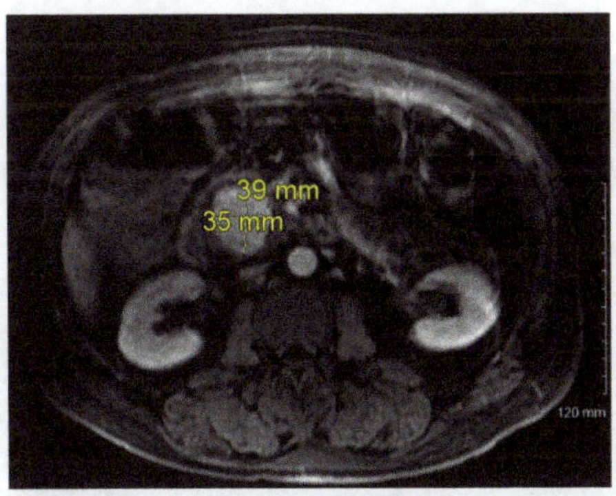

Figure 3: Magnetic resonance imaging with measurement of pseudoaneurysm.

Postoperatively, the patient did well and only required one week of monitoring before discharge. At the time of discharge, he was ambulating, having bowel movements, eating a normal diet, and had all drains removed. His pain was controlled with oral medications, and he had negative blood cultures. He was instructed to follow-up with his primary care physician and hepatobiliary surgeon within two weeks of discharge.

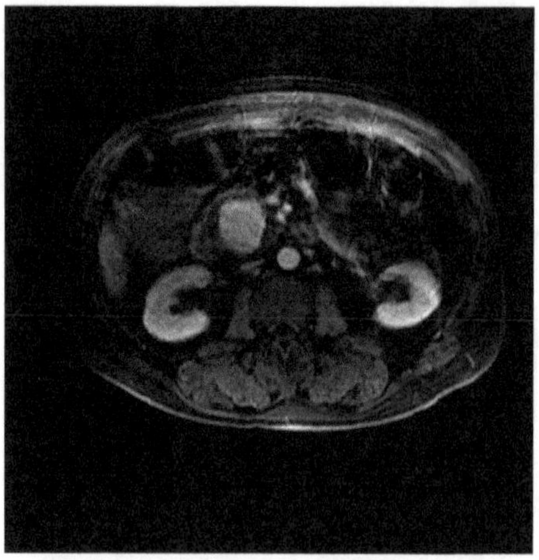

Figure 4: Magnetic resonance imaging without measurement of pseudoaneurysm.

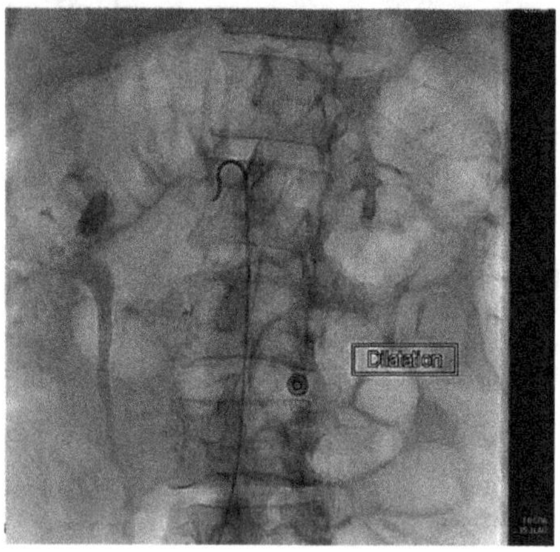

Figure 5: Dilatation evident during procedure.

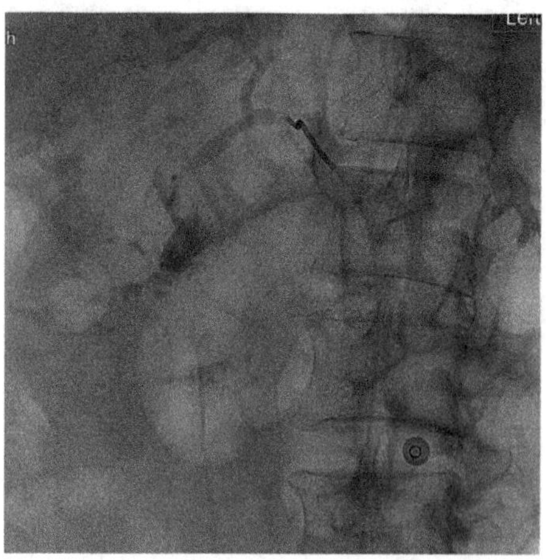

Figure 6: Contrast-enhanced image during the embolization.

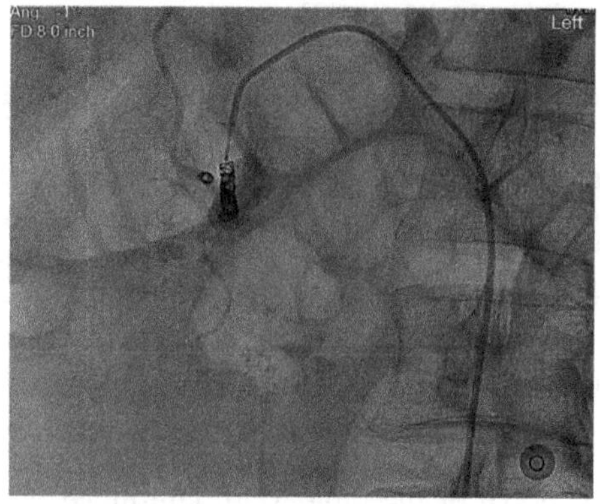

Figure 7: Multiple coils delivered at the side of the pseudoaneurysm during embolization.

3. Discussion

Pancreatic pseudoaneurysm is a rare but potentially fatal complication that can follow pancreatitis. In chronic pancreatitis patients who underwent imaging, incidence is estimated to be up to 10%, and notably, when associated with a concurrent pseudocyst, the bleeding risk is estimated at 15–20% [1]. While difficult to diagnose due to vague presenting symptoms, early localization and identification is important. Since chronic pancreatitis is a known risk factor for pseudoaneurysms, it is important to follow-up with these patients closely. However, as the clinical presentation of chronic pancreatitis can be vastly different, there is difficulty in following these patients on a regular basis. The American Pancreatic Association released guidelines in 2014 which offer direction in management of the patient with chronic pancreatitis [4]. Primarily, when chronic pancreatitis is clinically suspected, a contrast-enhanced CT is recommended along with lifestyle modifications such as the cessation of smoking and alcohol intake, as well as a low-fat diet [4]. Pain is the most common symptom that accompanies chronic pancreatitis, and thus, it is vital to manage the pain appropriately [5]. When symptoms of malabsorption or steatorrhea appear, it may be indicated to initiate pancreatic enzyme replacement [6]. If strictures, stones, or pseudocysts arise and are symptomatic, they can often be treated with endoscopy or if larger disease is present within the ducts, decompressive surgery such as a Whipple procedure might be indicated [6]. Often, pseudoaneurysms can manifest as asymptomatic anemia with or without melena, or silent bleeding into the peritoneal cavity [7].

While pancreatic pseudocysts resolve spontaneously in up to 60% of cases, it is important to rule out underlying pseudoaneurysms [8]. Small pseudoaneurysms can go undetected, but angiography is the gold standard for identifying both bleeding pseudoaneurysms as well as pseudocysts [9]. In 1976, White et al. identified the importance of differentiating between pseudoaneurysms and carcinoma of the pancreas in which unnecessary clinical biopsy can often worsen the progression if it is not a carcinoma [10]. In a study conducted by Zabicki, et al, the splenic artery was ruled as the most common site of pseudoaneurysm, followed by the hepatic artery and then right gastroepiploic artery [11].

Various endovascular procedures are used in the management of pseudoaneurysms, depending upon the hemodynamic stability of the patient as well as the vessel involved [11]. Coil embolization is often used, though this can lead to splenectomy due to splenic ischemia. Stent grafts can be used in surrounding arteries to maintain the integrity of viscera but carry risk of stent-related thrombosis. Thrombin injections, or thrombin-related injections, with ultrasound guidance can be used when primary involved vessels cannot be easily identified [11]. Further research is needed on the optimal management of this potentially lethal complication of pancreatitis.

References

[1] G. Mathew and H. Ahmad, "Pancreatic pseudoaneurysm," in *StatPearls*StatPearls Publishing, Treasure Island, FL, USA, 2019.

[2] T. Dörffel, T. Wruck, R. I. Rückert, P. Romaniuk, Q. Dörffel, and W. Wermke, "Vascular complications in acute pancreatitis assessed by color duplex ultrasonography," *Pancreas*, vol. 21, no. 2, pp. 126–133, 2000.

[3] R. P. Evans, M. M. Mourad, G. Pall, S. G. Fisher, and S. R. Bramhall, "Pancreatitis: preventing catastrophic haemorrhage," *World Journal of Gastroenterology*, vol. 23, no. 30, pp. 5460–5468, 2017.

[4] D. L. Conwell, L. S. Lee, D. Yadav et al., "American pancreatic association practice guidelines in chronic pancreatitis," *Pancreas*, vol. 43, no. 8, pp. 1143–1162, 2014.

[5] C. E. Forsmark, "Management of chronic pancreatitis," *Gastroenterology*, vol. 144, no. 6, pp. 1282–1291, 2013.

[6] K. Barry, "Chronic pancreatitis: diagnosis and treatment," *American Family Physician*, vol. 97, no. 6, pp. 385–393, 2018.

[7] J. T. Hsu, C. N. Yeh, C. F. Hung et al., "Management and outcome of bleeding pseudoaneurysm associated with chronic pancreatitis," *BMC Gastroenterology*, vol. 6, p. 3, 2006.

[8] A. Y. B. Teoh, V. Dhir, M. Kida et al., "Consensus guidelines on the optimal management in interventional EUS procedures: results from the Asian EUS group RAND/UCLA expert panel," *Gut*, vol. 67, no. 7, pp. 1209–1228, 2018.

[9] S. Balachandra and A. K. Siriwardena, "Systematic appraisal of the management of the major vascular complications of pancreatitis," *The American Journal of Surgery*, vol. 190, no. 3, pp. 489–495, 2005.

[10] A. White, S. Baum, and S. Buranasiri, "Aneurysms secondary to pancreatitis," *American Journal of Roentgenology*, vol. 127, no. 3, pp. 393–396, 1976.

[11] B. Zabicki, N. Limphaibool, M. Holstad, and R. Juszkat, "Endovascular management of pancreatitis-related pseudoaneurysms: a review of techniques," *PLoS One*, vol. 13, no. 1, Article ID e0191998, 2018.

18

A Case of Systemic AL Amyloidosis Diagnosed by Screening Colonoscopy

Lynna Alnimer,[1] Ali Zakaria,[2] Jalpa Patel,[2] Yazan Samhouri,[3] Samira Ahsan,[1] Lyle Goldman,[4] and Serge Sorser[2]

[1]*Department of Internal Medicine, Ascension Providence Hospital, Michigan State University/College of Human Medicine, Southfield, MI, USA*
[2]*Division of Gastroenterology, Ascension Providence Hospital, Michigan State University/College of Human Medicine, Southfield, MI, USA*
[3]*Division of Hematology and Cellular Therapy, Allegheny Health Network Cancer Institute, Pittsburgh, PA, USA*
[4]*Department of Hematology/Oncology, Ascension Providence Hospital, Michigan State University/College of Human Medicine, Southfield, MI, USA*

Correspondence should be addressed to Lynna Alnimer; lynna.alnimer@ascension.org

Academic Editor: Yoshifumi Nakayama

Amyloidosis encompasses several diseases associated with deposition of low-molecular-weight proteins in an abnormal configuration. In light-chain amyloidosis (AL), monoclonal free lambda (λ) or kappa (κ) light chains are the amyloid proteins involved and can deposit in almost any organ. Symptoms vary depending on presence and extent of organ involvement, and thus, clinical presentation varies. Diagnosis requires biopsy of the affected tissue, and sometimes, fat pad or bone marrow biopsy is completed initially. Prognosis of AL amyloidosis depends on the presence of cardiac involvement. Treatment of AL amyloidosis involves systemic chemotherapy and evaluation for autologous stem cell transplant. Herein, we present a case report of an asymptomatic middle-aged female who was diagnosed with AL amyloidosis during an average-risk screening colonoscopy, which is an unusual setting. We discuss the workup involved, clinical presentation, and gastroenterology-related organ involvement.

1. Introduction

Amyloidosis refers to a broad group of diseases associated with extracellular deposition of protein fibrils characterized by beta-pleated sheet arrangement [1]. There are six known types of abnormal proteins associated with amyloidosis. The most common and most severe form is primary or light-chain-associated AL amyloidosis [1]. AA amyloidosis, also known as secondary amyloidosis (A refers to serum amyloid A protein (SAA), an acute phase reactant), has been described in inflammatory conditions. SAA is the protein that forms the amyloid fibril and deposits in the setting of chronic inflammatory states such rheumatoid arthritis and inflammatory bowel disease (IBD), with greater recognition in Crohn's disease (CD) [2]. Gastrointestinal (GI) manifestations are described in both AL amyloidosis and AA amyloidosis [3, 4]. Patients usually present with symptoms related to organ involvement; however, herein, we report a case of AL amyloidosis diagnosed incidentally during average-risk screening colonoscopy.

2. Case Presentation

A 67-year-old African American female with a medical history of hypertension, dyslipidemia, diabetes mellitus type II, and chronic kidney disease IIIa underwent age-appropriate average-risk screening colonoscopy which revealed one 10 mm sessile polyp (Paris II-a) in the sigmoid colon (Figure 1) [5]. Complete polypectomy was performed via hot snare, and histopathology showed colonic mucosa with hyperplastic changes, accompanied by submucosal accumulation of eosinophilic, paucicellular materials positive for

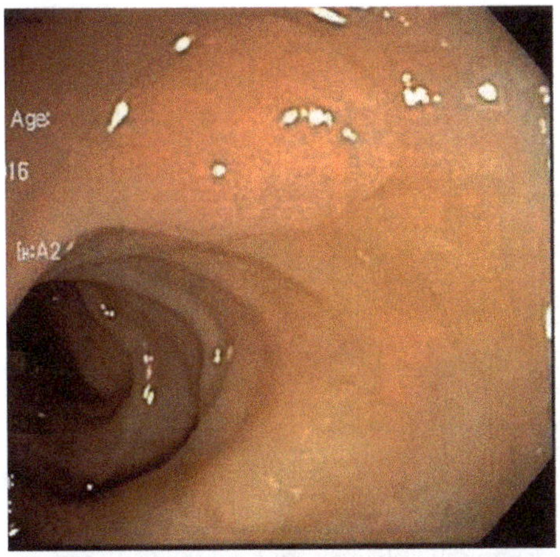

FIGURE 1: Colonoscopy showing a 10 mm sessile sigmoid colon polyp.

Congo red stain, with green birefringence, consistent with amyloids (Figure 2). Two other 3 mm ascending colon tubular adenomas, mild sigmoid colon diverticulosis, and nonbleeding mild internal hemorrhoids were found.

She complained of intermittent dyspnea on exertion but otherwise had no other symptoms. She denied any abdominal pain, nausea, vomiting, hematochezia, weight loss, or change in bowel habits. She was referred to evaluate this incidentally diagnosed amyloidosis, and a follow-up abdominal fat pad biopsy confirmed amyloid vascular deposition. Further workup by hematology revealed a faint IgG kappa monoclonal band on serum immunofixation. The free kappa light chain was elevated at 29.3 mg/dl with a kappa/lambda ratio of 9.54. B2-microglobulin was 3.0 mg/L. Bone marrow biopsy showed plasma cell neoplasm (10%) with no amyloid deposition. The myeloma fluorescence in situ hybridization (FISH) panel was negative for the specific mutations, and cytogenetics showed a normal female karyotype. Amyloid typing with liquid chromatography (mass spectrometry) confirmed the diagnosis of kappa AL amyloidosis.

Further workup was done to evaluate for other organ (cardiac and renal) involvement of amyloidosis particularly with her symptoms of dyspnea and presence of CKD IIIa. Serum biomarkers showed a troponin-I level of 0.06 ng/mL (normal range: 0.00–0.10 ng/mL) and N-terminal pro-B-type natriuretic peptide (NT-proBNP) level of 320 pg/mL (normal range: 50–137 pg/mL). Cardiac catheterization revealed mild coronary artery disease, and cardiac MRI was negative for particular characteristics related to amyloid deposition. Kidney biopsy was not done as a 24-hour urine collection did not show substantial proteinuria/Bence Jones protein.

There was a multidisciplinary discussion with amyloidosis specialists regarding whether the patient should be treated with a systemic regimen. The consensus opinion was to monitor expectantly as the patient did not have renal or cardiac involvement. She remained asymptomatic, and the kappa light chain, renal function, and cardiac status remained stable. The timing of her surveillance colonoscopy was based on the two low-risk tubular adenomas as no guidance is available on the follow-up of benign polyps with amyloid deposition.

3. Discussion

Epidemiological data on amyloidosis are scarce; however, a recent large study by Quock et al. reported a mean age at diagnosis of 63, with higher incidence and prevalence in males [6]. These findings are comparable to previous studies. The reported incidence varies between the types of amyloidosis; one study showed 6.13 per million person-years for AL amyloidosis vs. 1.21 per million person-years for AA amyloidosis [7]. Moreover, kappa light chain amyloidosis is considered relatively rare in comparison to that of lambda light chain as the reported incidence is lower [8].

Amyloidosis can affect almost any organ. Common systemic manifestations include weakness, fatigue, purpura, and marked weight loss. Macroglossia is considered pathognomonic of the disease, but tissue confirmation is required, which is often obtained with abdominal fat pad biopsy. Although cardiac involvement is the leading cause of morbidity and mortality, involvement of the GI tract is not uncommon and can be associated with debilitating nonspecific symptoms and complications [9]. Localized disease to the GI tract is rare as systemic involvement is more common [9]. The prognosis of patients with AL amyloidosis and GI involvement is worse than that in those without known GI involvement. Moreover, if GI involvement is diagnosed, then there is a higher probability that other organs are involved and advanced disease is expected. Thus, a prompt evaluation is warranted [10].

Amyloid deposition can be present throughout the GI tract including almost all luminal organs with the greatest involvement reported in the small bowel [11]. Symptoms from small bowel involvement include diarrhea, constipation, and steatorrhea which are attributable to malabsorption and motility dysfunction [12]. Abdominal computed tomography (CT) scans may show edematous wall thickening of the small bowel, and endoscopic findings include bulk depositions causing mucosal protrusions and thickened intestinal folds of the small bowel [13, 14]. Nutritional deficiencies secondary to malabsorptive diarrhea can be an issue to some patients, and supportive therapy with multivitamin supplementation plays a role [15]. When the vasculature is affected, more life-threatening symptoms can develop such as hemorrhage, bowel infarction, perforation, and mesenteric ischemia [16]. Fortunately, pseudo-obstruction resulting from dysmotility is less commonly encountered, as prognosis is usually unpromising and surgery can be unsafe [17]. One report suggested that 8% of patients with amyloidosis have gastric involvement by biopsy, but only 1% exhibited symptoms. Symptoms range from nausea and vomiting to hematemesis and gastric outlet obstruction [1, 18]. Two large studies by Lee et al. and James et al. described similar findings of gastrointestinal manifestations related to amyloidosis; both showing motility-related predominant symptoms [19].

Hepatic involvement is common, but symptoms are usually mild with the most common findings being hepatomegaly and elevated alkaline phosphatase [20]. When present, ascites in amyloidosis is usually from cardiac failure and hypoalbuminemia rather than liver disease involvement

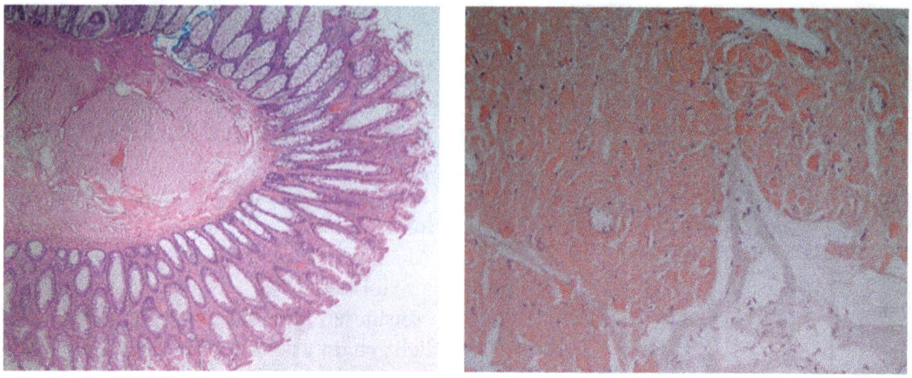

(a) (b)

Figure 2: Sigmoid colon polypectomy showing benign colonic mucosa with hyperplastic changes and submucosal accumulation of eosinophilic materials, which are S100, CD117, CD34, and SMA negative (excluding neuroma, GIST, and leiomyoma) (a). The material is positive for Congo red stain consistent with amyloids (b).

[1]. GI manifestations are nonspecific; thus, high clinical suspicion coupled with detailed investigation is necessary to make the diagnosis. When untreated, AL amyloidosis is associated with a median 1-year mortality rate around 50%; thus, timely diagnosis is essential [20].

In AL amyloidosis, amyloids tend to deposit in the form of a mass in the submucosal and muscularis propria layers of the GI tract [21]. However, in AA amyloidosis, the protein fibrils tend to deposit in the lamina propria mucosae and submucosal layer in a macular or perivascular form [22]. Given these differences, polypoid protrusions and thickening of the valvulae conniventes are more common in AL amyloidosis, while fine mucosal appearance and friable mucosa are classic findings in AA amyloidosis [22, 23]. In addition, the disease occurs more frequently in the descending and rectosigmoid regions of the colon [24]. This pattern is similar to that seen in our patient who had sigmoid colonic polyps. Similar to gastrointestinal complaints, endoscopic features of AL amyloidosis are not specific to the disease. Multiple findings have been described including thickened folds, erosions, ulcerations, friability, and edema [19].

There are several cases describing colon involvement in amyloidosis. Fukui et al. described a similar case in a 72-year-old patient who was incidentally diagnosed with AL amyloidosis caused by monoclonal gammopathy of undetermined significance (MGUS); however, the patient had a positive fecal occult blood test which prompted the colonoscopy [25]. Axelrad et al. described a case of amyloid deposition throughout the colon with negative fat pad biopsy [9]. Lee et al. presented a case of AL amyloidosis in a patient diagnosed with ulcerative colitis (UC) [23]. Our case is different compared to the former cases; the patient had a positive fat biopsy and was not diagnosed with IBD. James et al. described a distinctive finding of submucosal hematomas positive for AL amyloidosis, in the setting of gastrointestinal bleeding [19]. This should prompt physicians to suspect amyloidosis when encountering submucosal hematomas during endoscopy.

Differentiation between types of amyloidosis is essential as controlling the underlying disorder is of paramount importance in AA amyloidosis, while AL amyloidosis requires treatment with chemotherapy and hematopoietic stem cell transplant. Remarkably, the mortality is high in patients receiving transplant and the morbidity seen is commonly secondary to GI complications including GI bleeding and toxic megacolon [26].

The diagnosis of AL amyloidosis can be challenging, and it is based on the Mayo Clinic and the International Myeloma Working Group criteria [27]. Our patient met the four criteria as she had GI tract involvement, positive amyloid staining with Congo red in fat aspirate, light-chain-related disease as mass spectrometry confirmed AL amyloidosis, and smoldering myeloma (presence of 10% plasma cells in the bone marrow with the absence of the CRAB criteria (hypercalcemia, renal insufficiency, anemia, and bone lesions)).

It is important to identify the extent of the disease as indications for systematic therapy are specific. Mostly all patients with systemic AL amyloidosis require treatment at the time of diagnosis [28]. However, in asymptomatic patients who are incidentally diagnosed, initial therapy can be delayed until the first sign of organ involvement develops [28]. The prognosis of AL amyloidosis in the setting of gastrointestinal and, specifically, colonic involvement is unknown; however, pseudo-obstruction of the colon carries a grave prognosis [1].

It is essential, yet a clinical dilemma, to establish organ involvement by amyloidosis. Consensus criteria revised in 2011 on amyloid and amyloidosis state that direct biopsy verification with symptoms is considered as "GI tract involvement," while vascular only amyloid deposits biopsy verification without symptoms is not considered intestinal organ involvement [29]. Our patient had submucosal amyloid deposits but did not have any GI symptoms, which is why treatment was debatable and monitoring for symptoms or further organ involvement was the final plan. There is currently no established recommendation on the frequency of surveillance colonoscopy for polyps with amyloid deposition.

4. Conclusion

Endoscopic findings leading to a diagnosis of amyloidosis are uncommon; our patient is unique as she had no GI complaints, and her screening colonoscopy prompted the whole workup to be completed. If detected in an unusual setting, such as screening colonoscopy, it is important to refer patients for further evaluation as diagnosis can be time-sensitive. This case highlights the high-yield diagnostic value accompanying colonoscopy in diseases not necessarily belonging to the GI tract. It is important for gastroenterologists to consider amyloidosis amidst a background of nonspecific symptoms and refer patients to the appropriate subspecialist for further evaluation. There is currently no established recommendation on the frequency of surveillance colonoscopy for polyps with amyloid deposition.

References

[1] E. C. Ebert and M. Nagar, "Gastrointestinal manifestations of amyloidosis," *American Journal of Gastroenterology*, vol. 103, no. 3, pp. 776–787, 2008.

[2] P. T. Sattianayagam, P. N. Hawkins, and J. D. Gillmore, "Systemic amyloidosis and the gastrointestinal tract," *Nature Reviews Gastroenterology & Hepatology*, vol. 6, no. 10, pp. 608–617, 2009.

[3] R. A. Kyle and M. A. Gertz, "Primary systemic amyloidosis: clinical and laboratory features in 474 cases," *Seminars in Hematology*, vol. 32, 1995.

[4] R. A. Levine, "Amyloid disease of the liver," *American Journal of Medicine*, vol. 33, no. 3, pp. 349–357, 1962.

[5] R. Lambert, "The Paris endoscopic classification of superficial neoplastic lesions: esophagus, stomach, and colon: november 30 to December 1, 2002," *Gastrointestinal Endoscopy*, vol. 58, pp. S3–S43, 2003.

[6] T. P. Quock, T. Yan, E. Chang, S. Guthrie, and M. S. Broder, "Epidemiology of AL amyloidosis: a real-world study using US claims data," *Blood Advances*, vol. 2, no. 10, pp. 1046–1053, 2018.

[7] M. A. Aguirre, B. R. Boietti, E. Nucifora et al., "Incidence rate of amyloidosis in patients from a medical care program in buenos aires, argentina: a prospective cohort," *Amyloid: International Journal of Experimental & Clinical Investigation*, vol. 23, no. 3, pp. 184–187, 2016.

[8] E. Muchtar, M. A. Gertz, S. K. Kumar et al., "Improved outcomes for newly diagnosed AL amyloidosis between 2000 and 2014: cracking the glass ceiling of early death," *Blood*, vol. 129, no. 15, pp. 2111–2119, 2017.

[9] J. Axelrad, M. Lebwohl, and O. Lebwohl, "A rare finding in an inflammatory polyp," *Clinical Gastroenterology and Hepatology*, vol. 15, no. 5, pp. A35–A36, 2017.

[10] A. Y. Lim, J. H. Lee, K. S. Jung et al., "Clinical features and outcomes of systemic amyloidosis with gastrointestinal involvement: a single-center experience," *Korean Journal of Internal Medicine*, vol. 30, no. 4, p. 496, 2015.

[11] D. A. Legge, H. C. Carlson, and E. E. Wollaeger, "Roentgenologic appearance of systemic amyloidosis involving gastrointestinal tract," *American Journal of Roentgenology*, vol. 110, no. 2, pp. 406–412, 1970.

[12] J. M. French, G. Hall, D. J. Parish, and W. T. Smith, "Peripheral and autonomic nerve involvement in primary amyloidosis associated with uncontrollable diarrhoea and steatorrhoea," *American Journal of Medicine*, vol. 39, no. 2, pp. 277–284, 1965.

[13] S. Tada, M. Iida, T. Yao et al., "Endoscopic features in amyloidosis of the small intestine: clinical and morphologic differences between chemical types of amyloid protein," *Gastrointestinal Endoscopy*, vol. 40, no. 1, pp. 45–50, 1994.

[14] A. Azzam, R. Balasubramaniam, S. Safa, C. McIvor, and P. Mollee, "Malabsorption secondary to gout-induced amyloidosis," *ACG Case Reports Journal*, vol. 4, p. e32, 2017.

[15] K. Rowe, J. Pankow, F. Nehme, and W. Salyers, "Gastrointestinal amyloidosis: review of the literature," *Cureus*, vol. 9, no. 5, p. e1228, 2017.

[16] C. N. Andrews, J. N. Amar, M. M. Hayes, and R. A. Enns, "Systemic amyloidosis: a rare presentation of mesenteric angina," *Canadian Journal of Gastroenterology*, vol. 16, pp. 683–5, 2002.

[17] M. Deguchi, K. Shiraki, H. Okano et al., "Primary localized amyloidosis of the small intestine presenting as an intestinal pseudo-obstruction: report of a case," *Surgery Today*, vol. 31, no. 12, pp. 1091–1093, 2001.

[18] D. M. Menke, R. A. Kyle, C. R. Fleming, J. T. Wolfe, P. J. Kurtin, and W. A. Oldenburg, "Symptomatic gastric amyloidosis in patients with primary systemic amyloidosis," *Mayo Clinic Proceedings*, vol. 68, 1993.

[19] D. G. James, G. R. Zuckerman, G. S. Sayuk, H. L. Wang, and C. Prakash, "Clinical recognition of Al type amyloidosis of the luminal gastrointestinal tract," *Clinical Gastroenterology and Hepatology*, vol. 5, no. 5, pp. 582–588, 2007.

[20] K. A. Kyle and K. D. Bayed, "Amyloidosis: review op 236 cases," *Medicine*, vol. 54, no. 4, pp. 271–299, 1975.

[21] M. Yamada, S. Hatakeyama, and H. Tsukagoshi, "Gastrointestinal amyloid deposition in AL (primary or myeloma-associated) and AA (secondary) amyloidosis: diagnostic value of gastric biopsy," *Human Pathology*, vol. 16, no. 12, pp. 1206–1211, 1985.

[22] T. Iida, H. Yamano, and H. Nakase, "Systemic amyloidosis with gastrointestinal involvement: diagnosis from endoscopic and histological views," *Journal of Gastroenterology and Hepatology*, vol. 33, no. 3, pp. 583–590, 2018.

[23] B. S. Lee, Y. Chudasama, A. I. Chen, B. S. Lim, and M. T. Taira, "Colonoscopy leading to the diagnosis of AL amyloidosis in the gastrointestinal tract mimicking an acute ulcerative colitis flare," *ACG Case Reports Journal*, vol. 6, no. 11, Article ID e00289, 2019.

[24] T. D. Trinh, B. Jones, and E. K. Fishman, "Amyloidosis of the colon presenting as ischemic colitis: a case report and review of the literature," *Gastrointestinal Radiology*, vol. 16, no. 1, pp. 133–136, 1991.

[25] T. Fukui, Y. Tanimura, Y. Matsumoto, S. Horitani, T. Tomiyama, and K. Okazaki, "Incidentally detected amyloid light-chain amyloidosis caused by monoclonal gammopathy of undetermined significance: possible time-dependent change in colonic findings," *Case Reports in Gastroenterology*, vol. 12, no. 3, pp. 737–46, 2018.

[26] B. M. Hayes-Lattin, P. T. Curtin, W. H. Fleming et al., "Toxic megacolon: a life-threatening complication of high-dose therapy and autologous stem cell transplantation among

patients with AL amyloidosis," *Bone Marrow Transplantation*, vol. 30, no. 5, pp. 279–85, 2002.

[27] S. V. Rajkumar, M. A. Dimopoulos, A. Palumbo et al., "International myeloma working group updated criteria for the diagnosis of multiple myeloma," *Lancet Oncology*, vol. 15, no. 12, pp. e538–e548, 2014.

[28] M. A. Gertz, R. Comenzo, R. H. Falk et al., "Definition of organ involvement and treatment response in immunoglobulin light chain amyloidosis (AL): a consensus opinion from the 10th international symposium on amyloid and amyloidosis," *American Journal of Hematology*, vol. 79, no. 4, pp. 319–328, 2005.

[29] G. Merlini, D. C. Seldin, and M. A. Gertz, "Amyloidosis: pathogenesis and new therapeutic options," *Journal of Clinical Oncology*, vol. 29, no. 14, pp. 1924–1933, 2011.

19

Esomeprazole-Induced Chest Pain: A Case of an Unexpected Serious Adverse Reaction to a Proton Pump Inhibitor

Melanija Ražov Radas[1] **Aleksandar Knežević,**[2] **and Vladimir Trkulja**[3]

[1]*Department of Gastroenterology, Zadar General Hospital, Zadar, Croatia*
[2]*Department of Cardiology, Zadar General Hospital, Zadar, Croatia*
[3]*Department of Pharmacology, Zagreb University School of Medicine, Zagreb, Croatia*

Correspondence should be addressed to Melanija Ražov Radas; melanijarr@gmail.com

Academic Editor: Roberto Caronna

1. Introduction

Considering the high prevalence and chronic nature of the acid peptic disease, PPIs have been extensively used and their safety has attracted much attention. Esomeprazole has well-established efficacy and safety in treatment of all clinical manifestations of the acid peptic disease. As a group, PPIs inherently bear a potential for drug-drug interactions reflecting either on disposition of PPIs (e.g., their dependence on CYP-mediated metabolism, pantoprazole excepted) or on disposition of concomitant drugs (e.g., reduced gastrointestinal acidity may affect absorption of certain drugs; apart from pantoprazole, PPIs may inhibit CYP2C19). Clinically relevant drug-drug interactions with esomeprazole (or PPIs) have been only sporadic, likely also due to the awareness about this possibility. It is important to note that warnings have been issued regarding the potential of PPIs (including esomeprazole, but likely excluding pantoprazole) to reduce the efficacy of clopidogrel (inhibition of clopidogrel activation by CYP2C19), but this is not the subject of our presentation (our patient did not take clopidogrel). Also, the association between long-term use of PPIs and an increased risk of fractures has been recognized. Esomeprazole, as well as all marketed PPIs, has an overall excellent safety profile reflected by the fact that most of them have a world-wide over-the-counter status. In particular, cardiovascular safety of esomeprazole and omeprazole appears good and they seem not to increase the risk of adverse cardiac events. We present a patient with a condition that appears to be a case of esomeprazole-induced chest pain with changes that we recorded with the standard 12-lead electrocardiogram (ECG) which should be related to coronary ischemia but not typical for it.

2. Case Report

We present a patient with a condition that appears to be a case of esomeprazole-induced chest pain with ECG changes indicative of myocardial ischemia, albeit not typical for it.

Visit 1. In November 2004, a 57-year-old woman, nonsmoker with a 10-year history of hypertension (managed by atenolol 50 mg/day and aspirin 100 mg/day), presented with noncharacteristic chest pressure, palpitations, and shortness of breath during physical activity. Her sitting blood pressure (BP) was 140/90 mmHg, and physical examination, chest X-ray, and routine laboratory tests were unremarkable. Standard 12-lead electrocardiogram showed a sinus rhythm with 55 bpm, normal electrical axis, and shallow negative T-waves in V1–V3 leads, indicating possible myocardial ischemia. Echocardiography findings were normal. The exercise test showed a hypertensive reaction to strain, no rhythm disturbance, normal functional capacity, and a negative test of coronary reserve. However, since a negative coronary reserve test is possible even with a coronary vessel disease, coronarography was indicated that showed normal

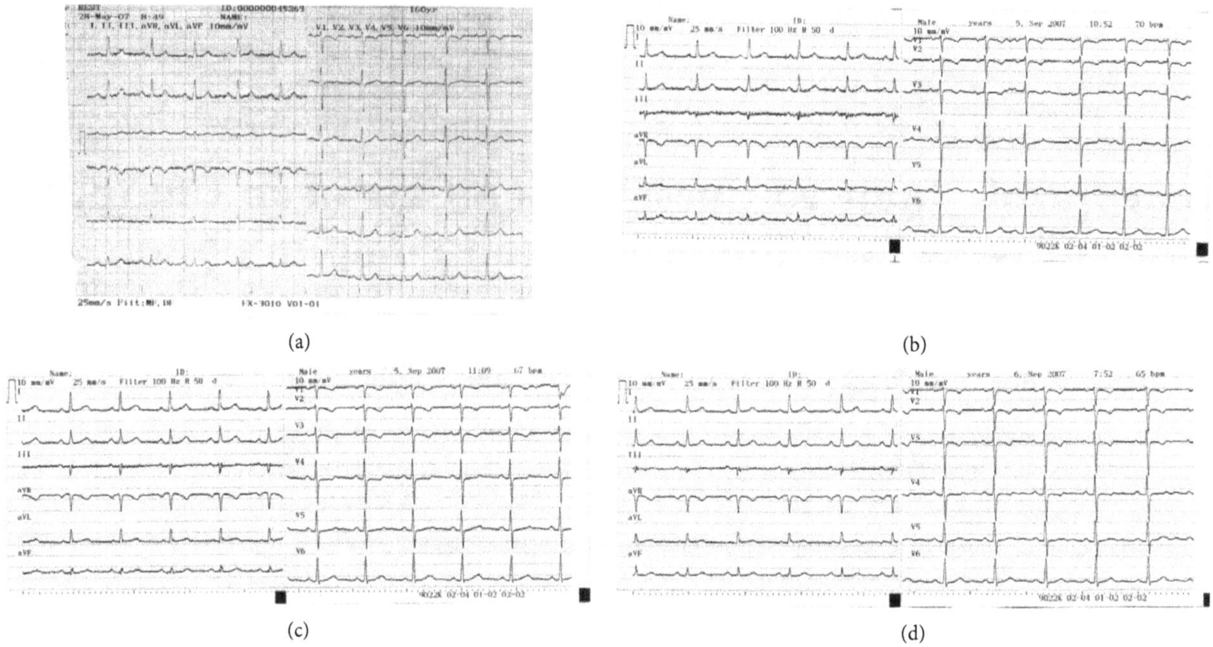

FIGURE 1: Standard 12-lead ECG recordings: (a) On May 28, 2007, no actual difficulties; (b) at 10 : 52 a.m., on September 5, 2007, before the chest pain episode; (c) at 11 : 09 a.m., on September 5, 2007, during the chest pain episode; (d) on September 6, 2007, at 7 : 52 a.m., no difficulties. Note that patient's sex was erroneously recorded as "male."

epicardial coronary vessels. Her difficulties were considered as a possible anginal discomfort. She was prescribed nitroglycerin spray to be used as needed in the case of remitting difficulties. In October 2006, in order to improve her BP control, antihypertensive treatment was changed to bisoprolol 5 mg/day, perindopril 2 × 4 mg/day, and aspirin 100 mg/day.

Visit 2. On May 28, 2007, she reported new complaints. Three weeks earlier, she had been diagnosed with gastroesophageal reflux disease (GERD) and started treatment with oral esomeprazole 20 mg/day. Since then, three to four hours after esomeprazole consumption (coinciding with "post-peak" esomeprazole concentrations [1]), she would feel chest constriction identical to anginal difficulties, which would stop after administration of nitroglycerin. Her sitting BP was 120/80 mmHg, and her physical examination, routine laboratory tests, and a 12-lead ECG (Fogure 1(a)) were unremarkable. She was advised to continue her treatment and to keep records of anginal difficulties.

Visit 3. Nineteen days later, on June 16, 2007, esomeprazole was withdrawn since the difficulties related to its consumption persisted.

Visit 4. On September 4, 2007, she reported no anginal difficulties since withdrawal of esomeprazole three months earlier. However, her GERD difficulties are prominent. Her BP is 140/95 mmHg, and she is clinically unremarkable. After a consultation with a clinical pharmacologist, 20 mg of esomeprazole is administered. She is observed for a day but only complains about a slight headache. She is advised to take esomeprazole the next morning and to refer to the cardiology unit for observation.

Visit 5. On September 5, 2007, she took 20 mg of esomeprazole at 6 a.m. At 10 a.m., her BP is 135/90 mmHg, and she is clinically unremarkable as is a 12-lead ECG taken at 10 : 52 a.m. (Figure 1(b)). However, at 11 : 05 a.m., she started feeling anginal discomfort. At that time (11 : 09 a.m.), ECG showed shallow negative T-waves with a milder ST-segment depression (by around 1 mm) in V1 – V4 leads (Figure 1(c)). The difficulties resolved a few minutes after administration of two sprays of nitroglycerin. Her BP measured on several occasions between 10 : 00 and 11 : 30 a.m. did not change. The next morning, she took no esomeprazole. Her ECG was unremarkable (Figure 1(d)).

3. Discussion

Esomeprazole is a potent selective inhibitor of the H^+/K^+ ATPase in the parietal cells of the gastric mucosa, i.e., a proton pump inhibitor. It is a pure *S*-enantiomer of omeprazole, a racemic mixture, the first marketed and prototypical PPI. Just as its ancestor, esomeprazole has well-established efficacy and safety in treatment of all clinical manifestations of the acid peptic disease [2]. Clearance of esomeprazole is apparently less dependent on CYP2C19 than that of omeprazole [3]. Proton pump inhibitors do not belong among known causes of ischemic or nonischemic chest pain [4]. But, it is important to note that warnings have been issued regarding the potential of PPIs (including esomeprazole, but likely excluding pantoprazole) to reduce the efficacy of clopidogrel (inhibition of clopidogrel activation by CYP2C19) [5]. A thorough evaluation of omeprazole and esomeprazole by FDA in 2007 concluded no association between the use of these two drugs and adverse cardiac events [6], and chest pain, as a possible side effect, is not part of the label of esomeprazole [1].

The mechanism(s) underlying the present observation remain(s) elusive: BP measurements did not indicate precipitation of chest pain by low or high BP; neither bisoprolol nor perindopril are known to affect disposition of esomeprazole and *vice versa*; esomeprazole is not known to affect disposition of bisoprolol or perindopril [2, 3]. PPIs are not among the known causes of ischemic or nonischemic chest pain [7]. The current dechallenge and rechallenge data strongly suggest a causal relationship between esomeprazole and the observed difficulties although the underlying mechanism(s) remain(s) elusive particularly since interactions between esomeprazole and coadministered treatments are not known [6]. Physical examination, of our patient, chest X-ray, and routine laboratory tests were unremarkable. Standard 12- lead electrocardiogram showed shallow negative T-waves in V1–V3 leads, indicating possible left atrial enlargement. Echocardiography findings were normal. The exercise test showed a hypertensive reaction. At the time, we were unable to determine troponin values. Coronarography was indicated and showed normal epicardial coronary vessels. Because the patient had ECG changes typical of transient myocardial ischemia and without myocardial damage, we characterized the reaction as microvascular dysfunction.

4. Conclusion

Esomeprazole was withdrawn permanently. Her GERD treatment continued with pantoprazole. Her antihypertensive treatment was not changed. Her BP has been successfully managed, and she has had no anginal discomfort since. This adverse reaction was reported to the Croatian agency for medicines and medical devices. In accordance with the criteria of the Council for International Organizations of Medical Sciences, it was judged as serious. Based on the rechallenge and dechallenge effects, the Croatian Agency judged its causal relationship to esomeprazole as certain.

Hence, the reported adverse reaction fulfills criteria of an unexpected or type B (atypical and idiosyncratic) adverse reaction.

Disclosure

This research was performed as part of the employment of the authors at Zadar General Hospital, 23000 Zadar, Croatia.

References

[1] Summary of Products Characteristics, "Nexium 20 mg & 40 mg tablets (esomeprazole)," Summary of products characteristics, Europe, 2010.

[2] K. McKeage, S. K. A. Blick, J. D. Croxtall, K. A. Lyseng-Williamson, and G. M. Keating, "Esomeprazole," *Drugs*, vol. 68, no. 11, pp. 1571–1607, 2008.

[3] H. Blume, F. Donath, A. Warnke, and B. S. Schug, "Pharmacokinetic drug interaction profiles of proton pump inhibitors," *Drug Safety*, vol. 29, no. 9, pp. 769–784, 2006.

[4] L. Erhardt, J. Herlitz, L. Bossaert et al., "Task force on the management of chest pain," *European Heart Journal*, vol. 23, no. 15, pp. 1153–1176, 2002.

[5] L. Laine and C. Hennekens, "Proton pump inhibitor and clopidogrel interaction: fact or fiction?" *American Journal of Gastroenterology*, vol. 105, no. 1, pp. 34–41, 2010.

[6] Food and Drug Administration, *Update of Safety Review–Follow-Up to the August 9, 2007, Communication About the Ongoing Safety Review of Omeprazole and Esomeprazole*, Food and drug administration, UK, 2010.

[7] A. B. R. Thomson, M. D. Sauve, N. Kassam, and H. Kamitakahara, "Safety of the long-term use of proton pump inhibitors," *World Journal of Gastroenterology*, vol. 21, no. 16, pp. 2323–2330, 2010.

20

Mucinous Signet-Cell Adenocarcinoma of the Ileum: A Diagnostic Challenge—Case Report and Review of the Literature

Tiago Martins[1] **Jalaluddin Umar,**[2] **Kevin Groudan,**[1] **Hariharan S. Bharadwaj,**[3] **and David Desilets**[2]

[1]*Baystate Medical Center, Internal Medicine Residency, 759 Chestnut Street, Springfield, MA 01199, USA*
[2]*Baystate Medical Center, Gastroenterology Department, 759 Chestnut Street, Springfield, MA 01199, USA*
[3]*Baystate Medical Center, Pathology Department, 759 Chestnut Street, Springfield, MA 01199, USA*

Correspondence should be addressed to Tiago Martins; tiago.martins@baystatehealth.org and David Desilets; david.desilets@baystatehealth.org

Academic Editor: Marcel Cerqueira Cesar Machado

Malignancies of the small intestine are rare. Signet-ring cell carcinoma (SRCC) is one of the rarest forms of adenocarcinoma that can arise in the small intestines. We present a case of a patient who originally presented with abdominal pain and radiographic findings suggestive of ileal congestion. The ileal biopsy specimens were nonspecific, and the patient began a trial of corticosteroid treatment for suspected Crohn's disease. A repeat colonoscopy yielded biopsies that were positive for malignancy. The patient then underwent an exploratory laparotomy which led to the diagnosis of SRCC. Given their similar presentations and the extreme rarity of this unusual malignancy, it can be difficult to differentiate between new-onset Crohn's disease and SRCC. A review of the literature was conducted to provide us with an improved understanding of previously documented cases of SRCC.

1. Introduction

Primary malignancies are detected only rarely in the small intestine. Small intestinal lesions represent only ~2.3% of all malignancies identified in the digestive system and ~0.42% of malignancies overall [1]. Signet-ring cell carcinoma (SRCC) is a rare subtype of adenocarcinoma that is identified most frequently in the stomach, where it accounts for 25% of all gastric cancers. SRCC has also been detected in the pancreas, breasts, bladder, ovaries, esophagus, lungs, and large intestine [2, 3]. The five-year survival rate of patients diagnosed with SRCC has been estimated at 20–30% [1]. While patients diagnosed with Crohn's disease (CD) have an increased risk of developing adenocarcinoma of the ileum compared to the general population, [4] the precise mechanisms underlying this observation remains unknown [4–7]. In this report, we present the case of a patient who was initially treated for presumed new-onset CD before receiving a correct diagnosis of SRCC, and so, we review how both diagnoses can present similarly and pose a diagnostic challenge.

2. Case

The patient was a 68-year-old woman with a prior hysterectomy and family history of CD who presented as a transfer from an outside hospital for the evaluation and treatment of recurrent severe lower abdominal pain.

The patient had initially presented to the outside hospital four weeks prior to this transfer with a chief complaint of constant lower abdominal pain without diarrhea, but with intermittent constipation. The patient also reported a four-pound weight loss. The patient's social history was negative for smoking, alcohol, or illicit drug use. She reported that her mother had been diagnosed with CD. An initial computed tomography (CT) scan revealed abnormal wall thickening and fat stranding within the terminal ileum consistent with an infectious or inflammatory process with no visible abscesses. The mesenteric lymph nodes in the right lower quadrant were also mildly prominent consistent with mesenteric adenitis, and neoplastic disease could not be ruled out. A follow-up colonoscopy revealed a redundant colon with normal mucosa except for superficial, linear erosions in the distal rectum, sigmoid diverticulosis, and an 8 mm polyp in the ascending colon. The terminal ileum appeared to be diffusely congested without any ulcerations or obvious inflammation.

No evidence of pathology was noted on biopsy specimens obtained from the ileocecal valve. Laboratory studies from the outside hospital included a complete blood count (CBC) that revealed slight anemia (hemoglobin at 12 g/L and hematocrit at 37.5%) with normal white blood cell (WBC; 10.2 cells/mcL) and platelet counts (338 cells/mcL). Her routine serum chemistry panel was also within normal limits. The patient had a negative T-spot for tuberculosis and a negative hepatitis panel; elevated levels of C-reactive protein (CRP; 45 mg/L) and calprotectin (408 μg/mL) levels were noted. Based on the family history, colonoscopy findings, and elevated levels of CRP and calprotectin, the patient was initially diagnosed with CD and began treatment with 60 mg methylprednisolone. Her symptoms initially improved on this regimen. She transitioned to oral prednisone and was discharged four days later.

Ten days after discharge, the patient returned to the same outside hospital with a recurrence of persistent abdominal pain. Results from a second CT scan were similar to those reported previously, including the possibility of an infectious process. The patient was hospitalized for an additional four days and was discharged with a treatment plan that included ciprofloxacin and metronidazole together with prednisone as previously prescribed. She was scheduled to complete a prednisone taper and begin treatment with 5 mg/kg infliximab on an outpatient basis.

Two days after the second hospital discharge, the patient returned with worsening abdominal pain. A third abdominal CT performed at this time revealed terminal ileal wall thickening with surrounding fat stranding. Free fluid was detected, and ileus was also documented. The CT report noted that a portion of the inflamed segment may have developed an abscess or phlegmon.

Given the ongoing complexity of this case, the patient was transferred to our tertiary care center. Upon arrival, she was hemodynamically stable (temperature, 36.7°C; pulse, 65 beats/min; blood pressure, 166/66 mmHg; SpO_2, 99% on room air; and respiratory rate, 21 breaths/min). Her CBC documented slight anemia with a normal WBC count and normal serum chemistries. Liver function tests, including serum lipase, were all unremarkable. The patient continued to experience abdominal pain without nausea or diarrhea. She denied any overt gastrointestinal bleeding, fever, or chills. Her initial diagnosis was an exacerbation of CD with ileus and a potential abscess/phlegmon. The gastroenterology team performed a repeat colonoscopy, and a biopsy of the terminal ileum was obtained; the specimen revealed mild inflammatory changes and congestion. Pathological analysis of this specimen revealed a malignant process. Microscopic evaluation revealed tubulovillous adenoma with high-grade dysplasia in Figure 1. This was then confirmed with immunohistochemistry. The cells were negative for cytokeratin 7 but positive for cytokeratin 20 and CDX 2. Although signet-ring cell carcinoma of the small bowel can occur, its relative rarity combined with lack of in situ tumor favored metastatic disease. However, biopsy specimens collected from a subsequent esophagogastroduodenoscopy were grossly negative for malignancy.

The patient underwent an exploratory laparotomy which resulted in the resection of the ileocolic mass; a right-sided colectomy, ileostomy, and abdominal washout were performed, and a mucous fistula was created. The mesentery and the mass adhered to the intestinal wall. An abscess with pus drainage and significant induration were also noted, which suggested an inflammatory process and/or lymphadenopathy. The tumor was 25 cm in length and poorly differentiated and was invading the visceral peritoneum and appendix. With this final resection, the pathology team confirmed the final diagnosis but was also able to find in situ components. The tumor was noted to be arising in a background of tubulovillous adenoma of the terminal ileum, with high-grade dysplasia. Based on the characteristics of this malignancy, the patient was deemed to be a good candidate for adjuvant chemotherapy. A FOLFOX (folinic acid, fluorouracil, and oxaliplatin) regimen was initiated. She is currently on her third cycle of chemotherapy and doing well. This treatment regimen aims to eliminate the disease, reduce the risk of its recurrence, and improve overall survival.

3. Discussion

The case presented in this report illuminates the diagnostic challenge presented by SRCC in the ileum. Of note, this diagnosis was reached only after multiple hospitalizations and ultimately required a multidisciplinary approach. SRCC is considered to be a diffuse type of malignancy with limited cell cohesion. This property permits the malignant cells to infiltrate the visceral wall and precludes the formation of a visible mass [8]. Primary gastric SRCC can spread to the colon through lymphatic vessels and can target the transverse colon via the gastrocolic ligament [9]. While a few case studies that describe SRCC in the ileum have already been published, this case has several unique features, including multiple admissions and specific diagnostic tests that were performed before reaching the correct diagnosis.

SRCC in the colon or small intestines may mimic the signs and symptoms of CD [10]. SRCC presents with many features that are similar to those of CD, including long segments of concentric small intestinal thickening, obstructions, and ulcerations as well as intraluminal masses [5, 10, 11]. Patients with SRCC may also experience nausea, vomiting, abdominal pain, fistulae, hemorrhage, and perforation [12–14]. Many of these symptoms overlap with those of CD, and it can be difficult to distinguish between CD and small intestinal malignancy based on these findings alone [14–16]. Nevertheless, malignancy should certainly emerge as more prominent in the differential diagnosis if these symptoms prove to be refractory to standard CD therapy and bowel obstruction becomes evident [13]. Finally, it is important to note that patients diagnosed with CD are most likely to develop colorectal malignancies at 45–50 years of age [12, 13]. By contrast, de novo small intestinal

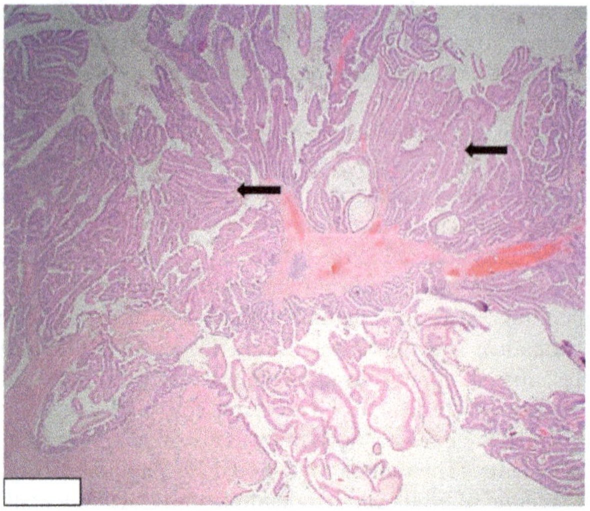

FIGURE 1: Tubulovillous adenoma with high-grade dysplasia. Ileal polyp showing slender, fingerlike projections formed by fibrovascular cores and lined by high-grade dysplastic epithelium (arrows) (H&E stain, 2×).

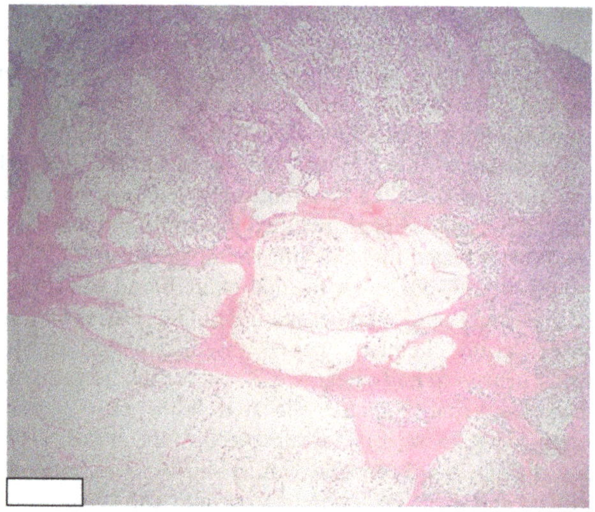

FIGURE 3: Invasive signet-ring cell carcinoma of the ileum with dissecting extracellular mucin pools. The tumor is seen invading the muscularis propria (H&E stain, 2×).

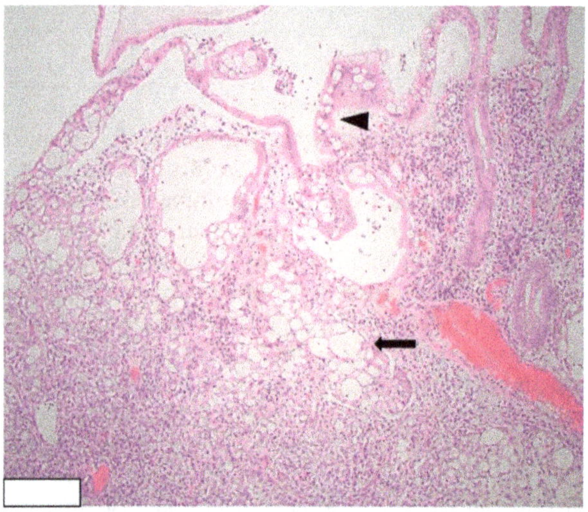

FIGURE 2: Invasive signet-ring cell carcinoma of the ileum (arrow) arising from dysplastic epithelium (arrowhead) (H&E stain, 20×).

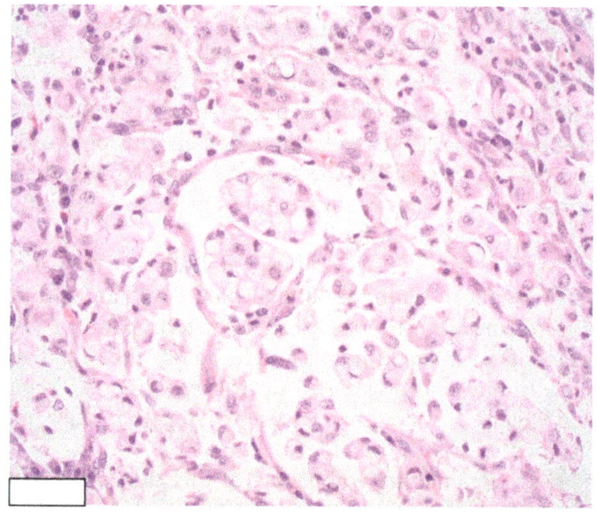

FIGURE 4: Image showing the signet-ring cell morphology at higher magnifications (H&E stain, 40×).

malignancies typically develop in patients within the 60–69 year age bracket [15]. The major risk factor for CD presented by this patient other than her symptoms was her positive family history, which has been reported to increase the risk of CD by 3.22-fold [16].

Given that the presenting signs and symptoms of SRCC can mimic those of CD, the most important diagnostic test leading to an accurate diagnosis is a colonoscopy and biopsy. The characteristic findings of SRCC include signet-ring cells, as shown in Figures 2–4. Histologically, SRCC cells produce mucin and have mucin vacuoles that displace the nucleus to the periphery of the cell [17]. It is important to note that approximately 50% of cases of poorly differentiated small intestinal malignancies that produce mucin, as in the case presented here, have a poor prognosis [4]. The current treatment options for small intestinal malignancies include wide resection that includes the mesentery and corresponding lymph nodes. The use of adjuvant chemotherapy has been described only in small retrospective studies [5].

This case report is important because it highlights the importance of considering malignancy in the differential diagnosis in cases of newly-diagnosed inflammatory bowel disease that do not respond to treatment. Despite its rarity, clinicians should maintain suspicion of SRCC even in the absence of immediate histological confirmation.

Authors' Contributions

Tiago Martins, DO, and David Desilets, MD, designed and directed the manuscript. Jalaluddin Umar, MD, collected the literature and provided the information for the initial draft. Kevin Groudan, MD, revised the manuscript and edited the language. Hariharan Bharadwaj, MD, assisted with the photos and pathology for the manuscript. All authors approved the final version of the manuscript. Jalaluddin Umar, MD, Kevin Groudan, MD, and Hariharan S. Bharadwaj, MD, have contributed equally to this work.

References

[1] A. Jemal, R. Siegel, E. Ward, Y. Hao, J. Xu, and M. J. Thun, "Cancer statistics, 2009," *CA: A Cancer Journal for Clinicians*, vol. 59, no. 4, pp. 225–249, 2009.

[2] S. Dogan, M. Celikbilek, E. Eroglu et al., "Signet ring cell carcinoma mimicking ileal Crohn's disease," *Gastroenterology Insights*, vol. 5, no. 1, pp. 7-8, 2013.

[3] F. Paparo, A. Piccardo, M. Clavarezza et al., "Computed tomography enterography and 18F-FDG PET/CT features of primary signet ring cell carcinoma of the small bowel in a patient with Crohn's disease," *Clinical Imaging*, vol. 37, no. 4, pp. 794–797, 2013.

[4] F. Valério, R. Cutait, A. Sipahi, A. Damião, and K. Leite, "Cancer in Crohn's disease: case report," *Revista Brasileira de Coloproctologia*, vol. 26, no. 4, pp. 443–446, 2006.

[5] C. Cahill, P. H. Gordon, A. Petrucci, and M. Boutros, "Small bowel adenocarcinoma and Crohn's disease: any further ahead than 50 years ago?" *World Journal of Gastroenterology*, vol. 20, no. 33, pp. 11486–11495, 2014.

[6] T. Jess, K. V. Winther, P. Munkholm, E. Langholz, and V. Binder, "Intestinal and extra-intestinal cancer in Crohn's disease: follow-up of a population-based cohort in Copenhagen County, Denmark," *Alimentary Pharmacology & Therapeutics*, vol. 19, no. 3, pp. 287–293, 2004.

[7] C. R. Ramos, P. Guillen, and M. J. Palomo, "Adenocarcinoma de intestine Delgado y enfermedad de Crohn," *Revista Española de Enfermedades Digestivas*, vol. 89, pp. 321–324, 1997.

[8] C. Hommel, M. Knoedler, C. Bojarski et al., "Diffuse gastric cancer with peritoneal carcinomatosis can mimic crohn's disease," *Case Reports in Gastroenterology*, vol. 6, no. 3, pp. 695–703, 2012.

[9] R. M. Katon, S. J. Brendler, and K. Ireland, "Gastric linitis plastica with metastases to the colon," *Journal of Clinical Gastroenterology*, vol. 11, no. 5, pp. 555–560, 1989.

[10] M. W. Winter, A. Dokmak, Z. Marnoy, S. Sinagare, and A. N. Levy, "Metastatic gastric signet ring cell carcinoma mimicking Crohn's disease," *ACG Case Reports Journal*, vol. 5, no. 1, p. e36, 2018.

[11] T. Zenda, K. Taniguchi, T. Hashimoto et al., "Metastatic colon cancer mimicking Crohn's disease," *Annals of Diagnostic Pathology*, vol. 11, no. 6, pp. 427–432, 2007.

[12] L. A. Dossett, L. M. White, D. C. Welch et al., "Small bowel adenocarcinoma complicating Crohn's disease: case series and review of the literature," *The American Surgeon*, vol. 73, no. 11, pp. 1181–1187, 2007.

[13] M. Widmar, A. J. Greenstein, D. B. Sachar, N. Harpaz, J. J. Bauer, and A. J. Greenstein, "Small bowel adenocarcinoma in Crohn's disease," *Journal of Gastrointestinal Surgery*, vol. 15, no. 5, pp. 797–802, 2011.

[14] A. J. Greenstein, "Cancer in inflammatory bowel disease," *The Mount Sinai journal of medicine, New York*, vol. 67, no. 3, pp. 227–240, 2000.

[15] E. Negri, C. Bosetti, C. La Vecchia, F. Fioretti, E. Conti, and S. Franceschi, "Risk factors for adenocarcinoma of the small intestine," *International Journal of Cancer*, vol. 82, no. 2, pp. 171–174, 1999.

[16] B. Shen, F. H. Remzi, J. P. Hammel et al., "Family history of Crohn's disease is associated with an increased risk for Crohn's disease of the pouch," *Inflammatory Bowel Diseases*, vol. 15, no. 2, pp. 163–170, 2009.

[17] Elsevier, *Elsevier's Integrated Pathology, by Thomas Charles King Mosby Elsevier*, pp. 217–246, Elsevier, Amsterdam, Netherlands, 2007.

A Rare Case of Gastric Lipoma Presenting with Gastric Outlet Obstruction Treated Endoscopically

Ahmad Sharayah,[1] Dileep C. Unnikrishnan,[1] Akhila Arya Perumangote Vasudevan,[2] Noor Hajjaj,[3] Rishi Raj,[1] and Kenneth Belitsis[4]

[1]*Internal Medicine Department, Monmouth Medical Center, Long Branch, NJ 07740, USA*
[2]*Internal Medicine Department, Govt Medical Collage, Kozhikode, India*
[3]*Faculty of Medicine, University of Jordan, Amman, Jordan*
[4]*Gastrointestinal Department, Monmouth Medical Center, Long Branch, NJ 07740, USA*

Correspondence should be addressed to Ahmad Sharayah; drsharayah@gmail.com

Academic Editor: Shiro Kikuchi

An 85-year-old male referred to the Gastroenterology (GI) clinic with three-month history of failure to thrive and three-week history of nausea, vomiting, and melanotic stools. Ulcerative mass obstructing gastric outlet was found on endoscopy and on follow-up CT abdomen a homogeneous submucosal mass in the gastric antrum was identified. Radiological diagnosis of giant gastric lipoma was established and patient was evaluated for surgery and, however, was rendered unfit for surgery due to his comorbid conditions. Patient was taken for endoscopic resection of the mass. On endoscopy, only partial resection was achieved due to the size of the mass, but endoloops were deployed at the stalk at the end of the procedure in hope of limiting blood supply to the lesion. On six-week follow-up endoscopy, patient's mass had completely disappeared with limited scar tissue at the site.

1. Introduction

Symptomatic gastric lipomas are rare neoplasms of GI tract. Bleeding due to mucosal erosions on top on the lipomas and mass effect leading to gastric outlet obstruction are some of the common presentations in such cases. Due to its rarity, there is no generalized consensus on the management. Surgical resection of the mass is the common approach in such cases, but in cases where debility or other comorbidities preclude surgery, endoscopic resection and debulking can be attempted. Here we present the case of a giant gastric lipoma where surgical resection was not feasible due to patient's comorbidities. Endoscopic resection was attempted; however due to the size and location of the lesion, only partial resection was achieved. At the end of the procedure, using a needle knife, base of the lesion was cut to create deep grooves at the stalk to prevent slipping of endoloops and an endoloop tightly encircling the stalk was left in place. On six-week follow-up, there was complete disappearance of the mass with minimal scarring of the site. Endoscopic loop placement to limit blood supply can be attempted in the management of large gastric lipoma to prevent major surgeries and its associated morbidity.

2. Case Presentation

An 85-year-old male was referred to GI clinic by his primary care physician for evaluation of anemia, weight loss, and positive stool occult blood. On obtaining a detailed history he admitted to having early satiety for the past three months and nonbilious vomiting and colicky epigastric abdominal pain for the past three weeks. His physical examination was pertinent for pallor and his abdomen was soft and nontender with no apparent swelling or hepatosplenomegaly. An esophagogastroduodenoscopy (Video 1) was performed which showed a large mass in the gastric antrum obstructing the gastric outlet with a nonbleeding but friable ulcer on top [Figure 1]. Biopsies were sent due to the concern for Gastrointestinal Stromal Tumor (GIST), gastric lymphoma,

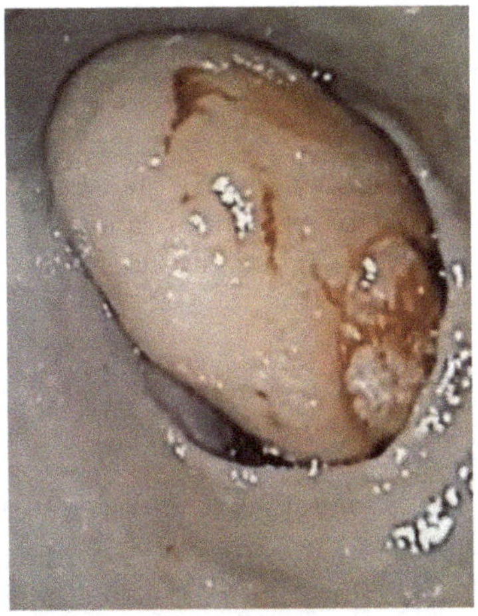

FIGURE 1: First endoscopy showing large gastric antral mass with friable ulcer at the top.

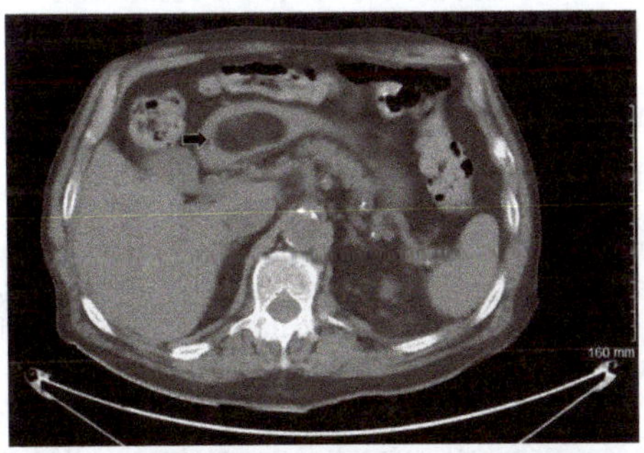

FIGURE 2: Computerized tomography abdomen. Black arrow showing gastric antral submucosal mass which is homogeneous in density and has sharp rounded borders. This is indicative of gastric lipoma.

or adenocarcinoma stomach. A Computerized Tomography (CT) abdomen was ordered to further look into the etiology of the mass and determine the size and presence of lesions elsewhere. The CT abdomen [Figure 2] revealed a homogeneous submucosal mass of 5 cm x 2.5 cm size. The lesion was in the gastric antrum, homogeneous, and well contained within the gastric wall. There were no lymphadenopathy or remote lesions in the abdomen. This together with endoscopic features of the mass was suggestive of benign gastric lipoma. Surgical referral was done for possible surgical removal; however, it was advised to try to endoscopically resect or at least debulk the mass for palliation of his symptoms before attempting a surgical removal because of patient's debility and comorbidities.

After the failure of initial attempts to do a complete resection, partial piecemeal resection was made with the aim of debulking the lesion to relieve symptomatic gastric outlet obstruction. To limit bleeding, endoloops were deployed at the base of the lesion prior to the start of resection. Because of the location and size of the lesion, only 2 cm by 2 cm of the mass was resected. At the end of the procedure, one of the endoloops remained deployed tightly at the base protecting the margins and limiting blood supply [Figure 3]. The base of the lesion was cut using a needle knife to create shelves

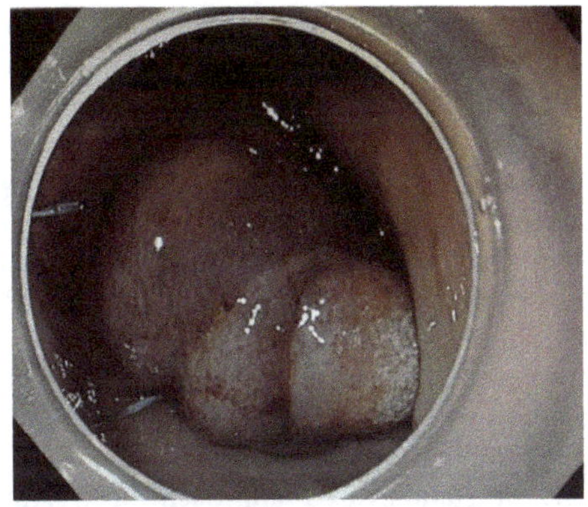

FIGURE 3: Endoscopic image of the mass after deployment of two gastric endoloops at the base.

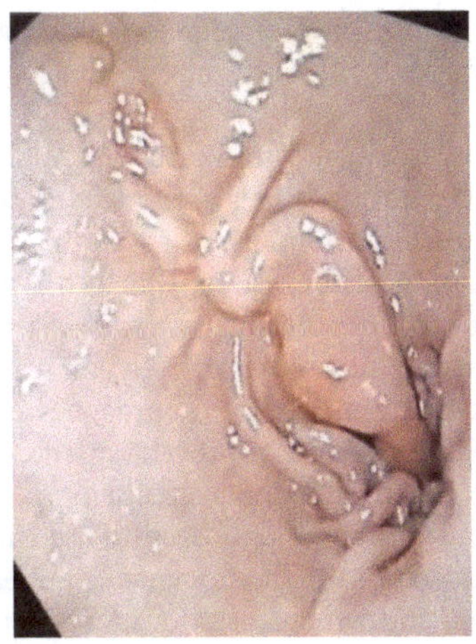

FIGURE 4: Near complete resolution of the mass with minimal scarring and residual tissue at the site on six-week follow-up endoscopy.

for the deployment of endoloops and prevent their slipping. After procedure, patient had good relief of symptoms. The pathology of the excision biopsy that came back positive for fatty tissue confirms the diagnosis of lipoma.

Repeated EGD (Video 2) at four-week interval revealed well-healed scar at the site of the lipoma without ulceration [Figure 4] and the patient at twelve-week follow-up remained asymptomatic.

3. Discussion

Lipomas of GI tract are rare in occurrence (1 in 600). These are the third common benign tumors in GIT after adenomas and hyperplastic polyps. These are intramucosal mesenchymal tumors of mature adipocytes and are often incidental findings on endoscopy or colonoscopy [1]. Lipomas occurring in stomach account only 1-3% of all gastric tumors. These are benign and slow growing lesions and commonly asymptomatic. When symptomatic, they can cause bleeding, abdominal pain, and intestinal intussusception. Gastric lipomas larger than four centimeter in size are more likely to be symptomatic and the common presenting symptoms are that of acute upper GI bleeding and gastric outlet obstruction.

In radiology, a well-defined and homogeneous mass in the stomach wall is suggestive of gastric lipoma. On endoscopic ultrasound, the lesion shows up as a homogeneous hypoechoic lesion. Biopsy is rarely needed for a diagnosis and endoscopic signs such as Cushing sign and tenting sign combined with EUS or CT scan are usually diagnostic.

In addition, because of the submucosal location, routine biopsies are never deep enough to secure tissue to make an accurate diagnosis [2].

Treatment for gastric lipoma is controversial. Because of its rarity, a standardized approach in treating large symptomatic lesions has not yet been established [3]. Generally asymptomatic small lipomas do not need surgical or endoscopic excision. Endoscopic polypectomy can be attempted for lipomas smaller than 3 cm; however larger broad based tumors have higher risk of perforation by endoscopic approach [4]. Surgical excision is resorted to in such cases.

Our patient, because of his cardiovascular risk factors, was not a candidate for surgery. The technique of limiting blood supply to the lesions using an endoloop resulted in complete resolution of the lesion. This technique which has already been used for other benign gastric lesions such as colonic polyps can be used effectively for cases of gastric lipoma as well. Such endoscopic approaches can be a good alternative to surgery and can prevent significant morbidity and mortality. Gastric lipomas are benign mesenchymal tumors of adipocytes commonly seen in the gastric antrum. They are diagnosed by the homogeneous appearance, well-defined borders, and submucosal location in imaging studies. In the rare situations where they cause symptoms, they can cause symptoms of upper gastrointestinal bleed or gastric outlet obstruction. Symptomatic gastric lipoma is a rare occurrence. Because of the rarity, there is no consensus on the treatment in such cases. Majority of cases are managed through surgical resection which can cause significant morbidity. In a systematic review of 32 cases of large gastric lipoma published by Cappell et al. [5] the vast majority of cases still opted for surgical resection of the tumor to endoscopic therapy. The various procedures performed in these cases included submucosal mass excision and enucleation of the lesion. Partial and in rare cases total gastrectomy accompanied these procedures depending on the degree of wall involvement by the tumor. In minority of cases, endoscopic and laparoscopic transgastric resection were performed. These methods cause less morbidity to the patient if successful, however has the risk of causing gastric perforation. Limiting blood supply to the mass using an endoloop applied at the base may lead to spontaneous resolution of the lesion as it was observed in our case. This can be attempted safely to avoid the morbidity of a surgery.

Conflicts of Interest

The authors whose names are listed in the article certify that they have no affiliations with or involvement in any organization or entity with any financial interest (such as honorarium; educational grants; participation in speakers' bureaus; membership, employment, consultancies, stock ownership, or other equity interests; and expert testimony or patent-licensing arrangements) or nonfinancial interest (such as personal or professional relationships, affiliations, knowledge, or beliefs) in the subject matter or materials discussed in this manuscript.

Supplementary Materials

Supplementary 1. Video 1: first endoscopy which shows a large gastric antral mass with friable ulcer at the top. The movement of mass with peristalsis in and out to the duodenum through the gastric outlet can be appreciated, which is leading to the gastric outlet obstruction.

Supplementary 2. Video 2: postprocedure endoscopy at six-week follow-up. There is near complete resolution of the mass with minimal scarring and residual tissue at the site.

References

[1] P. M. Y. Goh and J. E. Lenzi, "Benign tumors of the duodenum and stomach," in *Surgical Treatment: Evidence-Based and Problem-Oriented*, R. G. Holzheimer and J. A. Mannick, Eds., Zuckschwerdt, Munich, Germany, 2001.

[2] H. C. Kang, C. O. Menias, A. H. Gaballah et al., "Beyond the GIST: Mesenchymal tumors of the stomach," *RadioGraphics*, vol. 33, no. 6, pp. 1673–1690, 2013.

[3] R. K. Schmocker and A. O. Lidor, "Management of non-neoplastic gastric lesions," *Surgical Clinics of North America*, vol. 97, no. 2, pp. 387–403, 2017.

[4] S. Nakamura, M. Ida, H. Suekane, T. Mastsui, T. Yao, and M. Fujishima, "Endoscopic removal of gastric lipoma: Diagnostic value of endoscopic examination," *The American Journal of Gastroenterology*, vol. 86, pp. 619–621, 1991.

[5] M. S. Cappell, C. E. Stevens, and M. Amin, "Systematic review of giant gastric lipomas reported since 1980 and report of two new cases in a review of 117110 esophagogastroduodenoscopies," *World Journal of Gastroenterology*, vol. 23, no. 30, pp. 5619–5633, 2017.

22

Drug Induced Liver Injury Attributed to a Curcumin Supplement

Zaid Imam,[1] **Majd Khasawneh**,[1] **Diana Jomaa**,[2] **Hira Iftikhar**,[1] **and Ziad Sayedahmad**[1]

[1]*Departments of Internal Medicine, William Beaumont Hospital, Royal Oak, MI, USA*
[2]*Oakland University William Beaumont School of Medicine, Royal Oak, MI, USA*

Correspondence should be addressed to Zaid Imam; zaid.imam@beaumont.org

Academic Editor: Gregory Kouraklis

More severe reactions, higher acute liver failure rates, and higher recurrence rates on re-challenge occur with supplement-related Drug Induced Liver Injury (DILI) (Medina-Caliz et al., 2018). We report a case of curcumin-induced hepatocellular DILI in a 78-year old female admitted with jaundice, with a one-month latency. Extensive evaluation for alternative etiologies of hepatotoxicity was unremarkable. The Roussel Uclaf Causality Assessment Method (RUCAM) score of 6 for the supplement indicated a probable association (score >8: highly probable association). Peak levels of aspartate aminotransferase (AST) and alanine aminotransferase (ALT) were >20 times upper limit of normal. A 48% decrease in AST and ALT levels was observed 7 days after discontinuation of the supplement, and resolution of transaminitis was observed in 42 days. No re-challenge was performed. In conclusion, this case emphasizes the importance of recognizing curcumin supplements as DILI triggers. Furthermore, it reiterates the need for careful evaluation of herbal and dietary supplements (HDS) consumed by patients to identify potential DILI culprits, and to ultimately prevent DILI reactions with significant morbidity and mortality.

1. Introduction

It is challenging to diagnose DILI by primary care providers and specialists, as numerous alternative etiologies must be first excluded. Population surveys in France and Iceland estimate annual incidence between 14 and 19 per 100,000 inhabitants of DILI [1, 2]. Herbal and dietary supplements (HDS) accounted for 16% of DILI reactions in the Iceland population cohort [2]. In a Spanish DILI registry, HDS-associated DILI reactions had higher rates of acute liver failure than DILI caused by prescription medications and recurrence rates on re-challenge were higher [3].

Curcumin supplements are one of the most consumed herbal supplements in the United States (U.S.) [4] and have shown some promise in the treatment of osteoarthritis [5]. Curcumin is extracted from the plant turmeric (*Curcuma longa*). The content of curcuminoids in turmeric powder is 3.14%, which is used as a spice in cuisines of the Middle East and Indian subcontinent [6]. Much higher amounts of curcumin are present in over the counter supplements. This manuscript presents a case of Grade 3 DILI (severe hepatotoxicity) [7] attributed to a curcumin supplement with complete recovery on discontinuation of the supplement.

2. Case Presentation

A 78-year old Caucasian female with a history of well-controlled type 2 diabetes mellitus, and essential hypertension reported the presence of jaundice and acholic stools for one week. She denied any fever, abdominal pain, pruritus or changes in her bowel habits. She denied any consumption of alcohol as well as the use of any analgesics or antibiotics. She also denied any history of travel outside Michigan, United States of America. Her medications included aspirin (81 mg), citalopram, losartan, metformin, and oxybutynin, all of which she has taken for at least one year. She also took simvastatin for 2 years with no adverse effects but had replaced it a month prior to her presentation with a once daily over the counter curcumin supplement without seeking medical advice.

On physical examination, her blood pressure was 126/65 mmHg, her heart rate 66 beats/min, and her temperature 36.6°C. She appeared in no acute distress and was jaundiced. No hepatosplenomegaly, ascites, asterixis, encephalopathy, or other stigmata of chronic liver disease were noted on physical examination.

Her laboratory results showed a white blood cell count of 5,300 cells/mm^3 with a normal differential, hemoglobin of

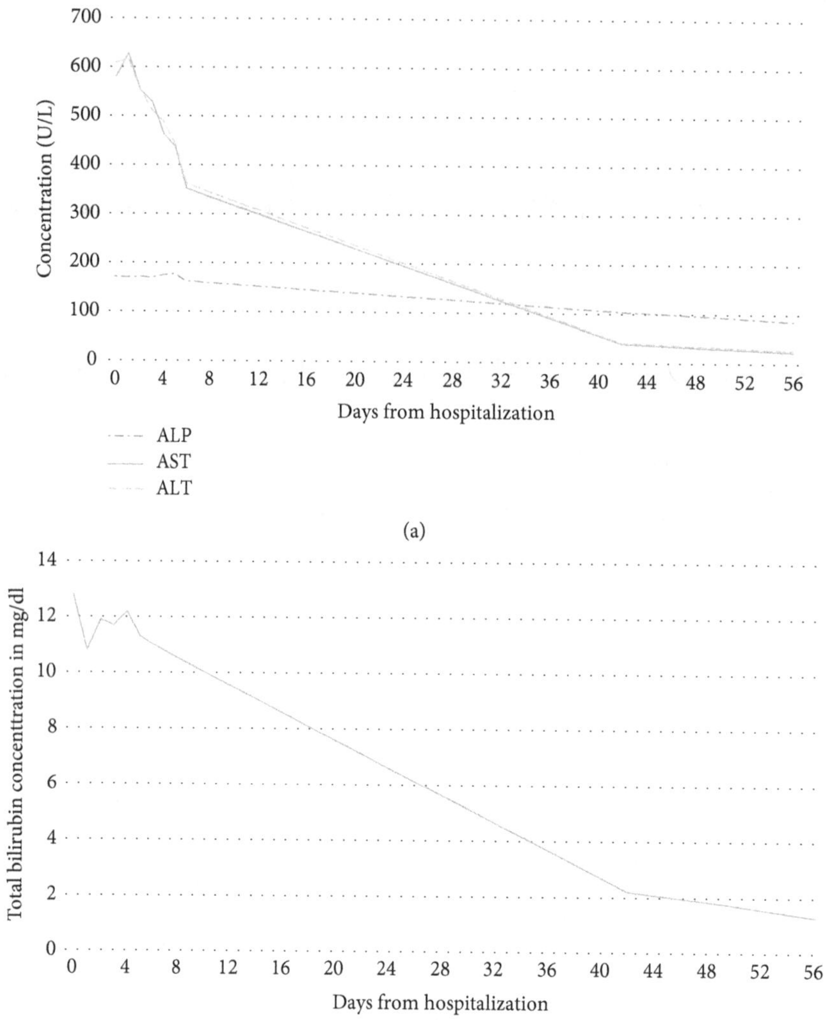

Figure 1: (a) Alkaline phosphatase, aspartate aminotransferase, and alanine aminotransferase levels trend since hospitalization. ALP: Alkaline phosphatase. AST: Aspartate aminotransferase. ALT: Alanine aminotransferase. (b) Total bilirubin levels trend since hospitalization.

12.6 g/dl, platelet count of 282,000 cells/mm^3, blood urea nitrogen of 11 mg/dl, creatinine of 0.59 mg/dl, alkaline phosphatase (ALP) of 171 U/L (lab normal: 33–120 U/L), aspartate aminotransferase (AST) of 581 U/L (lab normal: 0–34 U/L), alanine aminotransferase (ALT) of 609 U/L (lab normal: 9–47 U/L), total bilirubin of 12.8 mg/dl, direct bilirubin of 7.4 mg/dl, international normalized ratio (INR) of 1.1, serum albumin of 4.5 g/dl, and thyroid stimulating hormone (TSH) level of 1.99 mU/L. Liver chemistries from 5-years ago were normal (ALP: 101 U/L, AST 13 U/L, ALT 19 U/L, total bilirubin 0.3 mg/dl). Her R-factor was calculated at 15 consistent with a hepatocellular pattern of liver injury. Hepatitis A, B, C, and cytomegalovirus serologies were negative. Epstein-Barr virus and herpes simplex virus-1 serologies indicated previous exposures. Hepatitis E testing was not obtained given the patient had no exposure to jaundiced individuals, no recent travel history, and lived in a nonendemic country. Serum IgG level was 951 mg/dl (lab normal: 550–1650 mg/dl) with normal subclass levels. Antinuclear antibody (ANA) titers were 1 : 320 with a speckled pattern, and anti-smooth muscle antibody (ASMA) titers were 1 : 20. Anti-LKM (liver-kidney-microsomal) and antimitochondrial antibodies (AMA) were negative. Ferritin level was 689 ng/ml with a transferrin saturation of 32%. An abdominal ultrasound demonstrated a normal hepatic echotexture and incidental cholelithiasis. A magnetic resonance cholangiopancreaticogram (MRCP) revealed no additional findings.

A liver biopsy was planned if no improvement in the patient's liver chemistries was noted. Her liver function tests on day 7 of her admission showed an improvement of >40% in her ALT and AST, and so a biopsy was deferred. The curcumin supplement was discontinued on admission to the hospital, and the remainder of her medications continued except for simvastatin which wasn't restarted. A follow-up visit 42 days from the initial presentation showed complete resolution of her jaundice, and repeat labs showed normalization of her liver enzymes. The patient was instructed to avoid the curcumin supplement and no re-challenge was performed. No immunosuppressive treatments were initiated at any point during her management. The curcumin supplement the patient was taking was reviewed, and the label reported the following ingredients; 500 mg of curcumin; bovine gelatin; less than 2% of silica; and vegetable magnesium stearate. Follow-up liver enzymes two months and at 18 months from presentation remained normal. A trend of the patient's liver chemistries was summarized in Figures 1(a) and 1(b).

3. Discussion

HDS-related DILI is on the rise, with 20% of DILI reactions attributed to HDS in 2010–2012 compared to 7% in 2004–2005 in the U.S. [8]. Herbal product sales continue to rise in the U.S. [4], and while numerous herbs and supplements have been identified as DILI culprits, almost no reports exist on curcumin supplements. This manuscript highlights a case of DILI attributable to a curcumin supplement in a 78-year old female with a latency period of one month.

In the case reported, the patient's R-score was 15 consistent with a hepatocellular pattern of liver injury. DILI is a diagnosis by exclusion, and an extensive evaluation revealed no alternative etiology in our patient. A potential limitation was the lack of hepatitis C virus (HCV) RNA testing, and hepatitis E serologies. Testing for HCV-RNA and hepatitis E is recommended by the European Association for the Study of Liver (EASL) guidelines, particularly when there is no well-established causation between an agent and DILI [9]. Viral hepatitis serologies were negative or suggested previous exposure, the patient had no evidence of shock or hypotension, no evidence of biliary or hepatic pathology on MRCP, no evidence to support hemochromatosis, and autoimmune serologies argued against autoimmune hepatitis as detailed below. Hepatitis E testing was not obtained given the patient had no ill contacts, no recent travel history, and lived in a nonendemic country. The temporal association, and the marked improvement of the liver chemistries with discontinuation of the agent are consistent with the diagnosis of a supplement-induced DILI. An updated Roussel Uclaf Causality Assessment Method (RUCAM) score calculated for the supplement was 6 indicating a probable association (with scores >8 indicating a highly probable category, that is the highest association level on the score) [10].

In numerous reported cases on supplement-induced DILI, the actual supplement is often not identified. In the case reported, the supplement was identified as a supplement produced by a national pharmacy chain, and its label composition was reviewed clarifying the absence of other confounding hepatotoxic ingredients in the supplement. The Food and Drugs Administration (FDA) in the U.S. requests supplement labels to contain information regarding binders, colors, excipients, fillers, flavors, sweeteners, and other active ingredients in supplements. Ideally, a laboratory analysis on the supplement would have helped confirm the absence of inadvertent contaminants.

Lukefahr et al. reported a case of drug induced autoimmune hepatitis attributed to a turmeric containing supplement [11]. In the manuscript discussed, the patient's ANA titer is positive. However, more specific antibodies were unremarkable (ASMA titer $< 1:40$, negative anti-LKM antibodies) and no hypergammaglobulinemia is present. Furthermore, the spontaneous improvement with discontinuation of the supplement, and without any immunosuppressive treatment such as steroids argue against a picture of autoimmune hepatitis.

The pathogenesis of DILI is variable depending on the agent involved and that of herbal and supplement induced liver injury is poorly understood. Mechanisms of hepatotoxicity include; immune mediated; nonimmune; idiosyncratic; and direct hepatotoxicity [12, 13]. The ubiquity of curcumin in various cuisines, the rarity of reported hepatotoxic reactions in the literature, and the absence of convincing evidence for an immune mediated mechanism in the case reported, suggest an idiosyncratic reaction as a possible pathogenetic mechanism for the curcumin-induced DILI. Idiosyncratic reactions are believed to be mediated through the adaptive immune system and involve a complex interaction between predisposing genetic susceptibilities and immune responses [12].

More than two-thirds of patients do not disclose supplement use to their healthcare providers [14]. Numerous factors contribute to this incredibly high percentage including; lack of inquiry by physicians; patients' fears of being judged by their providers; and patients' inaccurate beliefs about the safety of these products [14].

In conclusion, this case illustrates the importance of recognizing curcumin supplements as DILI triggers by healthcare providers. It also reiterates the importance of a detailed evaluation of all over the counter agents and supplements that patients use by primary care providers, hospitalists, and hepatologists to identify potential DILI culprits, and educate patients about the risks involved. Strong relationships of trust between providers and patients, and a nonjudgmental approach to inquiries about complementary medicine use are both essential to allow providers to obtain critical information to prevent inadvertent DILI reactions that can lead to significant morbidity and mortality.

Authors' Contributions

Z.I., M.K., H.I. and D.J. have participated equally in preparing the manuscript. Z.S. has supervised and mentored the efforts of the other study members.

References

[1] C. Sgro, F. Clinard, K. Ouazir et al., "Incidence of drug-induced hepatic injuries: a French population-based study," *Hepatology* vol. 36, no. 2, pp. 451–455, 2002.

[2] E. S. Björnsson, O. M. Bergmann, H. K. Björnsson, R. B. Kvaran, and S. Olafsson, "Incidence, presentation, and outcomes in patients with drug-induced liver injury in the general population of Iceland," *Gastroenterology*, vol. 144, no. 7, pp. 1419–1425, 2013.

[3] I. Medina-Caliz, M. Garcia-Cortes, A. Gonzalez-Jimenez et al., "Herbal and dietary supplement-induced liver injuries in the Spanish DILI registry," *Clinical Gastroenterology and Hepatology*, vol. 16, no. 9, pp. 1495–1502, 2018.

[4] A. Lindstrom, C. Ooyen, M. E. Lynch, M. Blumenthal, and K. Kawa, "Sales of herbal dietary supplements increase by 7.9%

in 2013, marking a decade of rising sales: turmeric supplements climb to top ranking in natural channel," *HerbalGram*, vol. 103, pp. 52–56, 2014.

[5] J. W. Daily, M. Yang, and S. Park, "Efficacy of turmeric extracts and curcumin for alleviating the symptoms of joint arthritis: a systematic review and meta-analysis of randomized clinical trials," *Journal of Medicinal Food*, vol. 19, no. 8, pp. 717–729, 2016.

[6] R. F. Tayyem, D. D. Heath, W. K. Al-Delaimy, and C. L. Rock, "Curcumin content of turmeric and curry powders," *Nutrition and Cancer*, vol. 55, no. 2, pp. 126–131, 2006.

[7] Y.-c. Yu, Y.-m. Mao, C.-w. Chen et al., "CSH guidelines for the diagnosis and treatment of drug-induced liver injury," *Hepatology International*, vol. 11, no. 3, pp. 221–241, 2017.

[8] V. J. Navarro, H. Barnhart, H. L. Bonkovsky et al., "Liver injury from herbals and dietary supplements in the U.S. Drug-Induced Liver Injury Network," *Hepatology*, vol. 60, no. 4, pp. 1399–1408, 2014.

[9] R. J. Andrade, G. P. Aithal, E. S. Björnsson et al., "EASL clinical practice guidelines: drug-induced liver injury," *Journal of Hepatology*, vol. 70, no. 6, pp. 1222–1261, 2019.

[10] G. Danan and R. Teschke, "RUCAM in drug and herb induced liver injury: the update," *International Journal of Molecular Sciences*, vol. 17, no. 1, p. 14, 2016.

[11] A. L. Lukefahr, S. McEvoy, C. Alfafara, and J. L. Funk, "Drug-induced autoimmune hepatitis associated with turmeric dietary supplement use," *BMJ Case Reports*, vol. 2018, 2018.

[12] N. Noureddin and N. Kaplowitz, "Overview of mechanisms of drug-induced liver injury (DILI) and key challenges in DILI research," in *Drug-Induced Liver Toxicity. Methods in Pharmacology and Toxicology*, M. Chen and Y. Will, Eds., pp. 3–18, Humana Press, New York, NY, USA, 2018.

[13] M. P. Holt and C Ju, "Mechanisms of drug-induced liver injury," *AAPS Journal*, vol. 8, no. 1, pp. E48–E54, 2006.

[14] H. Foley, A. Steel, H. Cramer, J. Wardle, and J. Adams, "Disclosure of complementary medicine use to medical providers: a systematic review and meta-analysis," *Scientific Reports*, vol. 9, no. 1, 2019.

23

Delay in Diagnosis of Autoimmune Polyendocrine Syndrome Type 2 as a Consequence of Misinterpretation of Gastrointestinal Symptoms

Maciej Gonciarz,[1] Michał Krogulecki,[1] Dorota Brodowska-Kania,[2] Szczepan Cierniak,[3] and Grzegorz Kamiński[2]

[1]Military Institute of Medicine in Warsaw, Department of Gastroenterology and Internal Medicine, Warsaw, Poland
[2]Military Institute of Medicine in Warsaw, Department of Endocrinology and Radioisotope Therapy, Warsaw, Poland
[3]Military Institute of Medicine in Warsaw, Department of Pathology, Warsaw, Poland

Correspondence should be addressed to Maciej Gonciarz; mgonciarz@wim.mil.pl

Academic Editor: Olga I. Giouleme

Background. Type 2 autoimmune polyendocrine syndrome (APS-2) is characterized by the presence of at least two of three endocrinopathies: Addison's disease, autoimmune thyroiditis, and diabetes type 1. The prevalence of APS-2 is estimated to be 1 : 1000 to 1 : 20.000 in the general population. Diagnosis of APS-2 often is delayed due to its rarity and wide spectrum of clinical symptoms. *Case Presentation.* A 27-year-old presented with a 6-month history of abdominal pain, vomiting, diarrhea, weakness, fatigue, and 15 kg of weight loss. The patient was diagnosed with Crohn's disease in a local hospital and referred to our institution because of treatment failure. Colonoscopy performed in this hospital identified irregular mucosal erosions in terminal ileum, and the microscopy of biopsy specimens demonstrated nonspecific inflammation. On physical examination, the patient appeared cachectic. Blood pressure was 90/60 mmHg. Laboratory results were significant for severe hyponatremia and mild hyperkalemia. Morning cortisol was low, and adrenocorticotropic hormone (ACTH) concentration was high. An ACTH stimulation test did not present any increase in serum cortisol, which confirmed primary adrenal insufficiency. Antithyroid peroxidase antibody (anti-TPO) as well as both anti-21-hydroxylase antibodies and antiglutamic acid decarboxylase antibodies (GAD65) were positive. So, the diagnosis of APS-2 was made, and the replacement doses of hydrocortisone and fludrocortisone has brought a rapid improvement in all clinical symptoms; colonoscopy showed normal. *Conclusion.* The case presented herein highlights rapidly progressive nature of untreated APS-2 and that the diagnosis of APS-2 may be challenging.

1. Background

Autoimmune polyendocrine syndromes (APSs) also named polyglandular deficiency syndromes are rare disorders characterized by functional impairment of multiple endocrine glands due to loss of immune [1]. Three different clinical presentations can be distinguished:

(a) A very rare monogenic autoimmune polyendocrine syndrome type 1 (APS-1) that affects approximately 1 in 80 000 individuals in the general population. It is juvenile type inherited in an autosomal recessive manner and defined by the presence of 2 or more of the following: chronic mucocutaneous candidiasis, hypoparathyroidism, and adrenal insufficiency. Symptoms usually occur in young patients; however, other endocrine and nonendocrine disorders may appear until the age of 40 [1].

(b) A more common polygenic variety, autoimmune polyendocrine syndrome type 2 (APS-2) or Schmidt's syndrome named after Schmidt who originally described 2 cases of Addison disease and chronic lymphocytic thyroiditis in 1926 [2]. According to recent epidemiological data, the prevalence of APS-2 is estimated to be 1 : 1000 to 1 : 20000 in the general population [1]. APS-2 consists of Addison's disease, autoimmune thyroiditis, and/or diabetes type 1. At least two of these endocrinopathies are of diagnostic value. The complete triad of Addison's disease, autoimmune thyroiditis, and type 1 diabetes is termed Carpenter's syndrome [3]. APS-2 usually occurs in adults and more often affects women. It may occur alone or in association with other autoimmune disorders such as celiac disease, alopecia, vitiligo, premature ovarian insufficiency, pernicious anemia, and others [1].

(c) Type 3 autoimmune polyendocrine syndrome (APS-3) includes autoimmune thyroiditis and other autoimmune diseases except for Addison's disease [4].

A careful management of specific disorders can prevent complications; however, because of the wide spectrum of clinical symptoms of APS and its rarity, the diagnosis often is delayed for months resulting in errors in patient management.

2. Case Report

In June 2019, a 27-year-old patient was admitted to our department due to abdominal pain, vomiting, diarrhea, weakness, fatigue, and 15 kg of weight loss, all of 6 month's duration. In November 2018, when he began to experience a weakness and fatigue, complained of abdominal pain, and multiple loose nonbloody bowel movements per day, he was referred to a tertiary hospital's outpatient department. Basic laboratory testing revealed only slight hyponatremia. Other laboratory tests such as antibodies, tissue transglutaminase IgA (tTG-IgA), *Saccharomyces cerevisiae* (ASCA), and perinuclear antineutrophil (pANCA) antibodies were all negative. Stool samples for parasites, clostridium difficile toxins, occult blood, and calprotectin were also negative. There were no significant deviations from the normal state in the chest X-ray, ultrasound, and upper gastrointestinal endoscopy examinations. The colonoscopy identified irregular mucosal erosions in terminal ileum, and the microscopy of multiple biopsy specimens demonstrated nonspecific inflammation. Though the histopathological reassessment revealed heavy infiltration by extremely large quantities of lymphocytes and plasma cells (transmural inflammation) (Figure 1), a diagnosis of Crohn disease was also made. The patient was managed with budesonide 9 mg/day and mesalamine at a dose of 2.0 g/day. After two months, due to a result of treatment failure, azathioprine 100 mg/day was initiated. However, his bowel symptoms did not improve, while weakness and fatigue gradually aggravated, and the patient lost 15 kilograms of his weight. At this point, he was referred to our institution for further management.

His personal and family history was unremarkable, while only Hashimoto disease was recognized in the patient's mother and sister. On physical examination, the patient

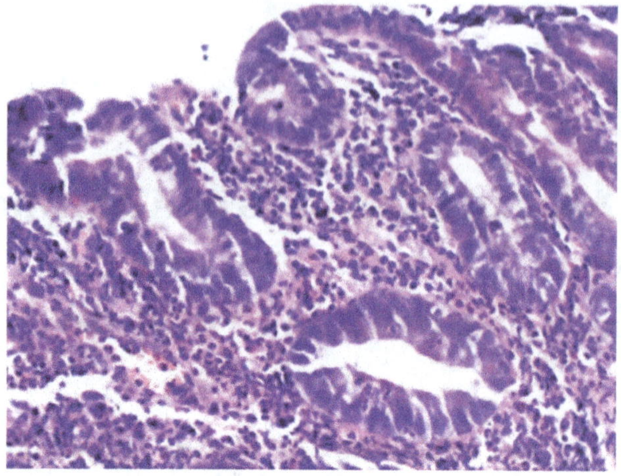

Figure 1: Ileum: the tissues are heavily infiltrated by extremely large quantities of inflammatory cells (transmural inflammation, lymphocytes and plasma cells). Hematoxylin-eosin, original magnification x 400.

appeared cachectic (56 kg, 165 cm), his epigastrium was tender, and the palms were with slightly increased pigmentation. Blood pressure was 90/60 mmHg, and heart rate was 100 beats/min. Otherwise, the physical examination was unremarkable. An ultrasound study of the abdomen and MR enterography were normal.

Laboratory results were significant for severe hyponatremia-sodium 119 mmol/l (reference: 135–145 mmol/l) and mild hyperkalemia-potassium 5.5 mmol/l (reference: 3.5–5.0 mmol/l). Laboratory tests showed the following results: the chloride concentration: 84 mmol/l (reference: 95–106 mmol/l), pH: 7.353, HCO_3^-: 21.3 mmol/l (reference: 22–29 mmol/l), and glucose: 4.38 mmol/l (reference: 3.9–5.5 mmol/l). Other biochemical tests including blood count, creatinine, and urea revealed no abnormalities. A morning cortisol was low at 6.63 μg/dl (reference: >10 μg/dl), and adrenocorticotropic hormone (ACTH) concentration was high at 1662 pmol/l (normal: 7.2–63.3 pmol/l). An ACTH stimulation test (short Synacthen (tetracosactide—a peptide representing the sequence of the first 24 (out of a total of 39)) amino acids of ACTH) did not present any increase in serum cortisol, which confirmed primary adrenal insufficiency. The tuberculin test and interferon-gamma release assay (IGRA) were negative. Dynamic contrast-enhanced magnetic resonance of the pituitary gland showed normal. We did not observe any other laboratory abnormalities (ANA, SM, ANCA, anti-LKM1, anti tGT-IgA, fT3, fT4, TSH, anti-TPO, ICA, IAA, and ICSA).

Antiglutamic acid decarboxylase antibodies (GAD65) were positive in titer of 158.1 IU/ml (positive ≥10 IU/ml). Given those findings, the diagnosis of autoimmune polyglandular syndrome type 2 was made, and the patient was started with replacement doses of hydrocortisone (35 mg per day) and fludrocortisone (0.1 mg per day). A week 12 colonoscopy and multiple colonic biopsies showed no abnormalities. At the 24-week follow-up, no signs of hypocortisolemia were present. In the 75 mg oral glucose tolerance test (OGTT), there were normal glucose concentration before (5.27 mmol/l) and after 120 min

(4.67 mmol/l), with signs of insulin resistance (inulin concentration too high, 51.8 μU/ml, after 2 hours in OGGT). This points to a risk of developing type 1 diabetes. Thyroid function remains normal with TSH 1.39 uUI/ml, fT4: 21.8 pmol/l (range: 10.3–30.9 pmol/l), and fT3: 5.38 pmol/l (range: 2.25–6.0 pmol/l). Sex hormone concentration remains within normal range, with testosterone concentration of 4.11 ng/ml (range: 2.8–8.2 ng/ml), FSH: 10.74 IU/l (range: 1.5–12.4 IU/l), and LH: 4.62 IU/ml (range: 1.7–8.6 IU/ml). Serum ACTH concentration is only 2.5 times increased, 163.6 pmol/ml, with normal sodium (Na, 135 mmol/l) and potassium (K, 4.2 mmol/l) concentration, what proves a good correction of hypocortisolemia in this case.

3. Discussion

This case highlights the nonspecific, varied presentation, and rapidly progressive nature of untreated APS-2. Immediate diagnosis and appropriate management are essential for a good outcome. The clinical presentation of APS type 2 includes a wide range of severity, from mild to seriously impaired patients. In our case, the degree of clinical symptoms could be placed in the high range. Symptoms can often be difficult to distinguish from gastroenterological etiologies, resulting in inaccurate diagnosis. In our case, the diagnosis of Crohn's disease made prior to admission was misleading. CRP and stool calprotectin were normal, and histology of ileal lesions showed no crypt distortion, cryptitis, crypt abscess, or granuloma. Misdiagnosis resulted in errors in patient management. The patient treated with mesalamine, budesonide, and azathioprine continued to be symptomatic, while the colonoscopy performed three months later with bare replacement doses of hydrocortisone showed no abnormalities.

The first clinical case showing difficulties of different diagnosis, Addison's and Crohn's disease, was described in 1958 [5]. All patients have gastrointestinal symptoms in Addison's disease. Usually, diagnosis is made with a delayed average at 6 months. The effect of this delay is an adrenal crisis, which it was in this case. A common feature of Addison's disease and Crohn's disease is progressive cachexia, anorexia, weight loss, vomiting, diarrhea, abdominal pain, depression, arthritis symptoms, and response to oral corticosteroids [6]. In Addison's disease, the most typical symptoms are hyperpigmentation, postural drop, muscle weakness, sex hormone, and electrolyte disturbances (hyponatremia and hyperkaliemia).

Our patient did not suffer from type 1 diabetes, but an antibody against GAD 65 for type 1 diabetes was positive with titers of 158.1 IU/ml. Other antibodies typical for type 1 diabetes were not detected. The presence of anti-TPO antibodies with a typical ultrasound image of the thyroid gland allows for an autoimmune thyroiditis diagnosis. However, the major clinical problem was severe hypoadrenocorticism associated with type 21-hydroxylase antibodies. Primary adrenal insufficiency, Addison's disease, is a life-threatening condition, so the early diagnosis and glucocorticoid therapy are crucial. In the case presented here, the delay in accurate diagnosis was about 6 months. The progressing autoimmune process resulted in adrenal crisis (hyponatremia, hyperkaliemia, hypotension, and hypoglycemia). Berkelhammer et al. [7] described a rare case of severe adrenal insufficiency complicating budesonide maintenance therapy for Crohn' disease. The authors cite the results of 11 studies which showed that patients with Crohn's disease on budesonide for maintenance of remission showed abnormal ACTH stimulation tests nearly three times more frequent than those of control groups. Our patient was on budesonide for several months before admission; thus, it could play an additional role in his adrenal dysfunction.

In this case, the coincidence of Addison's disease with autoimmune thyroiditis allowed for the diagnosis of the APS type 2 (Schmidt's syndrome). If diabetes appears, Carpenter's syndrome will be eligible [5, 6].

References

[1] E. S. Husebye, M. S. Anderson, and O. Kämpe, "Autoimmune polyendocrine syndromes," *New England Journal of Medicine*, vol. 378, no. 12, pp. 1132–1141, 2018.

[2] M. Schmidt, "Eine biglandulare Erkrankung (Nebennieren und Schilddrüse) bei Morbus Adisonii," *Verhandlungen der Deutschen Gesellschaft für Pathologie*, vol. 21, pp. 212–221, 1926.

[3] C. Betterle, F. Lazzarotto, and F. Presotto, "Autoimmune polyglandular syndrome Type 2: the tip of an iceberg?" *Clinical and Experimental Immunology*, vol. 137, no. 2, pp. 225–233, 2004.

[4] C. Betterle, S. Garelli, G. Coco, P. Burra, and P. Burra, "A rare combination of type 3 autoimmune polyendocrine syndrome (APS-3) or multiple autoimmune syndrome (MAS-3)," *Autoimmunity Highlights*, vol. 5, no. 1, pp. 27–31, 2014.

[5] F. T. Prunty, "Crohn's disease with features suggesting Addison's disease," *Proceedings of the Royal Society of Medicine*, vol. 51, pp. 719-720, 1958.

[6] P. Hall, "If it walks like Crohn's and talks like Crohn's, it must be," *BMJ Case Reports*, 2013.

[7] C. Berkelhammer, M. Trabolsi, J. Andrejic, and T. Yasmeen, "Severe adrenal insufficiency complicating budesonide therapy for Crohn's disease," *Inflammatory Bowel Diseases*, vol. 17, no. 4, pp. 1053-1054, 2011.

24

Endoscopic Repair of Gastrocolic and Colocutaneous Fistulas Complicating Percutaneous Endoscopic Gastrostomy Tube

Chukwunonso Chime, Ahmed Baiomi, Kishore Kumar, Harish Patel, Anil Dev, and Jasbir Makker

Department of Gastroenterology, Bronx Care Health Systems–Affiliate of Mount Sinai Hospital Systems, Bronx, NY 10457, USA

Correspondence should be addressed to Chukwunonso Chime; cchime@bronxleb.org

Academic Editor: Daniel C. Damin

Percutaneous endoscopic gastrostomy (PEG) tube feeding has become one of the options for supplemental feeding in a selected group of patients. It is a generally safe procedure usually undertaken by a gastroenterologist or a surgeon in most cases but with over 200,000 tubes being placed yearly, there is bound to be complications. Some of the encountered complications include bleeding, site infection, tube migration, and inadvertent creation of fistula. We present our index patient admitted from a long-term care facility for feculent vomiting and fecal material through the PEG tube. Imaging and colonoscopy confirmed the presence of both a gastrocolic and a colocutaneous fistula, both closed endoscopically with an over-the-scope and through-the-scope clips, respectively. Feeding through a nasogastric tube was resumed after 48 hours, and by the second week of admission, the patient was discharged back to the facility after placement of a new PEG tube.

1. Introduction

The use of a percutaneous endoscopic gastrostomy (PEG) tube for the maintenance of nutritional needs has gained increasing popularity since it was introduced in 1980s [1]. Compared to surgical gastrostomy tubes, PEG tubes have become the preferred method of gaining enteral access in patients that need feeding for a prolonged period [2]. There are still concerns for complications resulting from this route of enteral access. Complications, though rare, include bleeding, infection, inadvertent perforation of the bowel, and aspiration [3]. We present a case of an elderly male patient who had a PEG tube placed for long-term feeding, presented to our hospital with complaint of feculent vomiting and was noted to have a gastrocolic and a colocutaneous fistula, both repaired endoscopically.

2. Case Report

A 64-year-old male ventilator-dependent patient presented to the emergency department (ED) from a nursing home after he was noted with feculent emesis and fecal effluent from his gastrostomy tube. Two months earlier, the patient had a cardiac arrest in another hospital, resulting in anoxic brain injury. He required percutaneous endoscopic gastrostomy (PEG) tube insertion with tracheostomy prior to discharge to the nursing home. His other medical comorbidities were diabetes mellitus, chronic obstructive pulmonary disease, and right lower extremity deep vein thrombosis. In the ED, his vital signs were within normal limits. On physical examination, he was nonverbal and ventilator dependent through the tracheostomy tube with feculent material noted on PEG tube aspiration and rest of the examination was unremarkable. Laboratory investigations revealed hemoglobin of 9.1 g/dL, leukocyte count of 8.9 K cells/μL with neutrophil predominance, and platelet count of 619 K cells/μL.

He had a computed tomography (CT) scan done with oral contrast in the ED, and it showed a gastrostomy tube that appeared to be in the transverse colon (see Figure 1). On admission, he had an upper endoscopy showing feculent material in the stomach with evidence of a fistulous opening

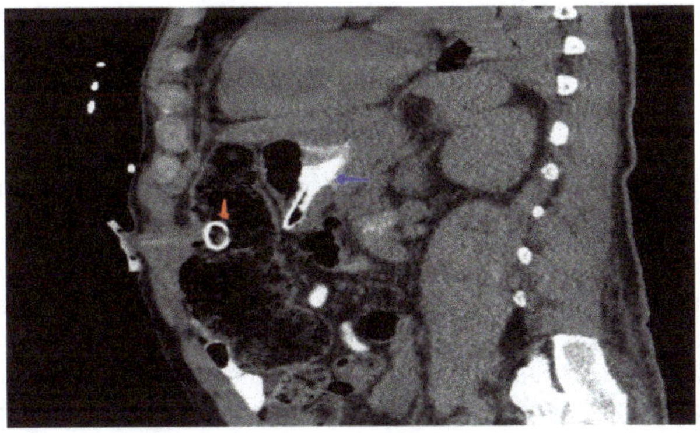

FIGURE 1: PEG tube in the transverse colon (red pointer) and contrast in the stomach (blue pointer) tracking through the fistula.

suspected to be in communication with the colon. The diameter was determined to be less than 10 mm, and this was repaired with an over-the-scope clip (OTSC) (see Figures 2 and 3). He also had a colonoscopy that revealed an internal bumper of the PEG tube located in the transverse colon, and this was cut externally at skin level and retrieved with a Roth net. The colocutaneous fistula could not be repaired with an OTSC as the location in the transverse colon could not be reached with a gastroscope, and this was subsequently repaired with through the scope clips using a pediatric colonoscope (see Figures 4 and 5). The success of the procedures was ascertained by adequate insufflation of the stomach and colon without air leak. Enteral feeding was resumed after 48 hours using a nasogastric tube access.

The patient was subsequently treated with antibiotics for a few days and had an unremarkable hospital course; 10 days after the repair of the fistulas, he had another PEG tube placed before being discharged back to the nursing home.

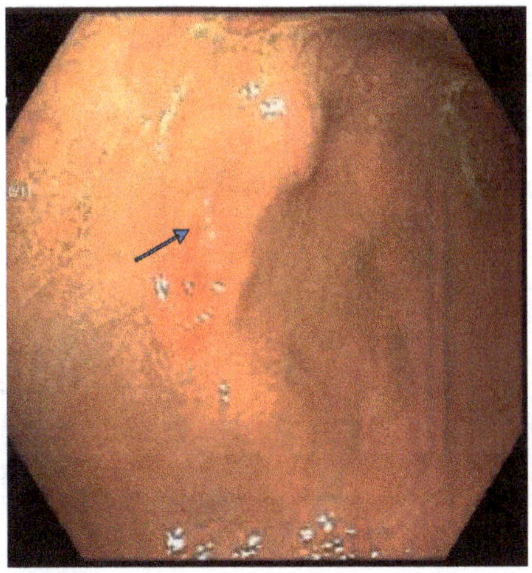

FIGURE 2: Gastrocolic fistula (blue arrow).

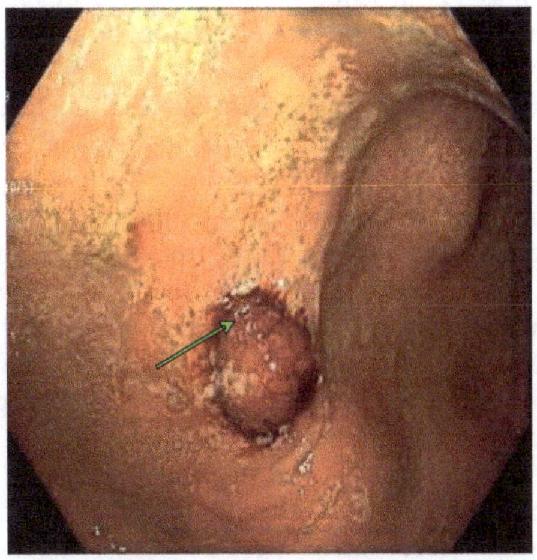

FIGURE 3: After over-the-scope repair (green arrow).

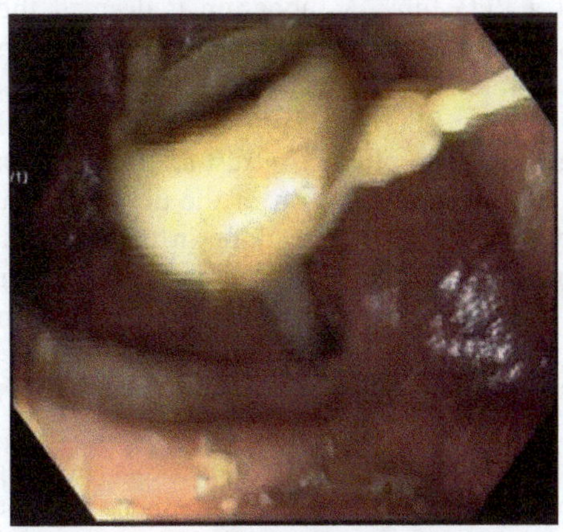

FIGURE 4: PEG tube internal bumper in the colon.

3. Discussion

Many patients with a spectrum of chronic medical illnesses and who are unable to meet their caloric needs through oral feeding require alternative means of achieving adequate nutrition through the enteral route. Nasogastric tubes can aid in creating access for nutrition with a drawback that they are short term, may cause irritation, bleeding, infection of nose, and throat, and may require the need to replace them when they dislodge. There was a need to create better long-term access, and PEG tubes have become a safe and effective means to achieve this need [4], with over 216,000 PEG tubes placed in the United States annually [5]. In general, there are two methods of PEG tube insertion and these utilize either the pull or push technique, resulting in the passage of a plastic tube through the skin to the stomach, anchored with an internal and external bumper. After placement of a PEG tube, a tract is usually formed from the skin, through subcutaneous tissue to the stomach. This tract begins to mature in 7 to 10 days, though in certain situations like immunosuppression or malnourishment, it may take longer [3].

Complications can be evident in the first few days due to lack of maturity of the PEG tract [1]. The incidence rate for major complications in adults after PEG tube placement has been reported to be 3% in one of the series [6]. These complications include bleeding, PEG site infection, dislodgement, aspiration, bowel trauma, and fistulous tracts [3, 7]. One of the major complications that could be

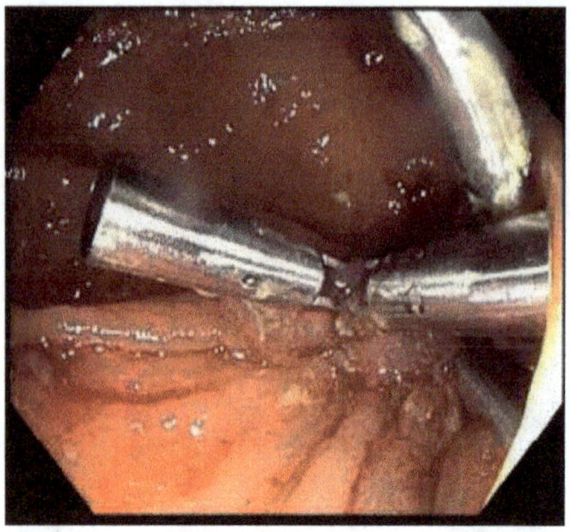

Figure 5: Repair of colocutaneous fistula.

encountered after PEG tube placement is formation of a false tract, such as a gastrocolic and/or colocutaneous fistula [8], as was the case with our patient. This is usually thought to result from juxtaposition of the colon between the stomach and the skin during the PEG insertion, resulting in a feeding tube passing through the colon, usually the transverse colon, before being anchored in the stomach [9]. Adequate air insufflation of the stomach can help prevent this complication by displacing the colon away from the path of the PEG tube [5]. Also, a two-step process that involves transillumination and finger indentation can help verify proper apposition of the abdominal wall with the gastric wall [10].

Suspicion for dislodged PEG with a resulting fistula should arise in patients with feculent vomiting or feculent material through the PEG as was the case in our patient. Recurrent postprandial diarrhea, though not present in our case, can also occur when the PEG tube is in the colon, resulting from direct feeding of the isotonic formula and has been described in literature [9]. Various modalities have been used to diagnose and delineate suspected misplacements of a PEG tube. A tubogram is deemed the test of choice as compared to colonoscopy or other imaging studies [11]. Caution should be exercised given the risk of contrast peritonitis if the PEG is in communication with the peritoneal cavity, water soluble contrast are therefore preferred [9]. In our case, the suspicion of the diagnosis was entertained by the initial CT scan done in the ED and confirmation made with an upper endoscopy demonstrating fecal material entering the stomach through a fistula and colonoscopy showing a PEG tube with internal bumper in the transverse colon, which could easily be mobilized through the colocutaneous fistula.

The management of an iatrogenic fistula resulting from a PEG tube would depend on the presence or absence of peritonitis, with the latter being managed successfully through a nonsurgical approach [12]. A conservative approach can be pursued with the drawback that it would take days or weeks for the fistula to heal, resulting in delays with reintroduction of feeding and increased hospital length of stay [13]. Attempts at endoscopic repair of the iatrogenic fistula resulting from a malpositioned PEG tube have been reported in the literature. Nici et al. reported closure of the gastrocolic fistula in a patient with partial colectomy for acute diverticulitis, using the scope resolution clips aided by fluoroscopy [14]. Our patient had repair of the 10 mm gastrocolic fistula with an over-the-scope padlock clip (US Endoscopy), while the colocutaneous fistula was closed with resolution clips (Boston Scientific). The colocutaneous fistula could not be repaired with an OTSC as the location in the transverse colon could not be reached with a gastroscope, and this was subsequently repaired with through the scope clips using a pediatric colonoscope. There are also limits to repair of these fistulas that can be extrapolated from a study by Matthes et al. They showed in animal studies that a single OTSC can be used to close defects in the stomach ranging from 5 to 20 mm and from 10 to 30 mm in the colon [15]. Other nonsurgical modalities that can be used to repair these fistulas include but not limited to endoloops, sutures, stents, injectables, and coagulants.

Closure of both fistulas was confirmed by air insufflation, and the patient tolerated the procedures with no further complications. This nonsurgical endoscopic repair enabled resumption of enteral feeding through the nasogastric tube 48 hours after procedure. The rest of his hospital course was uneventful, and 10 days later, he had another PEG tube placed at a different location. He was subsequently discharged back to a long-term care facility with no further concerns with the feeding tube during a seven-month follow-up.

4. Conclusion

With increasing use of the PEG tube for nutritional support in clinical setting, care should be taken to adhere to strict aseptic measures and other risk mitigating strategies that would help to reduce the chance of complications. Some of the encountered complications include but not limited to bleeding, infection, and iatrogenic fistula like a gastrocolic and colocutaneous as was the case in our index patient. The latter occurring especially when care is not taken to ensure that the colon is not juxtaposed between the stomach and abdominal wall. Nonsurgical repair is an option in patients without peritonitis and can be achieved with the use of over-the-scope and through-the-scope clips, aiding timely return to enteral feeding and subsequent discharge to home or to long-term care facilities.

Authors' Contributions

All authors have reviewed the literature and contributed to manuscript drafting. Chukwunonso Chime, Ahmed Baiomi, and Kishore Kumar were responsible for the revision of the manuscript for important intellectual content. Harish Patel, Jasbir Makker, and Anil Dev have critically reviewed the manuscript and figures. All authors issued final approval for the version to be submitted.

References

[1] M. R. Taheri, H. Singh, and D. R. Duerksen, "Peritonitis after gastrostomy tube replacement," *Journal of Parenteral and Enteral Nutrition*, vol. 35, no. 1, pp. 56–60, 2011.

[2] K. M. Dwyer, D. D. Watts, J. S. Thurber, R. S. Benoit, and S. M. Fakhry, "Percutaneous endoscopic gastrostomy: the preferred method of elective feeding tube placement in trauma patients," *Journal of Trauma and Acute Care Surgery*, vol. 52, no. 1, pp. 26–32, 2002.

[3] S. P. Schrag, R. Sharma, N. P. Jaik et al., "Complications related to percutaneous endoscopic gastrostomy (PEG) tubes. A comprehensive clinical review," *Journal of Gastrointestinal and Liver Diseases*, vol. 16, no. 4, pp. 407–418, 2007.

[4] J. J. Mamel, "Percutaneous endoscopic gastrostomy," *The American Journal of Gastroenterology*, vol. 84, no. 7, pp. 703–710, 1989.

[5] M. W. L. Gauderer, "Percutaneous endoscopic gastrostomy-20 years later: a historical perspective," *Journal of Pediatric Surgery*, vol. 36, no. 1, pp. 217–219, 2001.

[6] S. A. McClave and R. L. Neff, "Care and long-term maintenance of percutaneous endoscopic gastrostomy tubes," *Journal of Parenteral and Enteral Nutrition*, vol. 30, no. 1_suppl, pp. S27–S38, 2006.

[7] T. Sasaki, D. Fukumori, K. Sakai, M. Sato, H. Ohmori, and F. Yamamoto, "The safety and feasibility of percutaneous endoscopic gastrostomy placement," *Hepatogastroenterology*, vol. 51, no. 58, pp. 1062–1065, 2004.

[8] Y. Kinoshita, H. Udagawa, Y. Kajiyama et al., "Cologastric fistula and colonic perforation as a complication of percutaneous endoscopic gastrostomy," *Surgical Laparoscopy, Endoscopy & Percutaneous Techniques*, vol. 9, no. 3, pp. 220–222, 1999.

[9] G.-S. Lohiya, L. Tan-Figueroa, and V. Krishna, "Intermittent diarrhea as a delayed presentation of percutaneous endoscopic gastrostomy (PEG)-associated fistula," *The Journal of the American Board of Family Medicine*, vol. 23, no. 5, pp. 681–684, 2010.

[10] R. Friedmann, H. Feldman, and M. Sonnenblick, "Misplacement of percutaneously inserted gastrostomy tube into the colon: report of 6 cases and review of the literature," *Journal of Parenteral and Enteral Nutrition*, vol. 31, no. 6, pp. 469–476, 2007.

[11] R. Guloglu, K. Taviloglu, and O. Alimoglu, "Colon injury following percutaneous endoscopic gastrostomy tube insertion," *Journal of Laparoendoscopic & Advanced Surgical Techniques*, vol. 13, no. 1, pp. 69–72, 2003.

[12] C. Kilmartin, G. L. Brotzman, and P. Regan, "Colocutaneous fistula as a complication of PEG tube placement," *The Journal of Family Practice*, vol. 43, no. 1, pp. 76–78, 1996.

[13] H. S. Kim, D. K. Lee, S. K. Baik, and S. O. Kwon, "Endoscopic management of colocutaneous fistula after percutaneous endoscopic gastrostomy," *Endoscopy*, vol. 34, no. 5, p. 430, 2002.

[14] A. Nici, S. Hussain, M. Rubin, and S. Kim, "Repair of a gastrocolic fistula using a wire-guided, simultaneous dual scope approach," *Endoscopy*, vol. 45, no. S 02, pp. E307–E308, 2013.

[15] K. Matthes, Y. Jung, M. Kato, M. A. Gromski, and R. Chuttani, "Efficacy of full-thickness GI perforation closure with a novel over-the-scope clip application device: an animal study," *Gastrointestinal Endoscopy*, vol. 74, no. 6, pp. 1369–1375, 2011.

Menotrophin Induced Autoimmune Hepatitis

Shurouq H. Alqrinawi,[1] Nuralhuda Akbar,[2] Hind AlFaddag,[2] Shahrazad Akbar,[3] Lujayn Akbar,[3] Sohail A. Butt,[4] and Mohammed Aljawad[1]

[1]*Multiorgan Transplant Unit, King Fahd Specialist Hospital, Dammam, Saudi Arabia*
[2]*Department of Medicine, Dammam Medical Complex, Dammam, Saudi Arabia*
[3]*Department of Medicine, King Fahd Hospital of the University, Khobar, Saudi Arabia*
[4]*Blood Bank, Dammam Regional Laboratory, Dammam, Saudi Arabia*

Correspondence should be addressed to Mohammed Aljawad; mshj2013@hotmail.com

Academic Editor: Olga I. Giouleme

Menotrophin is a protein-based hormonal therapy. It is used as a fertility medication that is given as injection either subcutaneously or intramuscularly. Menotrophin has not been previously reported to cause drug-induced liver injury. Drug-induced liver injury (DILI) is commonly seen nowadays with the expansion of the drug industry. It is associated with prescribed medications, over the counter drugs, herbal and dietary supplements. We report the first case of Menotrophin-induced autoimmune hepatitis in a 26-year-old Caucasian woman who was diagnosed with primary infertility due to failure to conceive after five years of marriage. She had received several cycles of Menotrophin, then developed new onset jaundice and fatigue associated with increase in transaminases. She had normal baseline liver function and enzymes prior to receiving treatment with Menotrophin. Evaluation showed no evidence of viral hepatitis, metabolic, alcoholic or vascular causes of liver injury. Autoimmune screening was positive for antinuclear antibody (ANA) with titer of 1:640 fine speckled, immunoglobulin G (IgG) level was 1900 mg/dl. Antimitochondrial antibodies (AMA) and antismooth muscle antibodies were negative. Liver biopsy showed features of chronic hepatitis with interface hepatitis and prominence of plasma cells, which best reflects autoimmune hepatitis. Her liver enzymes and bilirubin completely normalized after discontinuation of further Menotrophin therapy and starting treatment with prednisolone and Azathioprine.

1. Introduction

Menotrophin is a female infertility gonadotropin treatment contains follicle stimulating hormone (FSH) and luteinizing hormone (LH) purified from the urine of postmenopausal women. It binds to the follicle stimulating hormone receptor (FSH), which results in ovulation in the absence of sufficient endogenous luteinizing hormone (LH). It also binds the LH receptor, thereby stimulating proper hormone release. Menotrophin is known to cause minor gastrointestinal symptoms such as abdominal pain, nausea, vomiting, and other unspecific symptoms. No other drugs or food interaction was found.

We here present first case of drug-induced autoimmune hepatitis (DIAIH) following treatment with Menotrophin requiring immunosuppressive therapy that has hitherto not been described to best of our knowledge.

The causality of autoimmune hepatitis (AIH) is uncertain, but the disease can be triggered in some patients by external factors such as viruses or drugs. DIAIH can mimic many liver diseases, and its effect can range from a mild elevation of liver enzymes to liver failure.

Many drugs have been linked to cause AIH, which sometimes persist after drug discontinuation, suggesting that they awaken latent autoimmunity. Drug-Induced Autoimmune hepatitis (DIAIH) is still a poorly defined and an under-reported liver disorder. Histologically distinguishing DILI from AIH remains a challenge.

2. Case Presentation

A 26-year-old Caucasian lady was diagnosed with primary infertility after failure to conceive despite ongoing attempts over five years. The patient received four cycles of treatment with Menotrophin within the last four years with approximate interval of 12 months in between cycles. Each cycle consisted of five doses of Menotrophin given as intramuscular injection every other day. One month after the last cycle, the patient started to develop yellowish discoloration of sclera and skin associated with pruritus, which was gradual and progressive with time. She also developed pale stool, and dark urine. There was no history of vomiting, nausea, abdominal pain, change in bowel habit, or weight loss. She had No history of alcohol consumption, and denied using recreational drug, other prescription or nonprescription drugs or herbal supplement. The patient is not known to have any prior medical conditions and no known autoimmune disorders.

On examination, vital signs were within normal limits. Despite being deeply jaundiced, she had normal level of consciousness and had no stigmata of chronic liver disease and negative abdominal finding. She had baseline investigations prior to starting Menotrophin that showed normal liver enzymes and liver synthetic functions. Her laboratory tests during this presentation showed Aspartate aminotransferase 590 U/L, Alanine aminotransferase 504 U/L, Total Bilirubin17.81 mg/dl, Gamma-glutamyl transferase 486 U/L, Direct Bilirubin 13.16 mg/dl, albumin 2.4 g/dl, alkaline phosphatase 366 U/L, International normalized ratio 1.3, Hemoglobin 11 g/dl, total white blood cells 9.25×10^9/L, platelets count 188×10^9/L. Further workup revealed immunoglobulin G (IgG) level 1900, B2 glycoprotein (IgG) 42.4 EU/ml, ANA 1:640 fine speckled.

AMA, antismooth muscle antibodies (ASMA), B2 glycoprotein (IgM), proteinase 3 antibodies (PR3), liver Kidney Microsomal antibodies (LKM), hepatitis B and C as well as EBV and CMV serology were all negative.

Liver ultrasonography showed coarse echotexture with lobulated surface and enlarged caudate lobe, no portal vein thrombosis, normal biliary, no stones. Unfortunately, there is no previous baseline liver ultrasound for comparison.

Liver biopsy revealed portal fibrosis with expansion and formation of portal-portal and portal-central bridging fibrosis. Marked mostly lymphocytic infiltrate containing plasma cells and occasional polymorphs & esosinophils were seen in portal tract, extending focally into the lobules with moderate interface & lobular hepatitis. No obvious hepatocyte rosette formation, though a few necrotic hepatocytes were present. The bile duct revealed focal injury through infiltration by polymorphs and lymphoid cells. The features of liver biopsy suggested chronic active hepatitis with interface hepatitis and prominence of plasma cells stage 3 (Figures 1, 2, 3(a) and 3(b)).

The diagnosis of autoimmune hepatitis was based on Simplified diagnostic criteria of International Autoimmune hepatitis Group with a score of 7 points, which make her case fall in the category of definite autoimmune hepatitis [1]. After establishing the diagnosis of AIH, she was started on prednisolone and Azathioprine. Her liver enzymes and synthetic function improved with time and then normalized after 4 weeks of treatment (Table 1). Her prednisolone was tapered down until complete discontinuation and maintained on Azathioprine monotherapy.

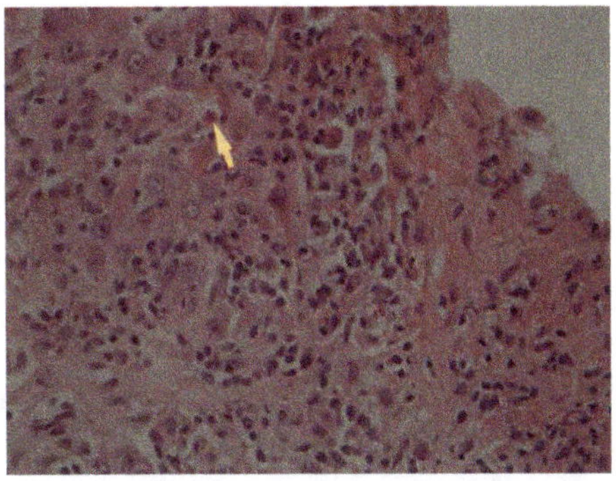

FIGURE 1: Liver biopsy showing Interface hepatitis revealing spillover of inflammation into adjacent liver parenchyma and necrotic hepatocytes. HE 10×20.

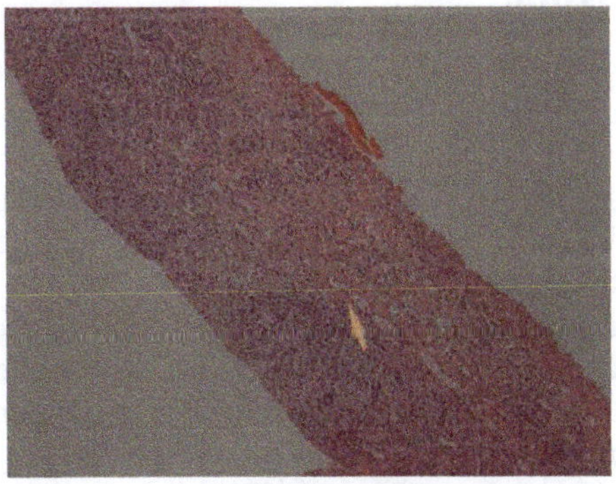

FIGURE 2: Liver biopsy showing portal expansion and bridging fibrosis. HE 10×10.

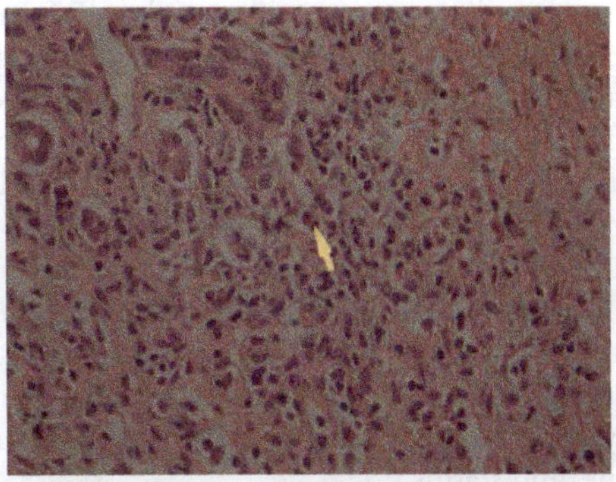

(a)

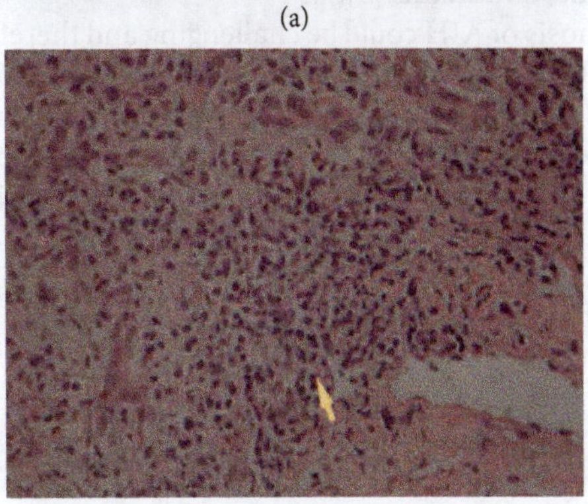

(b)

FIGURE 3: Liver biopsy showing moderate to marked portal tract mostly lymphoplasmacytic inflammatory cell infiltrate. HE: 10×20.

Table 1: Liver enzymes improved with the treatment.

	AST	ALT	ALP	Total bilirubin
Reference range	0–37 U/L	0–45 U/L	46–116 U/L	4–21 mmol/L
1st day of treatment	593	482	343	57.3
5th day of treatment	278	286	318	47.47
15th day of treatment	62	103	226	30.6
21st day of treatment	36.3	45	176	22.1
28th day of treatment	31	39	122	20.1

3. Discussion

Infertility has psychologic, emotional, and financial consequences on families. The prevalence of primary infertility in the United States in married women is between 15 and 44 years is 6% [2]. However, with medical development, advanced fertility treatment options are more numerous and variable than ever.

Menotrophin is a female infertility gonadotropin treatment which may induce minor gastrointestinal adverse effects such as abdominal pain, nausea, vomiting, and unspecific symptoms.

DILI is a common cause of liver disease that could be associated with prescribed medications, over the counter drugs, herbal and/or dietary supplements. Its manifestations can mimic many liver diseases, and its effect can range from a mild elevation of liver enzymes to liver failure. DILI accounts for 10%–50% of elevated liver enzymes in adults, and 10% of all acute hepatitis cases [3]. Risk factors include (a) age; adults are at higher risk than children except for that of valproic acid-induced DILI, which is more common in children; (b) women are at higher risk than men; (c) alcohol abuse; (d) malnutrition [4]. Few DILI cases may present with typical features of autoimmune hepatitis, which makes differentiating between the two challenging. DIAIH is still a poorly defined and an under-reported liver disorder. It can commonly be caused by minocycline, alpha-methyldopa, nitrofurantoin, hydralazine, and statins [5].

Diagnosis of AIH could be challenging and therefore several scoring systems have been developed to standardize the diagnosis. The Simplified diagnostic criteria of International Autoimmune hepatitis Group Score showed 81% sensitivity and 99% specificity when using a cutoff score ≥7 points as a definitive diagnosis of AIH [1].

In this case we present here, our patient scored 7 points; one point for positive ANA, two points for positive IgG, two points for liver histology & two points for absence of viral hepatitis, which qualify as definitive diagnosis of AIH.

DILI is still a diagnosis of exclusion especially with the lack of gold standard test or tool to establish the causality. The RUCAM (Roussel Uclaf Causality Assessment Method) or its previous synonym CIOMS (Council for International Organizations of Medical Sciences) score is a tool that could provide help in guiding a systematic and objective evaluation of patients suspected to have DILI [6,7]. RUCAM score ranges from −9 to +10 with higher score indicating higher likelihood of DILI [6]. The diagnosis of DILI in our patient is classified as probable based on RUCAM score of +6.

It is important to distinguish drugs as triggers of a self-perpetuating autoimmune liver disease from immune-mediated drug-induced liver injury (IM-DILI). Immune-mediated DILI nearly always resolves or becomes quiescent when drugs are withdrawn. Another possibility is that AIH was quiescent and remains undiagnosed until a drug triggered a new autoimmune process. Thus, to attempt to make a proper diagnosis of the type of immune process affecting the liver is challenging [5]. The presence of liver cirrhosis was surprising in this young patient which could suggest the possibility of unrevealed chronic liver disease with Menotrophin acting as a trigger to the recent inflammatory activity.

In addition, recognition and discontinuation of the drug causing DIAIH is the most crucial step in management, along with evaluating the severity and the characteristics of injury. Liver biopsy is not essential for diagnosis. The primary treatment is with corticosteroid therapy.

Clinical pictures and histopathological features of DILI and AIH are similar, but the key point of differentiation between the two is the response after cessation of immunosuppressive therapy. Successful cessation has been reported in DIAIH, while relapses has been reported in AIH [8].

4. Conclusion

This report describes a case of probable drug-induced autoimmune hepatitis following treatment with Menotrophin for infertility in a young female with no previous known liver disease and with documented normal liver enzymes prior to therapy. We suggest checking liver function test prior to staring and during such treatment, since there is a probability of serious DILI associated with its use.

References

[1] E. M. Hennes, M. Zeniya, A. J. Czaja et al., "Simplified criteria for the diagnosis of autoimmune hepatitis," *Hepatology*, vol. 48, no. 1, pp. 169–176, 2008.

[2] M. E. Thoma, A. C. McLain, J. F. Louis et al., "Prevalence of infertility in the United States as estimated by the current duration approach and a traditional constructed approach," *Fertility and Sterility*, vol. 99, no. 5, pp. 1324–1331, 2013.

[3] H. J. Zimmerman, "Drug-induced liver disease," *Clinics in Liver Disease*, vol. 4, no. 1, pp. 73–96, 2000.

[4] N. Chalasani and E. Björnsson, "Risk factors for idiosyncratic drug-induced liver injury," *Gastroenterology*, vol. 138, no. 7, pp. 2246–2259, 2010.

[5] A. Castiella, E. Zapata, M. I. Lucena, and R. J. Andrade, "Drug-induced autoimmune liver disease: a diagnostic dilemma of an increasingly reported disease," *World Journal of Hepatology*, vol. 6, no. 4, pp. 160–168, 2014.

[6] G. Danan and R. Teschke, "RUCAM in drug and herb induced liver injury: the update," *International Journal of Molecular Sciences*, vol. 17, no. 1, p. E14, 2015.

[7] R. J. Andrade, G. P. Aithal, E. S. Bjornsson et al., "EASL clinical practice guidelines: drug-induced liver injury," *Journal of Hepatology*, vol. 70, no. 6, pp. 1222–1261, 2019.

[8] J. S. Schneider, M. Montani, and F. Stickel, "Drug-induced autoimmune hepatitis following treatment with zoledronic acid," *Case Reports in Gastroenterology*, vol. 11, no. 2, pp. 440–445, 2017.

26

An Unfortunate Cause of Chronic Nausea and Vomiting: Mitochondrial Neurogastrointestinal Encephalomyopathy (MNGIE)

Neethi Dasu,[1] Brian Blair,[1] C. Jonathan Foster,[1] and Colin Smith[2]

[1]*Department of Gastroenterology, Jefferson Health New Jersey, Cherry Hill, NJ, USA*
[2]*Department of Gastroenterology, Jefferson Medical College of Thomas Jefferson University, Philadelphia, PA, USA*

Correspondence should be addressed to Neethi Dasu; dasu@rowan.edu

Academic Editor: Marcel Cerqueira Cesar Machado

We present a unique case of a 24-year-old male who was admitted for intractable nausea, emesis, weight loss, and abdominal discomfort. The patient underwent an extensive workup and was diagnosed with mitochondrial neurogastrointestinal encephalopathy. Early diagnosis is critical to proper management of this disease process. MGNIE is a difficult disorder to diagnose given the complexity of the disease, and this case provides clinicians the proper understanding and management of such a unique and difficult diagnosis.

1. Introduction

Mitochondrial neurogastrointestinal encephalomyopathy (MNGIE) is a progressive, autosomal recessive, degenerative disease which portends significant morbidity and mortality [1]. It is an extremely rare and devastating disease with a prevalence of 1–9 in 1000000 worldwide [1]. The average age of onset is 18, and the disease usually manifests in the first two decades of life [1]. Mutations in the TYMP gene lead to loss of function in thymidine phosphorylase activity which causes MNGIE [1, 2]. MNGIE is often misdiagnosed given the complexity in its presentation and subtle nonspecific symptoms. We present a case of a young male who was initially presented with chronic symptoms of malnutrition, nausea, and emesis, and he was subsequently diagnosed with MNGIE.

2. Case Report

A 24-year-old male with a medical history of anorexia, depression, clostridium difficile infection, weight loss, nausea, vomiting, diarrhea, and abdominal pain presented for evaluation of severe malnutrition and intractable nausea that had been occurring intermittently for three years as well as intermittent diarrhea and weight loss of seventy pounds. The patient was initially lost to follow-up in the outpatient setting and had underwent bidirectional endoscopy two years prior which revealed pangastritis with food in the stomach (Figure 1). Biopsies were negative for intestinal metaplasia, infiltrative disease, celiac disease, lymphoma, *H. pylori*, or inflammatory bowel disease. Ascending colon and rectum biopsies were positive for chronic inflammation and reactive changes.

On a physical exam, the patient was cachectic with bitemporal and diffuse muscle wasting, flexion contracture of left 5th metacarpal, and poor dentition. Initial lab work revealed the following: lactate of 6.8 (mg/dL), alkaline phosphatase of 198 (IU/L), aminotransferase of 42 (IU/L), alanine transferase of 58 (IU/L), prealbumin 12 (mg/dL), c-reactive protein of 27 (mg/L), gastrin of 67 (pg/mL), fecal calprotectin of 296 (μg/g), lactoferrin 313.40 (μg/g), and elastase (μg/g), within normal limits. Magnetic resonance enterography (MRE) was consistent with diffuse ileus (Figure 2). Due to his intractable symptoms, the patient underwent insertion of a gastrojejunostomy (GJ) tube and was started on tube feeds. A gastric emptying study was

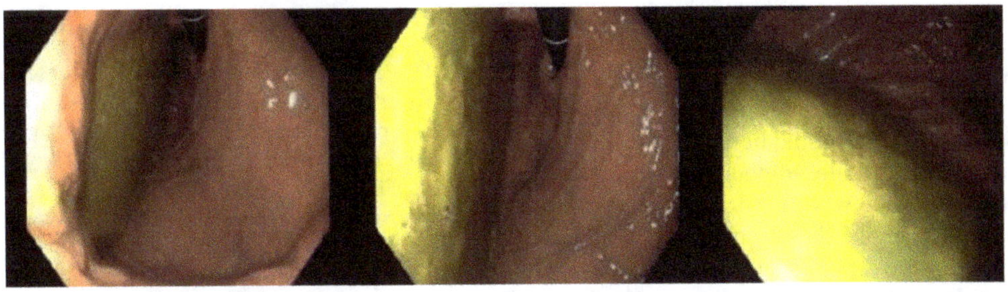

FIGURE 1: EGD with food in the stomach consistent with gastric atony.

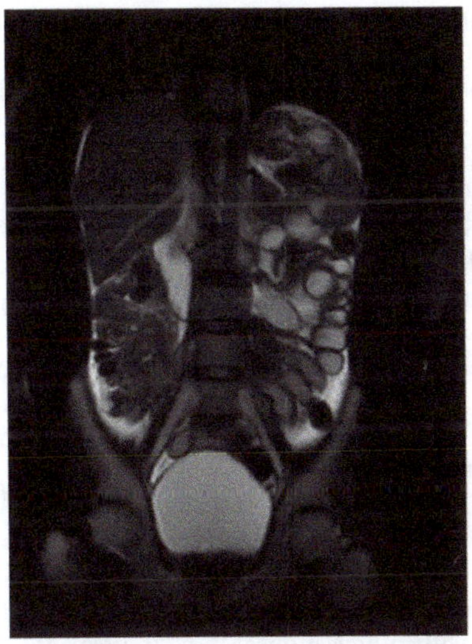

FIGURE 2: MRE showing diffuse ileus.

positive for delayed gastric emptying, and he was treated with metoclopramide and underwent esophagogastroduodenoscopy (EGD) with botulinum injection; stomach biopsies revealed a mild increase in intraepithelial T cells.

The patient's hospital course was complicated by aspiration pneumonia and malfunctioning of his GJ tube which required revision. Due to persistent elevated lactate levels, motility workup was ordered which included anticentromere antibody, aldolase levels, myositis specific antibodies, amino acid panel, RNA polymerase 3 antibody, scleroderma 70 antibody, thymidine phosphorylase (TP) enzyme analysis, plasma thymidine, and deoxyuridine analyte. The patient left against medical advice and was admitted to another hospital for aspiration pneumonia requiring intubation and eventual tracheostomy placement. The motility workup was negative except for thymidine and deoxyuridine analytes were noted to be elevated, revealing a thymidine phosphorylase deficiency, and the patient was diagnosed with MNGIE.

3. Discussion

MNGIE is a deadly mitochondrial multisystem disorder caused by mutations in the TYMP gene which leads to deficiency of thymidine phosphorylase activity [1, 2]. The TYMP gene is responsible for the degradation of thymidine and its dysfunction leads to a cascade of events including compromised mitochondrial DNA repair, loss of oxidative phosphorylation, nucleoside aggregation, and subsequent compounding of mutations [1, 2]. The TYMP gene is readily found throughout the human body, especially in the gastrointestinal tract, brain, blood, and nervous system. Epidemiologically, the prevalence of this disorder is less than ten in one million [1, 3]. The majority of individuals begin experiencing symptoms before the age of twenty with the mean age at onset being approximately 18 years [3]. MNGIE is distributed through multiple ethnic populations and is inherited in an autosomal recessive fashion [4].

The major clinical characteristics of MNGIE include progressive gastrointestinal dysmotility, leukoencephalopathy, peripheral neuropathy, and ocular manifestations [1, 3]. Gastrointestinal (GI) symptoms can present as diarrhea, nausea, emesis, cramping, gastroparesis and can lead to severe malnutrition and cachexia [1, 3]. Our patient presented with significant weight loss, malnutrition, postprandial abdominal discomfort, nausea, and emesis as well as delayed gastric emptying; these symptoms were consistent with the major GI characteristics of MNGIE; however, due to their nonspecificity, the diagnosis was somewhat delayed. Manifestations of leukoencephalopathy and peripheral neuropathy were also seen in our patient as he was profoundly weak and had contractures and progressive muscle wasting. Furthermore, he was diagnosed with depression multiple years ago which is a neurologic manifestation of MNGIE.

The clinical diagnosis of MNGIE disease is based on the presence of the major clinical characteristics or by detection of pathogenic mutations in TYMP, reduced levels of thymidine phosphorylase enzyme activity, or elevated plasma concentrations of deoxyuridine and thymidine [3]. In this case, plasma level of thymidine was noted to be 15.83 (normal $<0.25\,\mu$mol/L) and deoxyuridine was 25.92 (normal $<0.25\,\mu$mol/L), which was consistent with MNGIE. Some patients might have elevations in serum lactate which was a diagnostic clue in this case as the patient was noted to have persistently elevated lactate levels for months.

Treatment options are limited and based on symptom management including analgesics, antiemetics, probowel motility stimulant drugs, as well as treatment of malnutrition with parenteral nutrition or total parenteral nutrition [1]. Since many patients suffer from nausea, vomiting, weight loss, global dysmotility, and cachexia, treatment includes nutritional support, gastrostomy tube placement, and antibiotic treatment for bacterial overgrowth [5]. Medication regimens include domperidone for nausea and vomiting, as well as morphine, gabapentin, tricyclic antidepressants, and anticonvulsant medicines for relief of symptoms. Physical therapy and occupational therapy may help increase and preserve mobility [1, 5].

Drugs which are hepatically metabolized or that affect the mitochondrial metabolism should be avoided [3]. Drugs such as valproate, phenytoin, chloramphenicol, tetracycline, and antipsychotic medications can interfere with mitochondrial function and should also be avoided [5].

Currently, there are investigational therapies which include enzyme supplementation, stem cell transplantation (HPSCT), hemodialysis to decrease toxic metabolites, and liver transplantation [1, 6]. Liver transplant has been shown to be beneficial in certain patients. TP enzyme activity in the donor graft was sufficient to lower plasma thymidine to near-normal levels [7]. Posttransplant plasma thymidine levels were noted to be diminished in certain populations, with one study demonstrating that thymidine levels dropped more than 20 times lower than pretransplant levels with noted improvement in motility issues and neurologic deficits [7]. HPSCT can also be used to treat patients, and however, this treatment has a high mortality rate.

Gene therapy is currently experimental with promising murine studies. One study which utilized using viral DNA to deliver the TYMP gene to the liver reduced thymidine and deoxyuridine levels to normal levels in about half of the mice studied, showing potential that gene therapy can treat MNGIE [8].

As the disease progresses, patients die from GI complications, malnutrition, or infections, and the average age of death is 37 years [1]. Our patient chose to pursue hospice and died a few months later. Early diagnosis requires a high index of suspicion and recognition of symptoms before tissue damage and cachexia occurs. Treatment efficacy was higher in patients who did not have severe intestinal and peripheral nerve damage [9].

In conclusion, this case is important because it highlights a rare cause of common gastrointestinal symptoms. Most patients are often misdiagnosed due to the subtlety and nonspecificity of symptoms; thus, this case further emphasizes that gastroenterologists should be vigilant in recognizing rare disorders associated with GI dysmotility, especially in young patients. MNGIE should be suspected in all patients who present with both nervous system and gastrointestinal symptoms [10].

Disclosure

This manuscript has been previously submitted as a poster presentation and abstract at the American College of Gastroenterology 2021 Annual Scientific Conference.

Authors' Contributions

ND, BB, CJF, HS, and CS were responsible for the study concept and design, data collection, and drafting of the manuscript. ND, BB, and CJF edited the contents and grammar of the manuscript and supervised the entirety of the study.

References

[1] D. Pacitti, M. Levene, C. Garone, N. Nirmalananthan, and B. E. Bax, "Mitochondrial neurogastrointestinal encephalomyopathy: into the fourth decade, what we have learned so far," *Frontiers in Genetics*, vol. 9, 2018.

[2] M. Filosto, S. Cotti Piccinelli, F. Caria et al., "Mitochondrial neurogastrointestinal encephalomyopathy (MNGIE-MTDPS1)," *Journal of Clinical Medicine*, vol. 7, 2018.

[3] M. Hirano, "Mitochondrial neurogastrointestinal encephalopathy disease," 2016, https://www.ncbi.nlm.nih.gov/books/NBK1179/.

[4] O. Database, "Orphanet: mitochondrial neurogastrointestinal encephalomyopathy," 2021, https://www.orpha.net/consor/cgi-bin/OC_Exp.php?lng=EN&Expert=298.

[5] "Mitochondrial neurogastrointestinal encephalopathy syndrome: genetic and rare diseases information center (GARD)–an NCATS program," 2022, https://rarediseases.info.nih.gov/diseases/9920/mitochondrial-neurogastrointestinal-encephalopathy-syndrome.

[6] A. Tawk, M. Hussein Kamarreddine, M. Dagher et al., "Clinicopathology and diagnosis delay in a 40-year-old with mitochondrial neurogastrointestinal encephalomyopathy (MNGIE)," *Case Reports in Gastroenterology*, vol. 14, 2020.

[7] K. Kripps, W. Nakayuenyongsuk, B. J. Shayota et al., "Successful liver transplantation in mitochondrial neurogastrointestinal encephalomyopathy (MNGIE)," *Molecular Genetics and Metabolism*, vol. 130, no. 1, pp. 58–64, 2020.

[8] A. Melao, "Potential gene therapy may improve survival in MNGIE patients," 2022, https://mitochondrialdiseasenews.com/2018/03/05/tymp-gene-therapy-may-potentially-treat-patients-with-mngie-mouse.study/#:~:text=A%20gene%20therapy%20designed%20to,disease%2C%20a%20mouse%20study%20suggests.

[9] C. Giovanni, P. Cécile, H. Gaëlle, G. Besson, A. Lombès, and MNGIE Project, "MyoNeuroGastroIntestinal encephalopathy: natural history and means for early diagnosis," *Gastroenterology*, vol. 156, pp. 1525–1527, 2019.

[10] M. Scarpelli, A. Russignan, M. Zombor et al., "Poor outcome in a mitochondrial neurogastrointestinal: encephalomyopathy patient with a novel TYMP mutation: the need for early diagnosis," *Case Reports in Neurology*, vol. 4, 2012.

27

Hepatic *YAP1-TFE3* Rearranged Epithelioid Hemangioendothelioma

Mira M. Lotfalla,[1] Andrew L. Folpe,[1] Karen J. Fritchie,[1] Patricia T. Greipp,[1] Gretchen G. Galliano,[2] Kevin C. Halling,[1] Taofic Mounajjed,[1] Jorge Torres-Mora,[1] and Rondell P. Graham[1]

[1]*Department of Laboratory Medicine and Pathology, Mayo Clinic, Rochester, MN, USA*
[2]*Anatomic Pathology, Ochsner Health System, New Orleans, LA, USA*

Correspondence should be addressed to Rondell P. Graham; graham.rondell@mayo.edu

Academic Editor: Yoshifumi Nakayama

Epithelioid hemangioendothelioma (EHE) is an uncommon low-grade malignant vascular tumor that may arise in soft tissue/bone or visceral sites such as the liver and lung. As this tumor exhibits epithelioid morphology, it frequently causes diagnostic confusion with other epithelioid vascular neoplasms as well as carcinoma. While 90% of classic EHE are driven by a *WWTR1-CAMTA1* fusion gene, a histologically distinctive subset of EHE has been recently shown to harbor a different fusion gene, *YAP1-TFE3*. This variant is likely underrecognized given its rarity and only recent description. Notably, EHE frequently involves the liver but only one case of hepatic *YAP1-TFE3* rearranged EHE has been reported to date. We present the second case of *YAP1-TFE3* rearranged EHE affecting a 65-year-old woman and presenting as multiple liver masses, with characterization of the fusion gene at the transcriptomic and genomic levels. There are several educational points noted from this case. *YAP1-TFE3* rearranged EHE shows distinctly vasoformative foci, unlike classic EHE and mimicking angiosarcoma or epithelioid hemangioma. The tumors cells show a histiocytoid appearance with voluminous cytoplasm, similar to other *TFE3*-rearranged tumors. Finally, in the liver, this tumor may in part mimic focal nodular hyperplasia of the liver which is an underrecognized diagnostic pitfall. This report highlights the key diagnostic and genetic features of this newly recognized variant of hepatic EHE to aid pathologists in appropriately classifying these tumors.

1. Introduction

Epithelioid hemangioendothelioma (EHE) is an uncommon low-grade malignant vascular tumor that may arise in soft tissue/bone or visceral sites such as the liver and lung. As this tumor exhibits epithelioid morphology, it frequently causes diagnostic confusion with other epithelioid vascular neoplasms as well as carcinomas. While 90% of classic EHE are driven by a *WWTR1-CAMTA1* fusion gene, a histologically distinctive subset of EHE has been recently shown to harbor a different fusion gene, *YAP1-TFE3* [1]. This variant is likely underrecognized given its rarity and only recent description. Notably, EHE frequently involves the liver but only one case of hepatic *YAP1-TFE3* EHE has been reported to date [2]. We present an illustrative second case presenting as liver masses which shows the distinctive morphology and molecular features of this entity as well as the potential diagnostic pitfalls.

2. Case Presentation

A 65-year-old woman with multiple liver masses presented for transplantation following a diagnosis of EHE made on biopsy. Preoperative imaging revealed an enlarged liver with multifocal disease throughout the hepatic parenchyma. The lesions showed peripheral enhancement with central hypoattenuation on arterial phase and appeared isodense to the liver parenchyma on delayed phase imaging. Some of the masses showed calcifications (Figure 1). There was no significant interval change in size in the 10 months from initial diagnosis to transplantation. No chest or pelvic

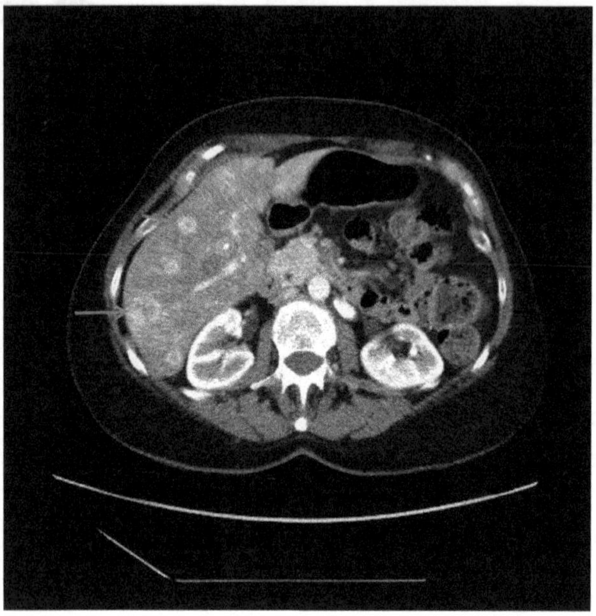

Figure 1: Computed tomography image showing multifocal hepatic lesions with peripheral enhancement and central hypoattenuation. Blue arrows point to calcifications.

masses were identified elsewhere during the preoperative workup.

Pathologic examination of the liver explant disclosed multiple tan discrete nodules ranging from 0.5 to 3.0 cm in greatest dimension and involving the bilateral lobes. Low power examination revealed 2 main histologic patterns. A subset of the nodules contained well-formed vascular channels and scattered cords of tumor cells embedded in an abundantly sclerotic hyalinized matrix (Figure 2(a)), while other areas of tumor were characterized by small, irregular central hyalinized scars containing small subtle foci of neoplastic cells and a mild bile ductular reaction (Figure 2(b)). On high magnification, the tumor cells in both components exhibited mild cytologic atypia and were characterized by abundant pale cytoplasm, nuclei bearing open chromatin and visible though not large nucleoli. Scattered intracytoplasmic vacuoles were noted in the tumor cells arranged in a linear pattern (Figure 2(c)). Mitotic figures were not observed; however, focal vascular invasion by single tumor cells was noted. There was stromal lymphocytic inflammation, and focal calcification was noted in one of the lesions. The surrounding liver parenchyma had a nodular architecture, reminiscent of focal nodular hyperplasia (Figure 2(b)).

Immunohistochemically, the tumor cells showed an endothelial phenotype with strong expression of CD31 (clone JC70A; 1/350; Dako) and ERG (clone EPR3864; predilute; Ventana) (Figure 2(d)). The tumor nuclei were positive for TFE3 (clone MRQ-37; 1/50; Cell Marque) (Figure 3(a)), but CAMTA1 (polyclonal; 1/300; Novus Biologicals) was negative (Figure 2(e)). Glutamine synthetase (clone GS-6; 1/2000; Millipore) showed a map-like pattern of distribution in the hepatocytes surrounding small irregular areas of scar mimicking focal nodular hyperplasia (Figure 2(f)).

RNA sequencing with fusion gene analysis from formalin-fixed paraffin embedded tissue revealed an in-frame *YAP1-TFE3* fusion gene joining exon 1 of *YAP1* to exon 4 of *TFE3* and a reciprocal *TFE3-YAP1* joining exon 3 of *TFE3* to exon 2 of *YAP1*, similar to the findings of Antonescu and colleagues [1], using a published lab-developed protocol [3]. No other fusion genes, including *WWTR1-CAMTA1*, were identified. Fluorescence in situ hybridization (FISH) was performed with lab-developed split apart probes for the *TFE3* locus (bacterial artificial chromosome clones RP11-416B14, CTD-2311N12, CTD-3009K20, and CTD-2173N15; all from Abbott Molecular, IL) and dual fusion probes for *YAP1-TFE3* loci (bacterial artificial chromosome clones RP11-635D24, RP11-451F15, RP11-90M3, and RP11-750P5 along with the previously mentioned clones for *TFE3*; all from Abbott Molecular, IL) using standard techniques as previously reported by our group [4]. Interphase FISH revealed rearrangement of the *TFE3* locus in all tumor cells and *YAP1-TFE3* fusion at the genomic level (Figure 3(b)). An image of intact CAMTA1 split apart FISH performed using the same method and probes to the CAMTA1 locus is also shown (Figure 3(c)). Based on the combination of morphologic, immunophenotypic, and genetic findings, this case was classified as a *YAP1-TFE3* rearranged EHE.

3. Discussion

EHE, a malignant vascular neoplasm first described by Enzinger and Weiss in 1982 [5], may arise at a variety of anatomic locations including bone, soft tissue, and viscera. Although this entity is well-recognized, EHE still represents a diagnostic challenge in routine practice due to its rarity and morphologic overlap with other epithelioid tumors, including other benign and malignant epithelioid vascular neoplasms and carcinomas, especially when these tumors present at visceral sites such as the liver. The vast majority (90%) of EHE harbor the *WWTR1-CAMTA1* fusion event [6, 7], which can be detected with molecular genetic methods or with the CAMTA1 immunostain, a reliable surrogate [8].

Recently, Antonescu and colleagues described a distinctive vascular neoplasm showing some features of EHE, but characterized by an alternate *YAP1-TFE3* fusion [1]. It is not yet entirely certain whether this unusual tumor represents a variant of EHE or an altogether unique tumor [1]. Although both tumors share epithelioid morphology and a corded growth pattern, tumors harboring the *YAP1-TFE3* fusion differ from conventional EHE inasmuch as they display overt vasoformation, consist of cells with voluminous cytoplasm, and lack the distinctive myxochondroid matrix of the latter tumor [1]. However, the natural history of conventional and *YAP1-TFE3* EHE seems to be similar, with significant potential for late distant metastasis [1].

Antonescu et al.'s seminal description of *YAP1-TFE3* EHE did not identify any tumors primary to the liver [1]. To the best of our knowledge, the only *bona fide* report of this rare tumor occurring in the liver is that of Kuo et al., who reported a morphologically typical, *TFE3*-rearranged EHE occurring

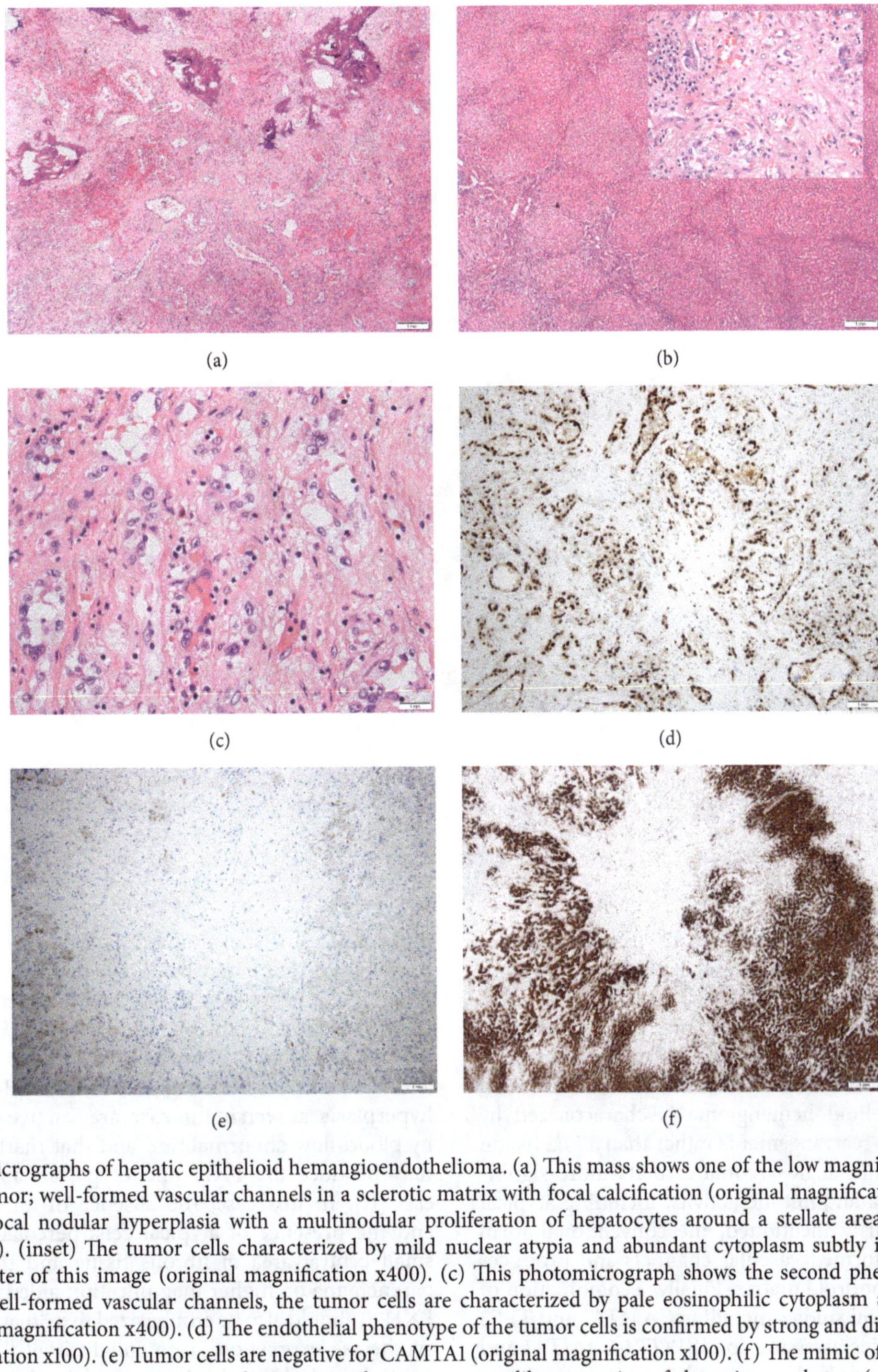

(a) (b) (c) (d) (e) (f)

FIGURE 2: Photomicrographs of hepatic epithelioid hemangioendothelioma. (a) This mass shows one of the low magnification morphologic patterns of this tumor; well-formed vascular channels in a sclerotic matrix with focal calcification (original magnification x 100). (b) Other areas resembled focal nodular hyperplasia with a multinodular proliferation of hepatocytes around a stellate area of fibrosis (original magnification x40). (inset) The tumor cells characterized by mild nuclear atypia and abundant cytoplasm subtly infiltrate the collagen as seen in the center of this image (original magnification x400). (c) This photomicrograph shows the second phenotype of the tumor cells. Instead of well-formed vascular channels, the tumor cells are characterized by pale eosinophilic cytoplasm and intracytoplasmic vacuoles (original magnification x400). (d) The endothelial phenotype of the tumor cells is confirmed by strong and diffuse expression ERG (original magnification x100). (e) Tumor cells are negative for CAMTA1 (original magnification x100). (f) The mimic of typical focal nodular hyperplasia extended beyond hematoxylin and eosin stained stains to a map-like expression of glutamine synthetase (original magnification x40).

in a 39-year-old woman [2]. Although another primary hepatic vascular tumor has been reported by Lee and coworkers as representing EHE showing "concomitant *YAP1-TFE3* and *WWTR1-CAMTA1* fusions," the morphologic and molecular genetic features of this lesion are not fully convincing, in our opinion [9].

Our case report highlights several diagnostic challenges of this variant of EHE. *YAP1-TFE3* rearranged EHE harbors areas with well-formed blood vessels, potentially mimicking a hemangioma, an entity much more common in the liver. The biphasic appearance, however, with a second component of tumor cells arranged in cords and containing scattered intracytoplasmic lumina should trigger pathologists to consider this variant of EHE. The epithelioid morphology of the neoplastic population may also raise the possibility of other epithelioid vascular tumors such as epithelioid hemangioma,

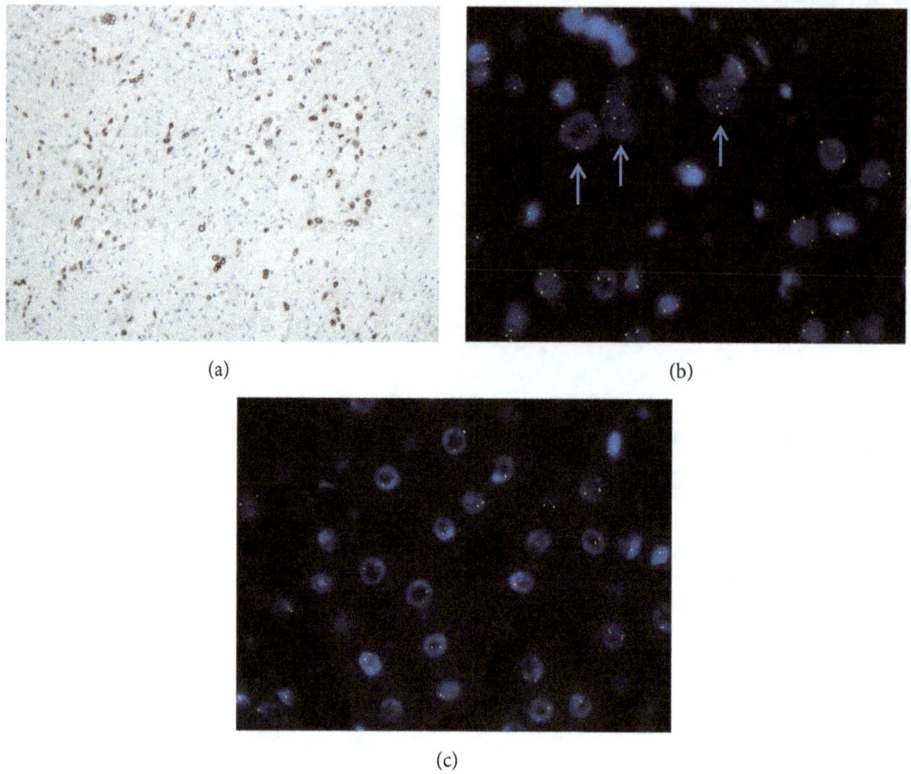

Figure 3: (a) Nuclear TFE3 expression by the neoplastic cells. (b) Dual fusion fluorescent in situ hybridization probes for *YAP1*- (spectrum green) *TFE3* (spectrum orange) showing fusion of the two loci highlighted by blue arrows. (c) Split apart fluorescent in situ hybridization showing intact CAMTA1.

epithelioid angiosarcoma, and the conventional form of EHE with *WWTR1-CAMTA1* fusion. Although the tumor cells of epithelioid hemangioma are plump and hobnailed, they lack significant atypia. Furthermore, these tumors are uniformly vasoformative and often containing numerous eosinophils. The latter feature was not seen in this case. Additionally, epithelioid hemangioma is characterized by frequent *FOSB* gene rearrangements rather than *TFE3* fusion genes [10]. Epithelioid angiosarcoma exhibits more significant cytologic atypia and mitotic activity, including atypical mitoses. As previously mentioned, the conventional form of EHE lacks well-formed vascular channels and produces distinctive myxochondroid matrix. Finally, a combination of immunohistochemical studies including CAMTA1 and TFE3 and molecular studies assessing for *WWTR1-CAMTA1* and *YAP1-TFE3* fusions aids in the correct diagnosis.

The epithelioid morphology of EHE may also mimic involvement by primary or metastatic carcinoma. Recognizing vasoformative areas is a helpful clue to endothelial lineage, but these areas may not always be present on biopsy material. The degree of atypia in *YAP1-TFE3* rearranged EHE is usually relatively mild, and pathologists should consider performing a battery of immunostains for endothelial markers (CD31, CD34, FLI-1, and ERG) on any epithelioid neoplasm lacking keratin expression or with a uniform cytologic appearance.

Finally, low magnification examination of the explanted specimen in our patient showed some masses with a striking resemblance to focal nodular hyperplasia (FNH). This low power architecture may be deceptive, potentially resulting in a failure to recognize the underlying vascular neoplasm as the tumor cells in our case were sparsely distributed within small irregular areas of fibrous tissue and in nearby sinusoids and vessels. It has been suggested that FNH and peritumoral hyperplasia, as seen in this case, are reactive processes unified by blood flow abnormalities, and that marked angiogenesis may produce the FNH phenotype, an appealing hypothesis [11]. In this case, the absence of an abnormal artery and the presence of atypical cells percolating through the small central area of fibrous tissue and the adjacent liver parenchyma on higher magnification aided distinction from FNH. It should also be emphasized that "map-like" glutamine synthetase expression, a potential pitfall illustrated by this case, should always be interpreted in the context of other clinical and morphological findings.

YAP1 and *WWTR1* are orthologues and are believed to function similarly in their respective fusion genes. A review of the biology of these genes is beyond the scope of this report but *YAP1-TFE3* and *WWTR1-CAMTA1* are believed to be oncogenic drivers. In brief, *YAP1* and *WWTR1* function via TEAD transcription factors to drive expression of proproliferative and antiapoptotic genes [12]. *TFE3* is one of the MiT family of transcription factors which bind to specific recognition sequences of DNA to alter gene expression. The available data indicate that, in *YAP1-TFE3*, the promoter of

YAP1 is juxtaposed to the key domains of *TFE3* to drive the development of tumors [1]. The specificity of the *YAP1-TFE3* and *WWTR1-CAMTA1* fusion genes makes them useful biomarkers for diagnosis as shown in this case.

4. Conclusion

In conclusion, we describe a second case of *YAP1-TFE3* hepatic EHE with complete characterization of the fusion gene at the transcriptomic and genomic levels. This case also exhibited findings reminiscent of focal nodular hyperplasia, which is an underrecognized potential pitfall. Pathologists should be aware of the morphologic features of this rare and recently described variant to avoid misclassification as other vascular tumors, carcinoma and focal nodular hyperplasia. Further clinicopathologic studies are necessary to determine the behavior of this variant, especially those arising in the liver.

References

[1] C. R. Antonescu, F. Le Loarer, J.-M. Mosquera et al., "Novel YAP1-TFE3 fusion defines a distinct subset of epithelioid hemangioendothelioma," *Genes, Chromosomes and Cancer*, vol. 52, no. 8, pp. 775–784, 2013.

[2] F.-Y. Kuo, H.-Y. Huang, C.-L. Chen et al., "TFE3-rearranged hepatic epithelioid hemangioendothelioma—a case report with immunohistochemical and molecular study," *APMIS-Acta Pathologica, Microbiologica et Immunologica Scandinavica*, vol. 125, no. 9, pp. 849–853, 2017.

[3] J. L. Winters, J. I. Davila, A. M. McDonald et al., "Development and verification of an RNA sequencing (RNA-Seq) assay for the detection of gene fusions in tumors," *The Journal of Molecular Diagnostics*, vol. 20, no. 4, pp. 495–511, 2018.

[4] R. P. Graham, A. A. Nair, J. I. Davila et al., "Gastroblastoma harbors a recurrent somatic MALAT1-GLI1 fusion gene," *Modern Pathology*, vol. 30, no. 10, pp. 1443–1452, 2017.

[5] S. W. Weiss and F. M. Enzinger, "Epitheloid hemangioendothelioma: a vascular tumor often mistaken for a carcinoma," *Cancer*, vol. 50, no. 5, pp. 970–981, 1982.

[6] C. Errani, L. Zhang, Y. S. Sung et al., "A novel WWTR1-CAMTA1 gene fusion is a consistent abnormality in epithelioid hemangioendothelioma of different anatomic sites," *Genes, Chromosomes and Cancer*, vol. 50, no. 8, pp. 644–653, 2011.

[7] M. R. Tanas, A. Sboner, A. M. Oliveira et al., "Identification of a disease-defining gene fusion in epithelioid hemangioendothelioma," *Science Translational Medicine*, vol. 3, no. 98, p. 98ra82, 2011.

[8] L. A. Doyle, C. D. M. Fletcher, and J. L. Hornick, "Nuclear expression of CAMTA1 distinguishes epithelioid hemangioendothelioma from histologic mimics," *The American Journal of Surgical Pathology*, vol. 40, no. 1, pp. 94–102, 2016.

[9] S. J. Lee, W. I. Yang, W.-S. Chung et al., "Epithelioid hemangioendotheliomas with TFE3 gene translocations are compossible with CAMTA1 gene rearrangements," *Oncotarget*, vol. 7, no. 7, pp. 7480–7488, 2016.

[10] S. C. Huang, L. Zhang, Y. S. Sung et al., "Frequent FOS gene rearrangements in epithelioid hemangioma: a molecular study of 58 cases with morphologic reappraisal," *The American Journal of Surgical Pathology*, vol. 39, no. 10, pp. 1313–1321, 2015.

[11] I. R. Wanless, "Epithelioid hemangioendothelioma, multiple focal nodular hyperplasias, and cavernous hemangiomas of the liver," *Archives of Pathology & Laboratory Medicine*, vol. 124, no. 8, pp. 1105–1107, 2000.

[12] B. Zhao, X. Ye, J. Yu et al., "TEAD mediates YAP-dependent gene induction and growth control," *Genes & Development*, vol. 22, no. 14, pp. 1962–1971, 2008.

28

Use of Lumen-Apposing Stents for the Treatment of Postsurgical Fluid Collections: A Case Series and a Review of Literature

Priyanka Priyanka,[1] **William Hsueh**,[2] **and John Nasr**[2]

[1]*Department of Medicine, WV University Hospital, Morgantown, WV, USA*
[2]*Department of Medicine, Division of Gastroenterology, WVU University Hospital, Morgantown, WV, USA*

Correspondence should be addressed to Priyanka Priyanka; priyanka.priyanka@hsc.wvu.edu

Academic Editor: I. Michael Leitman

Lumen-apposing metal stents (LAMS) use in gastrointestinal endoscopy has been on the rise for various indications for the last few years. Currently, LAMS is a well-established treatment for post-pancreatitis peri-pancreatic fluid collections and walled-off necrosis (WON), but it is still not a standard of care in the treatment of post-surgical fluid collections (PSFC). Most of the earlier studies for treatment of PSFC utilized double pigtail plastic stents (DPS). We present a series of 3 cases where LAMS was successfully used for PSFC drainage. The cases include a patient with perigastric abscess after Whipple's procedure, a case of peri-pancreatic collection after distal pancreatectomy, and a patient with peri-pancreatic fluid collection after right partial hepatectomy and splenectomy due to lacerations from a motor vehicle accident.

1. Introduction

Post-surgical fluid collections (PSFCs) can be an important cause of morbidity and mortality depending upon the nature of the surgery and site of the collection. Over the last few decades, percutaneous radiologic drainage (PCD) has been considered the first-line treatment of PSFC with a success rate of 80-100% [1, 2]. Due to its lower morbidity, mortality, and costs, percutaneous drainage has become widely accepted over open surgical drainage.

With advances in therapeutic endoscopy over the past few years, there has been increasing use of plastic and metal stents as an attractive alternative to PCD, especially in the treatment of pancreatic and peripancreatic fluid collections and walled-off necrosis (WON) [3, 4]. Recently, the use of these stents has been extended for postsurgical fluid collection drainage [5–7]. Newer studies have contributed to the understanding that endoscopic ultrasound guided drainage (EUS-GD) and PCD are equally effective and safe in treatment of PSFCs [2]. In addition, the advantages of endoscopic drainage over PCD include higher clinical success rate, lower complication rate, less procedure related mortality, lack of an external drain, improvement in quality of life, lower total costs, and fewer complications related to a drain such as fluid losses and bleeding. Most of the earlier studies used double pigtail plastic stents (DPS) [6, 7]. Lumen-apposing metal stents (LAMS) use in gastrointestinal endoscopy has been on the rise for the past 2-3 years for various indications since its first clinical use in 2012. Recent studies have suggested the superiority of LAMS to DPS for WON drainage; however the scientific literature available with regard to PSFCs is scarce with only one study reporting their use for this indication so far [3, 5]. We present a series of cases of successful use of LAMS for drainage of PSFCs.

2. Case Series

2.1. Patient 1. A 54-year-old male with a history of renal cell carcinoma, pancreatic adenocarcinoma stage II (T2 N1 3/5 lymph nodes positive), having previously received chemotherapy followed by stereotactic body radiation therapy (SBRT) presented 5 months after the Whipple's surgery with failure to thrive, fatigue, and nausea. Exam was unremarkable and laboratory investigations revealed albumin of 1.3 mg /dl, bilirubin of 2.8 mg/dl, mainly conjugated, serum alkaline phosphatase of 825 U/L, and CA 19-9 of 81.4

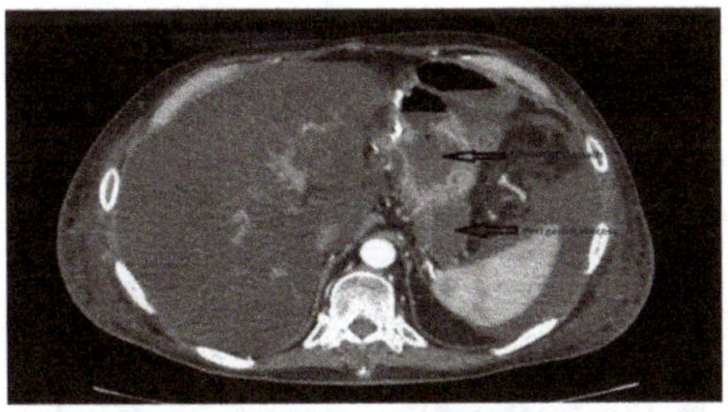

FIGURE 1: Patient 1, CT abdomen showing perigastric abscess.

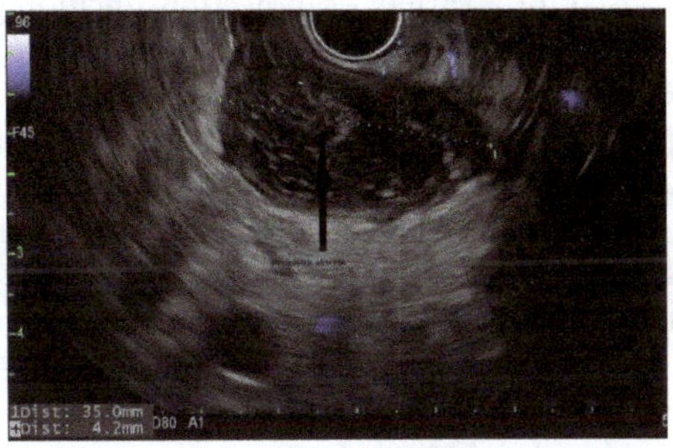

FIGURE 2: Patient 1, EUS confirming perigastric abscess in fundal area.

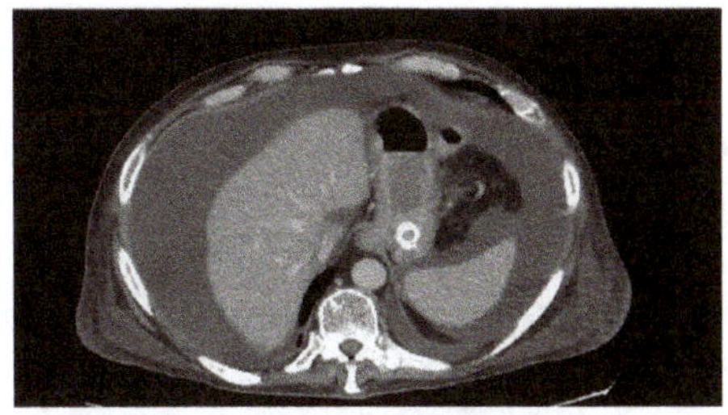

FIGURE 3: Patient 1, CT scan abdomen showing resolution of perigastric abscess.

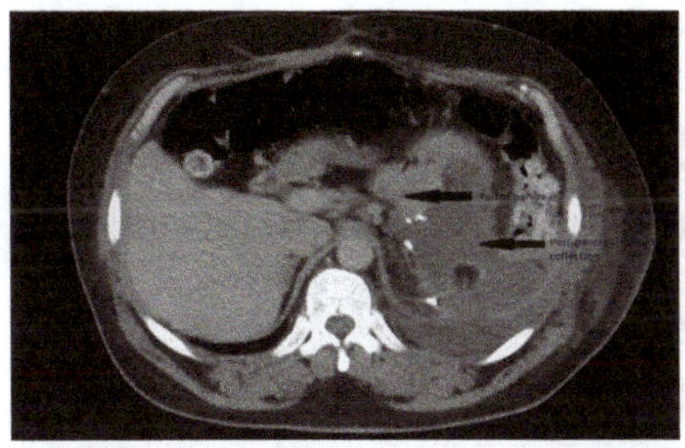

FIGURE 4: Patient 2, CT scan abdomen showing fluid collection around the tail of pancreas.

(normal <37 U/ml). Computed tomography scan (CT) of abdomen showed a perigastric abscess adjacent to the fundus (Figure 1). Endoscopic ultrasound (EUS) was suggestive of 35 mm anechoic, heterogeneous, well-circumscribed fluid collection in the immediate perigastric area surrounding the fundus (Figure 2). Under endosonographic, fluoroscopic, and Doppler guidance, a 10 x 10 mm LAMS was placed from the stomach into the fluid collection with drainage of pus.

The patient improved clinically along with significant improvement in his bilirubin and alkaline phosphatase after the procedure. Repeat CT abdomen after one week of stent placement showed a near-complete resolution of the abscess (Figure 3), although he had developed ascites by this time, likely due to presence of severe hypoalbuminemia. Removal of the stent was planned after 3 weeks of placement. However, the patient was readmitted 3 weeks later with respiratory failure and altered mental status. His family elected to provide supportive care only and he died shortly thereafter.

2.2. Case 2. 54-year-old male underwent distal pancreatectomy with splenectomy for treatment of pancreatic neuroendocrine tumor. In the immediate postoperative period, patient developed a pancreatic fluid leak from the tail of pancreas and an intra-abdominal drain was placed that was removed after it stopped draining. CT scan showed interval increase in the size of the rim enhancing fluid collection around tail of pancreas 1 month after drain removal (Figure 4). ERCP was performed for suspected pancreatic duct (PD) leak and confirmed a leak from the tail of the pancreas. Endoscopic pancreatic sphincterotomy was done with placement of a 5 Fr x 13 cm pancreatic duct stent with internal barbs. Subsequently, EUS showed a well demarcated, hypoechoic, heterogeneous collection, adjacent to the tail of the pancreas about 6.5 cm in the largest dimension (Figure 5). Under endosonographic guidance, a 15 mm x 10 mm LAMS was placed from the stomach into the fluid collection with drainage of a large amount of pus. CT scan of abdomen after 1 month showed decrease in the size of the previously demonstrated LUQ rim-enhancing fluid collection (Figure 6). Unfortunately, patient later had a neurological event that led to his demise, prior to stent removal.

2.3. Case 3. A 34-year-old male presented to hospital after a motor vehicle accident. Patient was hypotensive on arrival and underwent exploratory laparotomy, splenectomy, embolization of hepatic vessels, and right-sided partial hepatectomy due to grade V liver laceration. Postoperatively, the patient developed bilious drainage from an intra-abdominal drain and underwent ERCP for suspected bile leak. ERCP revealed a leak from the right biliary system; therefore a 10 Fr x 5 cm plastic biliary stent was placed. A week later, the patient continued to have high output of amylase-rich fluid from a separate intra-abdominal drain which was suspicious for a pancreatic duct leak. Repeat ERCP with pancreatogram revealed a leak from the pancreatic tail for which a 5 Fr x 13 cm pancreatic duct stent was placed and the biliary stent was upsized to a 10 mm x 4 cm covered self-expanding metallic stent (SEMS) due to a persistent biliary leak.

After 1 month, the patient became septic and was found to have a peri-pancreatic abscess on CT abdomen. IR performed a percutaneous drainage of the peripancreatic abscess with minimal drainage through the drain, without any clinical improvement. EUS was then performed by one of the authors

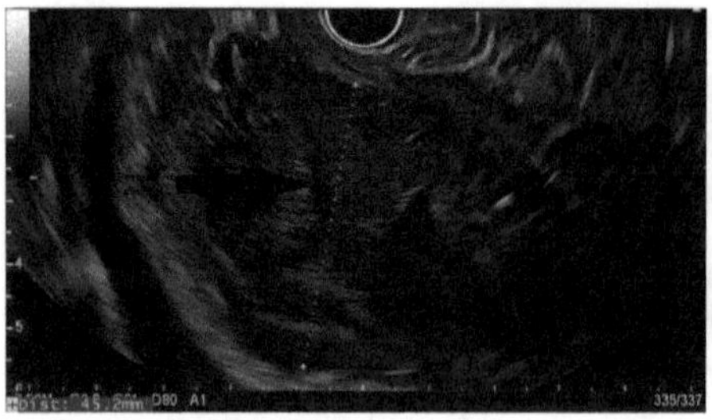

FIGURE 5: Patient 2, EUS confirming peripancreatic fluid collection around tail of pancreas.

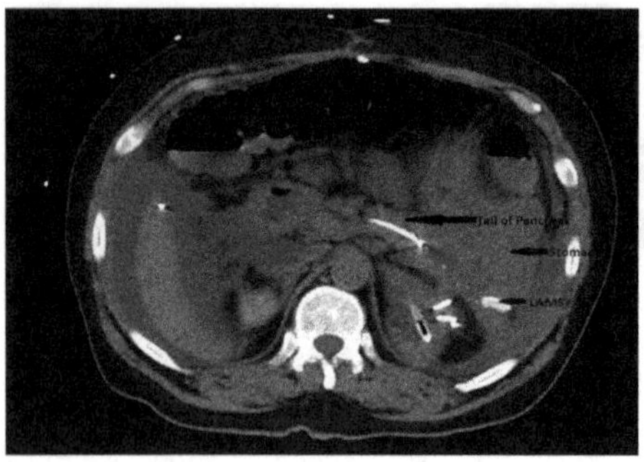

FIGURE 6: Patient 2, CT scan showing resolution of peripancreatic fluid collection.

(JN) that revealed a 55 mm, oval, heterogeneous peripancreatic fluid collection which had hyperechoic material consistent with the solid debris. A 10mm x 10mm LAMS was then placed from the stomach into the fluid collection with subsequent drainage of pus and debris. The patient clinically improved and was discharged home with improvement of the fluid collection. A follow-up CT Abdomen 4 weeks later showed interval decrease in the size of the previous small fluid collection. The LAMS was uneventfully removed endoscopically at 8 weeks after the initial placement.

3. Discussion

Current treatment options for postoperative fluid collections include percutaneous drainage, EUS-guided drainage, and open surgical drainage. Of these, PCD is the current standard of care. Despite its success rate of more than 80%, PCD has numerous disadvantages. Although good results can be achieved with surgery, it is not preferred these days due to relatively higher morbidity and costs [8]. Increasing evidence is accumulating in the literature suggesting EUS-GD as an attractive first-line option due to limitations of PCD.

Limitations of PCD include higher costs compared to EUS-GD due to need for regular monitoring by health care providers, tendency to get obstructed, repeated need for use of disposable health supplies, increased radiation from multiple CT scans, and longer median hospital stay [9–11]. Significant fluid and electrolyte losses, risk of infection, increased morbidity and patient discomfort with an external drain, need for frequent repositioning and drain exchanges, need for repeated drain flushing to maintain patency, and increased risk of long term cutaneous fistula and thereby leading to worse quality of life for patients are some of other disadvantages of PCD [9, 10, 12]. In addition, not all collections are accessible through PCD and PCD could be less successful in infected collections.

3.1. Use of Stents for Drainage of PSFC (Table 1). Currently, there are a large number of studies supporting the use of stents in the treatment of pancreatic pseudocysts and WON [3, 4, 13–15]. Most of the earlier studies involving PSFC treatment have used DPS [6, 7]. More recently, LAMS have been used for a variety of indications including biliary drainage, gallbladder drainage, gastrojejunostomy in gastric outlet obstruction (GOO), EUS-directed transgastric ERCP, drainage of liver abscess, mediastinal abscess, and malignant fluid collections [16–19]. LAMS address the need for larger diameter lumens which can provide direct endoscopic access into a cyst cavity and provide adequate drainage. Specifically, it is becoming more preferred by endoscopists for cystogastrostomy and pancreatic necrosectomy procedures [4, 5].

There are multiple studies in the literature supporting successful use of LAMS for pancreatic fluid collections drainage, but the only study that is available at this time for the use of LAMS in PSFCs of all etiologies is a US multicentre, retrospective analysis of 47 patients by Mudireddy et al. [5]. The authors concluded that the use of LAMS for PSFCs is an attractive alternative option to surgery or PCD for collections situated close to stomach, duodenum, and rectum. The characteristics of collections in this series were inflammation (n=24), abscesses (n=19), and bilomas (n=4). This is similar to our patients who had perigastric abscesses and excellent resolution of abscess cavities was noted. In this study, the clinical success rates were different depending on the site of LAMS placement with highest success rates with transgastric (91.2%), followed by transrectal (87.5%) and then transduodenal (80%) [5]. Notably, the technical and clinical success rates in postpancreatic surgery collections were higher at 100% and 96%, respectively. Another subgroup with high technical and clinical success rates in this study was pelvic fluid collections, which could be attributed to large inner diameter of LAMS allowing better drainage without catheter placement, less chance for stent obstruction by fecal matter, and ability to do debridement as needed [5].

LAMS has many potential advantages compared to plastic stents in PSFC drainage including obviating the need for fluoroscopic guidance as the stent is well visualized under EUS. The possibility of performing the entire procedure under EUS guidance alone is a major advance in therapeutic endoscopy. LAMS are also technically easier to deploy and extract thereby reducing the procedure time and has higher technical success rates [20, 21]. There is reduced risk of leakage with LAMS compared to plastic stents. Due to dual flange anchors and fully covered nature of LAMS, close apposition between the collection and GI lumen can be created minimizing the risk of leakage of secretions into the peritoneum. Saddle shaped design of LAMS makes it less prone to stent migration. LAMS may be more useful in the presence of necrosis due to their wider lumen especially with newer 20 mm diameter stent and providing the endoscopist

Table 1

Authors, Year, Place	Number of patients, Study design	Indication	Stent type and route, size	Average size of collection Success rate (TS, CS)	Time to resolution (TRL) and stent removal (TRO)	Average follow up	Complication rate	Complications
Mudireddy et al. 2018 US	Multi center, retro spective, n=47	Pancreatic surgery Extra pancreatic surgery Previous failed PCD or surgical drainage (13/47)	LAMS Hot 76% Cold 24% TG 72% TR 17% TD 11% 15mm 70% 10 mm 30%	78.6 mm TS-93.6% (overall) TS- 100% (pancreatic) CS-89.3% (overall) CS- 96% (pancreatic) Necrosectomy 6	TRL- 27.4 d TRO- 36 d	1-8 weeks	Intra-procedural 4.25% Post-procedural 6.4%	Intra-procedural Stent mis deployment N=2, Post procedural Perforation, N=1 Stent migration N=1 Infection N=1
Donatelli et al 2017	Single center, Retrospective, N=32	Post pancreatic N=10 (31%)	DPS	TS 100% CS 93.4%		13.5 months	Immediate 12.5 %	Bleeding N=1 Stent migration N=3(all rectal)
Tellez-Avilla 2015	Retrospective N=43	Pancreatic 4/13 (30.8%) Prior PCD 2/13	DPS Mean size 6.5 cm TG 87.5% TD 12.5 %	TS 100% CS 100%			None	
Gupta 2012 Europe	Retrospective, N=43	Pancreatic surg 57% Extrapancreatic surgery Previous failed PCD or surgical drainage 13/47	DPS TG 85.7% TD 6%	TS CS 80% -8 weeks CS 90% later follow up		60 weeks	14.6%	Early: Bleeding N=4 Stent migration Late: Colonic fistula N=1
Azeem 2012 Mayo	Retrospective, Total N=48 PCD N= 33 EUS GD N=15	Post pancreatic tail resection	DPS FCSEMS(n=1) TP 12/21 TG 13 /21 TD 3/21 Debridement 2/48	7 cm TS 100% CS 80%			9.6%	Delayed bleeding n=2 Stent migration n=1
Varadarajulu 2009 Alabama	Prospective, case series. N=10	Post-distal pancreatectomy Prior PCD N=1	DPS TG 9 /10 TO 1/10	91.4mm TS 100% CS 90%	TRL 8 wk TRO 8 wk	151		Stent migration n=1
Varadarajulu, 2011 Alabama	Retrospective, N=20	Post-distal pancreatectomy Prior PCD or pancreatic stents 10/20	DPS TG 85% TO 15%	78.5 mm TS 100% CS 100%		199 days	None	

Table 1: Continued.

Authors, Year, Place	**Number of patients, Study design**	**Indication**	**Stent type and route, size**	**Average size of collection Success rate (TS, CS)**	**Time to resolution (TRL) and stent removal (TRO)**	**Average follow up**	**Complication rate**	**Complications**
Kwon 2013 MSKCC	Retrospective Total N=23 PCD N= 12 EUS –GD N= 9 including (3 with prev PCD)	Post-distal pancreatectomy Previous PCD 3/23	DPPS TG Necrosectomy 4/12	89 mm TS 100% CS 100%	TRL 57 days			Intra-procedural none Post-procedure Small bowel obstruction N=1 Bleeding gastric ulcer N=1

TS: technical success, CS: clinical success, TRL: time to resolution, TRO: time to removal, PCD: percutaneous drainage, LAMS: lumen-apposing metal stent, TG: transgastric, TD: transduodenal, TR: transrectal, TO: transesophageal, DPS: double pigtail stent, FCSEMS: fully covered self-expanding metal stent, and EUS-GD: endoscopic ultrasound-guided drainage.

with direct access for necrosectomy [4, 11]. Superior success rate of LAMS for transrectal drainage of PSFCs was found in one study [7]. Due to the frequent coexistence of solid necrotic component inside the cavity in transrectal fluid collections, these authors did not achieve satisfactory results with the use of DPS and switched to LAMS deployment after the first six cases that were included in their study.

The drawbacks of LAMS include paucity of experience in the use of these stents but that is changing quickly with the wider acceptance of this stent. Higher costs of LAMS at the time of placement is a deterrent compared to PCD [10]. Secondly, due to their wider lumens, LAMS may be more prone to occlusion by necrotic debris and food, thereby increasing the risk of secondary infection. A possible solution to this situation is placement of multiple pigtail stents simultaneously within the lumen of metal cystogastrostomy stents thereby making it difficult for solid particles to pass while continuing to allow for drainage of liquid secretions around the pigtail stents [11, 17]. In addition, LAMS were also found to be associated with higher bleeding rate, including late bleeding at 3-5 weeks in the treatment of postpancreatitis pancreatic fluid collections [22]. EUS guidance with the use of Color Doppler may reduce the risk of intraprocedural bleeding but would not affect delayed bleeding [7]. One hypothesis is that LAMS remained in place even after collapse of the collection without any movement and this causes friction to surrounding vasculature around the necrotic cavity causing increased propensity to bleed [22]. This prompted these authors to change their practice of repeating imaging at 3 weeks to assess the cavity resolution instead of 6 weeks, followed by stent removal if the fluid collection is resolved. Another explanation for increased bleeding events with the use of LAMS is the easier access of low pH fluid with gastric acid into the cyst cavity due to wider lumen of LAMS, thereby causing irritation of exposed intracavitary vessels and increased tendency for bleeding [23]. Notably, no bleeding events were seen in the only study available in the literature on the use of LAMS in PSFCs [5].

Stent migration (both spontaneous and during direct necrosectomy) has also been noted with LAMS possibly due to rapid decompression of cysts with LAMS [14]. Maldeployment of stent was also noted by Siddiqui et al. [4]. In another study of LAMS use in pancreatic collections, pneumoperitoneum and perforation was also reported [5]. Another risk of LAMS is buried stent syndrome usually seen at 3-4 months after placement. LAMS are fairly short (10mm) and immobile. After resolution of PSFCs, due to its lumen apposing nature, the stent may get deeply embedded in the gastric wall with mucosal overgrowth and its removal may be technically challenging requiring an additional endoscopic procedure with sedation [22].

Finally, authors acknowledge that although the procedure was technically successful in all the cases, the final outcome of the patients did not improve in 2 out of the 3 cases, primarily due to the underlying diagnosis of malignancy that adversely affected their prognosis. Therefore, appropriate patient selection is very important in deciding who would benefit from the procedure.

3.2. Conclusions and Future Directions. In conclusion, EUS-GD using LAMS is an equally effective but safer and cost-efficient alternative to PCD for treatment of PSFCs. With the increased availability of forward viewing echoendoscopes, the therapeutic possibilities have increased including accessing perisplenic collections and collections around modified anatomy such as Roux-en–Y gastric bypass. With availability of 20 mm diameter LAMS, the efficacy of drainage of PSFCs may even improve further. Further studies for PSFC treatment with EUS-GD using LAMS are warranted for understanding their full scope of use and possibly becoming an established standard of care.

References

[1] I. Marano, P. P. Mainenti, G. Selva, M. Cannavale, and A. Sodano, "CT-guided percutaneous aspiration and drainage of postoperative abdominal fluid collections," *La Radiologia Medica*, vol. 97, no. 3, pp. 160–165, 1999.

[2] F. Téllez-Ávila, G. J. Carmona-Aguilera, F. Valdovinos-Andraca et al., "Postoperative abdominal collections drainage: Percutaneous versus guided by endoscopic ultrasound," *Digestive Endoscopy*, vol. 27, no. 7, pp. 762–766, 2015.

[3] R. Z. Sharaiha, A. Tyberg, M. A. Khashab et al., "Endoscopic therapy with lumen-apposing metal stents is safe and effective for patients with pancreatic walled-off necrosis," *Clinical Gastroenterology and Hepatology*, vol. 14, no. 12, pp. 1797–1803, 2016.

[4] A. A. Siddiqui, T. E. Kowalski, D. E. Loren et al., "Fully covered self-expanding metal stents versus lumen-apposing fully covered self-expanding metal stent versus plastic stents for endoscopic drainage of pancreatic walled-off necrosis: clinical outcomes and success," *Gastrointestinal Endoscopy*, vol. 85, no. 4, pp. 758–765, 2017.

[5] P. R. Mudireddy, A. Sethi, A. A. Siddiqui et al., "EUS-guided drainage of postsurgical fluid collections using lumen-apposing metal stents: A multicenter study," *Gastrointestinal Endoscopy*, 2017.

[6] T. Gupta, A. Lemmers, D. Tan, M. Ibrahim, O. Le Moine, and J. Devière, "EUS-guided transmural drainage of postoperative collections," *Gastrointestinal Endoscopy*, vol. 76, no. 6, pp. 1259–1265, 2012.

[7] G. Donatelli, J.-. L. Dumont, F. Cereatti et al., "EUS-guided transrectal evacuation of organized pelvic collection following roux-en-y gastric bypass after failure of radiological and surgical approach," *Obesity Surgery*, vol. 28, no. 2, pp. 595-596, 2018.

[8] C. G. Cronin, D. A. Gervais, C. Fernandez-Del Castillo, P. R. Mueller, and R. S. Arellano, "Interventional radiology in the management of abdominal collections after distal pancreatectomy: A retrospective review," *American Journal of Roentgenology*, vol. 197, no. 1, pp. 241–246, 2011.

[9] A. Tilara, H. Gerdes, P. Allen et al., "Endoscopic ultrasound-guided transmural drainage of postoperative pancreatic collections," *Journal of the American College of Surgeons*, vol. 218, no. 1, pp. 33–40, 2014.

[10] N. Azeem, T. H. Baron, M. D. Topazian, N. Zhong, C. J. Fleming, and M. L. Kendrick, "Outcomes of endoscopic and percutaneous drainage of pancreatic fluid collections arising after pancreatic tail resection," *Journal of the American College of Surgeons*, vol. 215, no. 2, pp. 177–185, 2012.

[11] Y. M. Kwon, H. Gerdes, M. A. Schattner et al., "Management of peripancreatic fluid collections following partial pancreatectomy: A comparison of percutaneous versus EUS-guided drainage," *Surgical Endoscopy*, vol. 27, no. 7, pp. 2422–2427, 2013.

[12] S. Varadarajulu, J. M. Trevino, and J. D. Christein, "EUS for the management of peripancreatic fluid collections after distal pancreatectomy," *Gastrointestinal Endoscopy*, vol. 70, no. 6, pp. 1260–1265, 2009.

[13] R. J. Shah, J. N. Shah, I. Waxman et al., "Safety and efficacy of endoscopic ultrasound-guided drainage of pancreatic fluid collections with lumen-apposing covered self-expanding metal stents," *Clinical Gastroenterology and Hepatology*, vol. 13, no. 4, pp. 747–752, 2015.

[14] S. Chandran, M. Efthymiou, A. Kaffes et al., "Management of pancreatic collections with a novel endoscopically placed fully covered self-expandable metal stent: A national experience (with videos)," *Gastrointestinal Endoscopy*, vol. 81, no. 1, pp. 127–135, 2015.

[15] E. Rinninella, R. Kunda, M. Dollhopf et al., "EUS-guided drainage of pancreatic fluid collections using a novel lumen-apposing metal stent on an electrocautery-enhanced delivery system: a large retrospective study (with video)," *Gastrointestinal Endoscopy*, vol. 82, no. 6, pp. 1039–1046, 2015.

[16] J. S. Bank, "Lumen apposing metal stents: A review of current uses and outcomes," in *Gastrintestinal Intervention*, D. G. Adler, Ed., vol. 6, p. 14, 9, 2017.

[17] C. Musumba, N. Tutticci, K. Nanda, and V. Kwan, "Endosonography-guided drainage of malignant fluid collections using lumen-apposing, fully covered self-expanding metal stents," *Endoscopy*, vol. 46, no. 8, pp. 690–692, 2014.

[18] C. F. Consiglieri, I. Escobar, and J. B. Gornals, "EUS-guided transesophageal drainage of a mediastinal abscess using a diabolo-shaped lumen-apposing metal stent," *Gastrointestinal Endoscopy*, vol. 81, no. 1, pp. 221-222, 2015.

[19] S. Varadarajulu, C. M. Wilcox, and J. D. Christein, "EUS-guided therapy for management of peripancreatic fluid collections after distal pancreatectomy in 20 consecutive patients," *Gastrointestinal Endoscopy*, vol. 74, no. 2, pp. 418–423, 2011.

[20] T. Itoi, K. F. Binmoeller, J. Shah et al., "Clinical evaluation of a novel lumen-apposing metal stent for endosonography-guided pancreatic pseudocyst and gallbladder drainage (with videos)," *Gastrointestinal Endoscopy*, vol. 75, no. 4, pp. 870–876, 2012.

[21] N. Yamamoto, H. Isayama, H. Kawakami et al., "Preliminary report on a new, fully covered, metal stent designed for the treatment of pancreatic fluid collections," *Gastrointestinal Endoscopy*, vol. 77, no. 5, pp. 809–814, 2013.

[22] J. Y. Bang, M. Hasan, U. Navaneethan, R. Hawes, and S. Varadarajulu, "Lumen-apposing metal stents (LAMS) for pancreatic fluid collection (PFC) drainage: May not be business as usual," *Gut*, vol. 66, no. 12, pp. 2054–2056, 2017.

[23] S. Seewald, T. L. Ang, H. Richter et al., "Long-term results after endoscopic drainage and necrosectomy of symptomatic pancreatic fluid collections," *Digestive Endoscopy*, vol. 24, no. 1, pp. 36–41, 2012.

Pernicious Anemia and Vitiligo in an HIV Patient: An Unfamiliar Case Presentation

Katongo Mutengo,[1] Francis Mupeta,[2] and Owen Ngalamika[3]

[1]*Department of Internal Medicine, Livingstone Central Hospital, Ministry of Health, Livingstone, Zambia*
[2]*Infectious Diseases Unit, Department of Internal Medicine, University Teaching Hospital, Lusaka, Zambia*
[3]*Dermatology and Venereology Section, University Teaching Hospital, University of Zambia, School of Medicine, Lusaka, Zambia*

Correspondence should be addressed to Owen Ngalamika; owen_ngalamika@yahoo.com

Academic Editor: Hirotada Akiho

Pernicious anemia (PA) is a rarely considered cause of anemia in HIV-infected population and is seldom on the list of differential diagnoses. However, PA can have serious consequences if misdiagnosed or left untreated. We present the case of a 38-year-old HIV-positive man who was diagnosed with PA, which was preceded by a one-year history of vitiligo. Our case is a reminder for clinicians to have a high index of suspicion for an autoimmune process as a potential cause of anemia in HIV-infected individuals.

1. Introduction

Anemia is one of the commonest presentations among human immunodeficiency virus- (HIV-) infected individuals. However, due to the diversity of etiological factors in the HIV-infected population such as poor diet, medications, secondary infections, or the virus itself, anemia is rarely attributed to an autoimmune process [1]. More so, in resource-limited settings, the high cost of workup coupled with a low index of suspicion makes it almost impossible to investigate for autoimmune causes of anemia such as PA. Yet, if left untreated, PA can have seriously debilitating effects including irreversible neurologic damage and susceptibility to gastric tumors associated with the disease [2].

Scientific evidence shows that autoimmune activation can be triggered by environmental and infectious agents [3], including HIV. But, the decline in immunity associated with HIV would often make the autoimmune process occult while the converse holds true as well [4]. Despite PA generally contributing close to 90% of vitamin B12 deficiency in Africa [5], it is rarely investigated for as a cause of vitamin B12 deficiency in the HIV population, which may present as a macrocytic anemia. In fact, extensive literature research yields scanty information on PA occurring in HIV population to date. The antipathy of PA and HIV disease processes, therefore, presents a diagnostic enigma to clinicians especially when the autoimmune process is coexisting in the setting of a low immune status. Here, we present the case of an HIV-positive Zambian man of African descent diagnosed with PA, who presented with vitiligo a year before the diagnosis of macrocytic anemia. This case highlights the need of screening for an autoimmune process as a cause of anemia even in the presence of an underlying disease with contrasting pathogenesis such as HIV.

2. Case Presentation

A 38-year-old Zambian man of African descent presented to Livingstone Central Hospital, a tertiary institution in the southern province of Zambia, with a history of spontaneous loss of skin pigmentation on the face for 20 months and progressive lethargy for 8 months. The skin hypopigmentation started as small pink patches on his cheeks and nose but progressively increased in size. He was said to be in good health, was energetic, and was able to carry out his usual activities despite the facial hypopigmentation. However, about 12 months after the onset of this condition, he described feeling weak and tired on minimal exertion such as walking a distance of about 6 meters. He, however, denied any history of constitutional symptoms, cough, body swelling, orthopnea, paroxysmal nocturnal dyspnea, or joint pains. He also denied any history of sensory paresthesias. He was diagnosed with HIV-1 about 4 years prior to presentation. However, he initially declined initiation of combined antiretroviral therapy (cART) and opted for traditional herbal medication which he took for 4 years. There was no history of any other comorbidities.

The symptoms of lethargy were ongoing for one month when he first presented to the general practitioner (GP). After a full clinical assessment, a complete blood count was done, and he was found to have a hemoglobin concentration of 6.9 g/dL with a mean cell volume (MCV) of 121 fl and mean cell hemoglobin (MCH) of 42.5 pg/cell. Other parameters on the hemogram were unremarkable. His renal biochemistry and liver biochemistry were normal. He was prescribed folic acid 5 mg once a day by his GP. He was also recounselled and initiated on cART comprising Tenofovir disoproxil fumarate 300 mg once daily, lamivudine 150 mg once daily, and dolutegravir 50 mg once daily (TLD). His baseline CD4 count at the start of cART was 350 cells/μL, and HIV viral load was 76,118 copies/ml. No further workup was done. He continued on this treatment for 7 months. However, despite this therapy, he stated that he continued getting weaker, and the weakness was throughout the day until he was no longer able to get up from his sitting position and often required help to move. He was, therefore, referred to our medical clinic for further assessment.

On examination, he was of fair nutritional status and was lethargic and breathless at rest. He could not get up from his sitting position without assistance. His blood pressure was 123/88 mmHg in an erect position, radial pulse was 112 beats per minute, respiratory rate was 24 breaths per minute, and peripheral oxygen saturation was 98% at room air. He had obvious conjunctival and palmar pallor, but there was no icterus, hyperpigmentation of palmar creases, lymphadenopathy, or peripheral edema. The oral cavity was normal. Local examination revealed hypopigmented, well-demarcated patches on the nose, lips, cheeks, eyebrows, part of the ears, and forehead in a symmetrical distribution consistent with vitiligo (Figure 1(a)). Examination of the lower limbs did not reveal any dysesthesia, proprioception disturbance, spastic paraparesis, or tetraparesis. Further systemic examination was only significant for a resting tachycardia on the cardiovascular system with a heart rate of about 110 beats per minute. Subsequent laboratory workup was noteworthy for severe macrocytic anemia with a hemoglobin level of 3.9 g/dl and MCV of 115.5 fl, very low serum vitamin B12 levels at <61 pmol/l, and positive intrinsic factor (IF) antibodies test. His repeat CD4 count was 920 cells/μL, and HIV viral load was undetectable. Endoscopy and biopsy of the gastric mucosa were not done due to nonavailability of the service at our institution at the time of presentation. A summary of laboratory results before and after treatment is shown in Table 1.

A diagnosis of pernicious anemia was made based on the results, and the patient was started on vitamin B12 (hydroxocobalamin) injections at 1000 mcg once daily for one week, followed by 1000 mcg weekly for 4 weeks and thereafter 1000 mcg once monthly for life. He was also started on prednisolone 40 mg once daily for 5 days, tapered down by 10 mg every 5 days, and finally maintained at 5 mg once daily, not exceeding 3 months. He showed marked improvement in his serum vitamin B12 levels after 3 weeks of treatment as well as improvement on his hemogram (Table 1). There was also notable repigmentation of the parts of skin affected by vitiligo (Figure 1(b)). Our patient was able to resume his normal duties 3 weeks after treatment.

3. Discussion

PA, also known as Biermer disease or Addison anemia, is an autoimmune disease presenting as vitamin B12 (cobalamin) deficiency [2]. It results from a deficiency of intrinsic factor (IF), a protein responsible for binding and transport of dietary cobalamins [2, 6]. Studies indicate that PA is the commonest cause of vitamin B12 deficiency worldwide, and in Africa, PA contributes close to 90% of vitamin B12 deficiency [5, 7]. It is, however, uncommon to find PA as a cause of vitamin B12 deficiency in HIV as was the case with our patient.

Generally, anemia in HIV is attributed to poor appetite accompanying chronic illness, coinfections such as tuberculosis, and drugs such as zidovudine, co-trimoxazole, and fluconazole commonly used in the management of HIV [1]. More so, in resource-limited settings, the diagnosis of PA is likely to be overshadowed by a low index of suspicion as well as the lack of readily available resources for investigations. With the coexistence of immunosuppressive conditions such as HIV, the suspicion index may further be masked by the fact that the two conditions require two disparate pathways for their pathogenesis.

Infections have been known to trigger immune activation leading to autoimmune diseases [3]. Therefore, HIV, as an infectious etiology can also trigger an autoimmune process. However, the decline in immunity associated with HIV would often make the autoimmune process occult [4]. It would be expected that unmasking of the autoimmune disease process would often occur after the resurgence of immunosuppressive status. In the case of PA, autoimmunity has been postulated to be initiated by pathogenic autoreactive CD4 T-lymphocytes which do not express CD25 receptors, a T-cell-activation marker expressed by regulatory T-lymphocytes. These gastric-derived pathogenic autoreactive CD4 T-lymphocytes are specifically directed against H+/K+ ATPase pump and IF [6, 8]. Large populations of these pathogenic autoreactive CD4 T-lymphocytes have been found infiltrating the gastric parietal cells in PA leading to autoimmune gastritis by promoting local cytotoxicity and B-cell immune activation [8]. This case may, therefore, shade light on immune dysregulation associated with HIV, especially that CD4 T-lymphocytes are the major target for HIV-1 infection [9]. Studies have shown that gut-associated lymphoid tissue (GALT) is a site of early viral seeding and establishment of the proviral reservoir which causes a distorted activation pattern of lymphocytes [10]. Our patient had a CD4 count of 350 cells/μL with an HIV viral load of

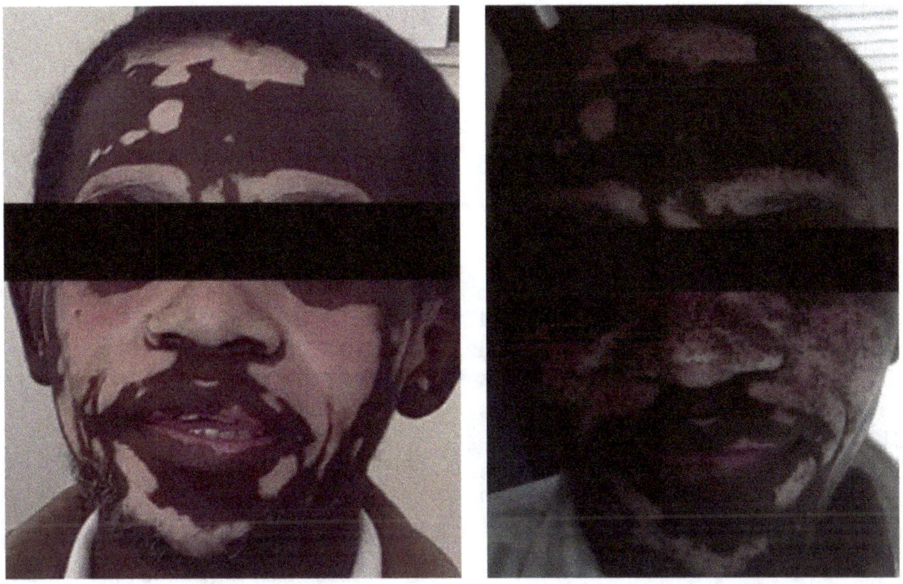

(a) (b)

FIGURE 1: (a) Before treatment with parenteral vitamin B12. Hypopigmented, well-demarcated patches on the nose, lips, cheeks, eyebrows, part of the ears, and forehead in a symmetrical distribution. (b) Repigmentation of affected parts of the skin 3 weeks after treatment.

TABLE 1: Laboratory test and results before and after treatment.

	7 months before presentation	At time of presentation	3 weeks after treatment	References
White cell count ($\times 10^9$/L)	4.1	8.0	7.7	4.0–10.0
Hemoglobin (g/dl)	*6.9	*3.9	*11.0	14.3–18.3
Mean cell volume (Fl)	*121	*155.5	*101.4	79.1–98.9
Mean corpuscular hemoglobin (pg/cell)	*42.5	*35.9	*30.5	27.0–32.0
Platelet count ($\times 10^9$/L)	288	*107	292	142–375
CD4 count (μL)	*350	920		500–1,400
Viral load (copies per ml)	76,118	Undetectable		<20
S-vitamin B12 (pmol/L)	Not done	*<61	>1476	>138
Intrinsic factor antibodies (IFA) (AU/ml)	Not done	*>153		0.93–<1.20
Parietal cell antibodies (PCA)	Not done	Negative		
TSH (μIU/mL)	Not done	2.14		0.27–4.20
FT4 (pmol/L)	Not done	15.5		10.16–22.0
FT3 (pmol/L)	Not done	5.0		2.8–12.0
Serum 9am cortisol (mmol/L)	Not done	295		101–535
Fasting blood glucose (mmol/L)	Not done	5.1		4.0–5.4

*Above or below the reference range

76,118 copies/ml when he first presented. This would place the patient in stage II HIV disease (CD4 count of 200–499 cell/μL), in which according to Zandmann-Goddard et al., autoimmune diseases are unlikely [4]. Could it be possible, therefore, that the GALT HIV-1 infected CD4 T-lymphocytes may have been the pathogenic autoreactive CD4 T-lymphocytes in this patient? Indeed, more studies are needed.

The anemia in our patient was highly attributed to PA due to positive intrinsic factor antibodies (IFA), low levels of vitamin B12, macrocytosis, and co-occurrence of vitiligo. This was further consolidated by the improvement of clinical and laboratory parameters with parenteral vitamin B12 replacement. Scientific evidence also indicates the frequent association of PA with other autoimmune diseases such as autoimmune vitiligo, thyroid disease, and type 1 diabetes [2, 11]. This could explain the presence of vitiligo in our patient. Our patient was further screened for thyroid hormone disorders, diabetes mellitus, and Addison's disease, but the tests were normal.

In the gastric mucosa of PA patients, there is a high proportion of autoreactive activated CD4+ T cells that specifically recognize intrinsic factor [2, 8]. Hence, there is a strong association between PA and autoimmune gastritis which may progress to gastric atrophy and may eventually result in malignant transformation [8, 12]. It is therefore highly recommended to perform an endoscopy and biopsy to diagnose or rule out these changes. On the other hand, *Helicobacter pylori* (*H. pylori*) infection is associated with both PA and vitamin B12 deficiency [2, 8, 13]. This association is reported to result from the triggering of autoantibodies by a mechanism of molecular mimicry. A direct test on an endoscopic biopsy would have led to the definitive diagnosis of *H. pylori* in our patient. Unfortunately, endoscopy was not available at our center at the time the patient was seen. Nevertheless, there was enough evidence to suggest a diagnosis of PA in our patient.

Our patient responded well to parenteral vitamin B12 and steroid therapy. Vitamin B12, given as hydroxocobalamin, has also been shown to reduce the gastric inflammatory process as well as retard the development of immune dysfunction associated with HIV/AIDS [14, 15]. On the other hand, short course steroid therapy was given as adjunct treatment, as it has been shown that corticosteroids improve vitamin B12 absorption by reducing gastric inflammation [16]. Steroid therapy, given as a short term course of not more than 158 days, has been known to be well tolerated and reasonably safe in HIV infection [17].

At his latest review 3 weeks later, our patient had shown great improvement in both his clinical and laboratory markers. He reported complete resolution of the clinical symptoms of anemia as well as partial repigmentation of the skin and had since gone back to his usual activities. He was counselled on the need for lifelong vitamin B12 injections and need for twice-yearly endoscopy for gastric malignancy surveillance at a different institution providing the service in a different town.

Our case is a reminder of the likely cause of macrocytic anemia in the HIV population. A perfunctory view in most of our healthcare settings showed that the immediate care plan for a patient presenting with macrocytic anemia is usually folic acid replacement as was the case with this patient. However, due to the pathophysiological basis of the disease, parenteral vitamin B12 replacement and not folate is needed in the management of PA to avert deleterious effect. To the best of our knowledge, this is the first case reported of PA in HIV infection in Zambia. We, therefore, recommend an autoimmune screen in HIV patients who present with either vitiligo alone or in combination with macrocytic anemia.

4. Conclusion

PA is a difficult autoimmune condition to diagnose as a cause of anemia especially in the setting of HIV infection. Clinicians need to have a high index of suspicion for PA in patients presenting with macrocytic anemia, as treatment will often require vitamin B12 replacement rather than folate or blood transfusion. Any delay in treatment is detrimental to the patient.

Acknowledgments

The authors wish to thank the patient for his co-operation and his relentless willingness to give all the relevant information provided in this manuscript. Without his support, this manuscript would not have been possible.

References

[1] P. S. Sullivan, D. L. Hanson, S. Y. Chu, J. L. Jones, J. W. Ward, and Adult/Adolescent Spectrum of Disease Group, "Epidemiology of anemia in human immunodeficiency virus (HIV)-infected persons: results from the multistate adult and adolescent spectrum of HIV disease surveillance project," *Blood*, vol. 91, no. 1, pp. 301–308, 1998.

[2] E. Andres and K. Serraj, "Optimal management of pernicious anemia," *Journal of Blood Medicine*, vol. 3, pp. 97–103, 2012.

[3] A. Vojdani, "A potential link between environmental triggers and autoimmunity," *Autoimmune Diseases*, vol. 2014, Article ID 437231, 18 pages, 2014.

[4] G. Zandman-Goddard and Y. Shoenfeld, "HIV and autoimmunity," *Autoimmunity Reviews*, vol. 1, no. 6, pp. 329–337, 2002.

[5] C. Maktouf, A. Bchir, H. Louzir et al., "Megaloblastic anemia in north Africa," *Haematologica*, vol. 91, no. 7, pp. 990-991, 2006.

[6] B.-H. Toh, I. R. van Driel, and P. A. Gleeson, "Pernicious anemia," *New England Journal of Medicine*, vol. 337, no. 20, pp. 1441–1448, 1997.

[7] S. P. Stabler and R. H. Allen, "Vitamin B12 deficiency as a worldwide problem," *Annual Review of Nutrition*, vol. 24, no. 1, pp. 299–326, 2004.

[8] A. Troilo, A. Grassi, L. Petrone et al., "Intrinsic factor recognition promotes T helper 17/T helper 1 autoimmune gastric inflammation in patients with pernicious anemia," *Oncotarget*, vol. 10, no. 30, pp. 2921–2929, 2019.

[9] X. Pan, H.-M. Baldauf, O. T. Keppler, and O. T. Fackler, "Restrictions to HIV-1 replication in resting CD4+ T lymphocytes," *Cell Research*, vol. 23, no. 7, pp. 876–885, 2013.

[10] A. Biancotto, S. J. Iglehart, C. Vanpouille et al., "HIV-1-induced activation of CD4+ T cells creates new targets for HIV-1 infection in human lymphoid tissue ex vivo," *Blood*, vol. 111, no. 2, pp. 699–704, 2008.

[11] A. Van den Driessche, V. Eenkhoorn, L. Van Gaal, and C. De Block, "Type 1 diabetes and autoimmune polyglandular syndrome: a clinical review," *The Netherlands Journal of Medicine*, vol. 67, no. 11, pp. 376–387, 2009.

[12] T. Banhock, I. R. V. Driel, and P. A. Gleeson, *Mechanisms of Disease Pernicious Anemia*, Vol. 337, Massachusetts Medical Society, MA, USA, 1997.

[13] H. B. Gowdappa, M. Mahesh, K. V. K. S. N. Murthy, and M. G. Narahari, "*Helicobacter pylori* associated vitamin B12 deficiency, pernicious anaemia and subacute combined degeneration of the spinal cord," *Case Reports*, vol. 2013, no. sep29 1, Article ID bcr2013200380, 2013.

[14] T. R. Elliott and A. L. Guildford, "An in vitro model of gastric inflammation and treatment with cobalamin," *International Journal of Inflammation*, vol. 2017, Article ID 5968618, 8 pages, 2017.

[15] B. Liang, S. Chung, M. Araghiniknam, L. C. Lane, and R. R. Watson, "Vitamins and immunomodulation in AIDS," *Nutrition*, vol. 12, no. 1, pp. 1–7, 1996.

[16] S. Ardeman and I. Chanarin, "Steroids and addisonian pernicious anemia," *New England Journal of Medicine*, vol. 273, no. 25, pp. 1352–1355, 1965.

[17] G. A. McComsey, C. C. Whalen, S. D. Mawhorter et al., "Placebo-controlled trial of prednisone in advanced HIV-1 infection," *AIDS*, vol. 15, no. 3, pp. 321–327, 2001.

30

Intestinal Diffuse Large B-Cell Lymphoma in a Patient with Systemic Lupus Erythematosus

Masaya Iwamuro,[1] Takahide Takahashi,[2] Yoko Ota,[3] Takehiro Tanaka,[4] Noboru Asada,[5] Shuya Yano,[6] Mayu Uka,[7] Rei Nakamura,[8] Yuki Baba,[1] Seiji Kawano,[1] Yoshiro Kawahara,[9] and Hiroyuki Okada[1]

[1]*Department of Gastroenterology and Hepatology, Okayama University Graduate School of Medicine, Dentistry, and Pharmaceutical Sciences, Okayama 700-8558, Japan*
[2]*Division of Medical Support, Okayama University Hospital, Okayama 700-8558, Japan*
[3]*Department of Pathology & Experimental Medicine, Okayama University Graduate School of Medicine, Dentistry, and Pharmaceutical Sciences, Okayama 700-8558, Japan*
[4]*Department of Pathology, Okayama University Graduate School of Medicine, Dentistry, and Pharmaceutical Sciences, Okayama 700-8558, Japan*
[5]*Department of Hematology and Oncology, Okayama University Hospital, Okayama 700-8558, Japan*
[6]*Department of Gastroenterological Surgery, Okayama University Graduate School of Medicine, Dentistry, and Pharmaceutical Sciences, Okayama 700-8558, Japan*
[7]*Department of Radiology, Okayama University Hospital, Okayama 700-8558, Japan*
[8]*Department of Nephrology, Rheumatology, Endocrinology and Metabolism, Okayama University Graduate School of Medicine, Dentistry, and Pharmaceutical Sciences, Okayama 700-8558, Japan*
[9]*Department of Practical Gastrointestinal Endoscopy, Okayama University Hospital, Okayama 700-8558, Japan*

Correspondence should be addressed to Masaya Iwamuro; pr145h2k@okayama-u.ac.jp

Academic Editor: Yoshihiro Moriwaki

A 44-year-old Japanese woman with systemic lupus erythematosus (SLE) presented to our hospital with abdominal pain. Radiological and endoscopic examinations led to the diagnosis of diffuse large B-cell lymphoma of the jejunum, which was subsequently resected. Patients with SLE reportedly have an increased risk of non-Hodgkin lymphoma, as demonstrated by our patient. Hence, lymphoma should be considered in the differential diagnosis of neoplastic lesions emerging in SLE patients. In addition, flow cytometry using endoscopically biopsied fragments is useful for the immediate diagnosis of lymphoma, leading to timely and accurate preoperative staging.

1. Introduction

Systemic lupus erythematosus (SLE) is a multifactorial autoimmune disease that affects various organs in the body. SLE occasionally affects the gastrointestinal tract, leading to bowel wall thickening, hemorrhage, obstruction, perforation, infarction, or pancreatitis owing to serositis and mesenteric vasculitis [1, 2]. In addition to inflammation, SLE is reportedly linked to an increased risk of malignant diseases such as cancers of the esophagus, stomach, hepatobiliary complex, cervix, vagina/vulva, kidney, bladder, lung, oropharynx, larynx, skin, and thyroid [3–5]. SLE patients have a particularly increased risk of lymphoproliferative disorders. Malignant diseases are one of the major causes of morbidity and mortality in SLE patients, and prompt diagnosis and treatment are keys to their successful management.

We report a case of an SLE patient who presented with postprandial abdominal pain. Radiological, endoscopic, and pathological examinations led to the diagnosis of diffuse large B-cell lymphoma in the jejunum. Of note, double balloon enteroscopy and flow cytometry analysis using endoscopically biopsied fragments were useful for the immediate diagnosis of lymphoma, leading to timely and accurate preoperative staging.

2. Case Presentation

A 44-year-old Japanese woman presented with postprandial abdominal pain since 2 months. She had been diagnosed with SLE at the age of 37 years. The patient also had lupus nephritis, Basedow's disease, steroid diabetes, idiopathic thrombocytopenic purpura, and hypertension, for which she had been taking tacrolimus, azathioprine, hydroxychloroquine, prednisolone (10 mg/day), nifedipine, eplerenone, hydralazine, lansoprazole, propylthiouracil, alfacalcidol, and sodium ferrous citrate. She was a social drinker and an ex-smoker who smoked 30 cigarettes/day for 10 years. On examination, her body temperature was 36.7°C, blood pressure was 123/80 mmHg, and pulse rate was 103 bpm. Her height was 148.5 cm and weight was 42.4 kg. Physical examination revealed conjunctival anemia, exophthalmos, enlarged thyroid, and distended abdomen with hyperactive bowel sounds, but there was no palpable mass or tenderness in her abdomen. Laboratory tests showed decreased values for hemoglobin concentration (9.0 g/dL) and hematocrit (28.3%). The C-reactive protein (4.11 mg/dL), erythrocyte sedimentation rate (104 mm/h), and soluble interleukin-2 receptor (779 U/mL) levels were elevated. The white blood cells, platelets, lactate dehydrogenase, creatine phosphokinase, anti-double stranded DNA IgG antibody, complements, carcinoembryonic antigen, and carbohydrate antigen 19–9 were within the normal range. Urinalysis revealed proteinuria, leukocytes (20–29 cells/high power field), and tubular epithelium. Hematuria was absent.

Computed tomography scanning showed whole circumferential thickening of the jejunum with aneurysmal dilatation, which is a typical feature of malignant lymphomas of the intestine (Figure 1). On positron emission tomography scanning, tracer uptake was observed in the thickened intestinal wall (Figure 2). Double balloon enteroscopy revealed circumferential ulcer and necrotic debris in the jejunum (Figure 3). A contrast study during enteroscopy showed dilated jejunal lumen (Figure 4). Based on the morphology of the jejunal lesion, we suspected small intestinal lymphoma rather than cancer. Thus, we performed flow cytometry analysis with 2 endoscopically biopsied fragments, as described previously (Figure 5) [6]. The κ/λ ratio of CD19 + CD20+ cells was 3.3 (53.36/16.39), indicating monoclonal proliferation of the B cells producing the κ light chain. The isolated cells were negative for CD5 and CD10 on flow cytometry analysis. Bone marrow biopsy and cytology revealed no lymphoma cell invasion. Biopsy of the jejunal lesion showed infiltration of atypical, large lymphoid cells that were positive for CD20 and BCL2 and negative for CD3, CD5, CD10, and cMYC (Figure 6). The cells were diffusely positive for Ki-67. The results of in situ hybridization for Epstein–Barr virus-encoded small RNA-1 were also positive. The jejunal tumor, which had invaded the transverse colon, was surgically resected. Lymphadenopathies of the mesentery were observed intraoperatively. Consequently, a diagnosis of diffuse large B-cell lymphoma in the jejunum at stage II_{1E} (large intestine) was made. Chemotherapy with cyclophosphamide, adriamycin, vincristine, and prednisone plus rituximab was administered postoperatively.

3. Discussion

Patients with SLE and other rheumatic diseases have an increased risk of malignant diseases, of which lymphoma is the most common neoplasm [7–9]. A nationwide population-based study in Taiwan revealed that among the 16,417 patients with SLE, 512 developed cancers (3.1%), including 34 with non-Hodgkin lymphoma (0.2%) [10]. The standardized incidence ratio was the highest for non-Hodgkin lymphoma (4.2, 95% CI: 2.9–5.9) on site-specific cancer risk analysis. A meta-analysis also showed that the pooled standardized incidence ratio for non-Hodgkin lymphoma in patients with SLE was 4.93 (95% CI: 3.81–6.36). SLE is considered to be correlated with an increased risk of non-Hodgkin lymphoma, and the risk is estimated to be 4–7 times greater than that in the general population [7]. In addition, diffuse large B-cell lymphoma is the most common subtype of lymphoma, accounting for 37–62% of all lymphomas in SLE patients [11–13]. Therefore, diffuse large B-cell lymphoma should be considered a probable diagnosis when tumorous lesions are found in patients with SLE.

Several mechanisms can be hypothesized in the pathogenesis of non-Hodgkin lymphoma in SLE patients. First, chronic inflammation may lead to hyperactivity and proliferation of B lymphocytes, resulting in autonomous, monoclonal expansion [14]. Second, dysregulation of the immune system may cause a defective clearance of apoptotic cells [7, 15]. Third, it has been reported that immunosuppressants such as cyclophosphamide are partly responsible for the increased incidence of lymphoma in patients with SLE [16]. Fourth, the Epstein–Barr virus infection may be a common trigger factor for SLE and non-Hodgkin lymphoma [10]. Previous studies have revealed that patients with SLE have an elevated viral load, increased Epstein–Barr virus mRNA expression, elevated levels of Epstein–Barr virus-directed antibodies, and decreased cell-mediated immunity against the virus when compared to healthy controls [17]. The Epstein–Barr virus infection results in the production of the viral protein "Epstein–Barr virus nuclear antigen-1" (EBNA-1). Antibodies against EBNA-1 cross react with the autoantigens found in SLE, including Ro, Sm B/B′, and Sm D1 [18]. Thus, molecular mimicry may play a crucial role in the pathogenesis of SLE. Simultaneously, the Epstein–Barr virus can also promote lymphomagenesis [19]. We believed that the Epstein–Barr virus played a pivotal role in the development of diffuse large B-cell lymphoma in our patient because the in situ hybridization for Epstein–Barr virus-encoded small RNA-1 was positive.

It was also noteworthy that flow cytometry analysis using 2 endoscopically biopsied fragments was useful for the prompt diagnosis of lymphoma in our patient. Since B-cell lymphomas typically arise from a massive expansion of a B-cell clone,

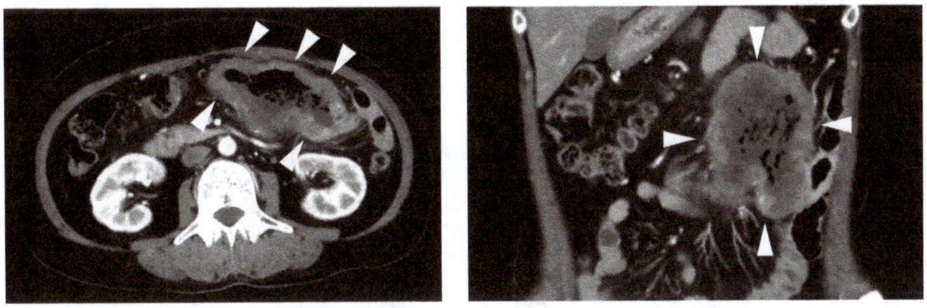

(a) (b)

FIGURE 1: Computed tomography scanning images. Whole circumferential thickening of the jejunum is shown (arrows) (a), (b).

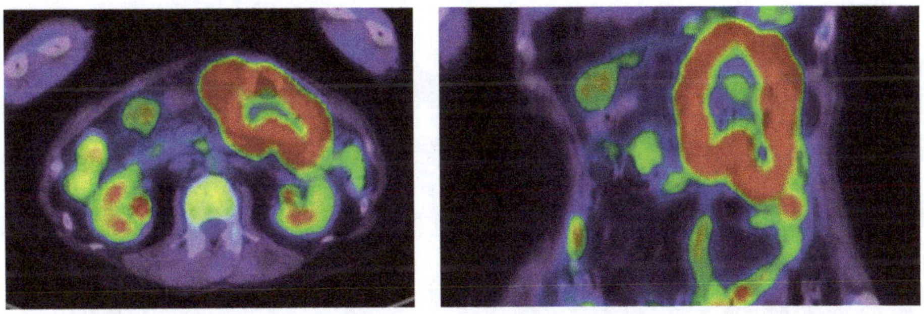

(a) (b)

FIGURE 2: Positron emission tomography scanning images. Tracer uptake is observed in the thickened intestinal wall.

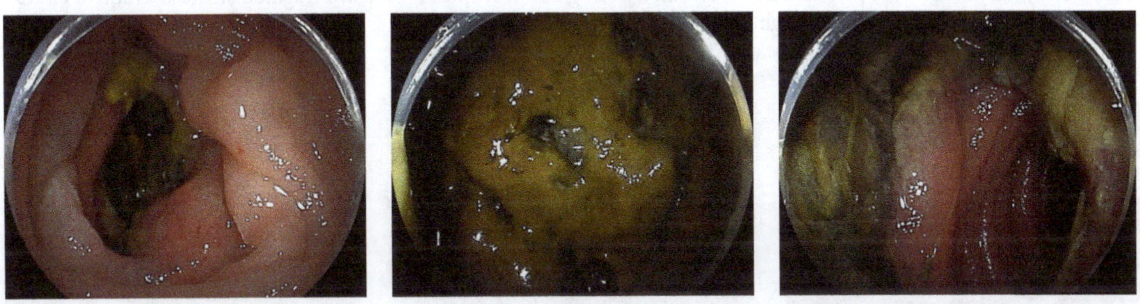

(a) (b) (c)

FIGURE 3: Double balloon enteroscopy images. A circumferential ulcer with necrotic debris in the jejunum is shown.

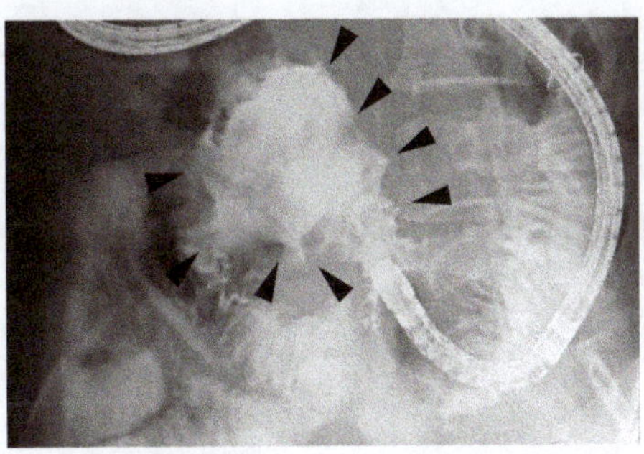

FIGURE 4: A contrast study image during enteroscopy. An irregularly dilated jejunal lumen is observed (arrows).

neoplastic cells express only 1 class of immunoglobulin light chain, which is either κ or λ chain. Thus, immunoglobulin light-chain expression can be used as a surrogate marker for clonality. However, flow cytometry has not been widely used in routine clinical practice for the diagnosis of gastrointestinal lymphoma, mainly because an appropriate protocol is absent. We have recently established lymphocyte isolation techniques and revealed that light chain expression analysis could be performed with 2 endoscopic biopsy fragments obtained from 10 patients (6). Although pathological analysis is still a standard for the diagnosis of lymphoma subtype, flow cytometry analysis has the advantage of delivering faster results; while several

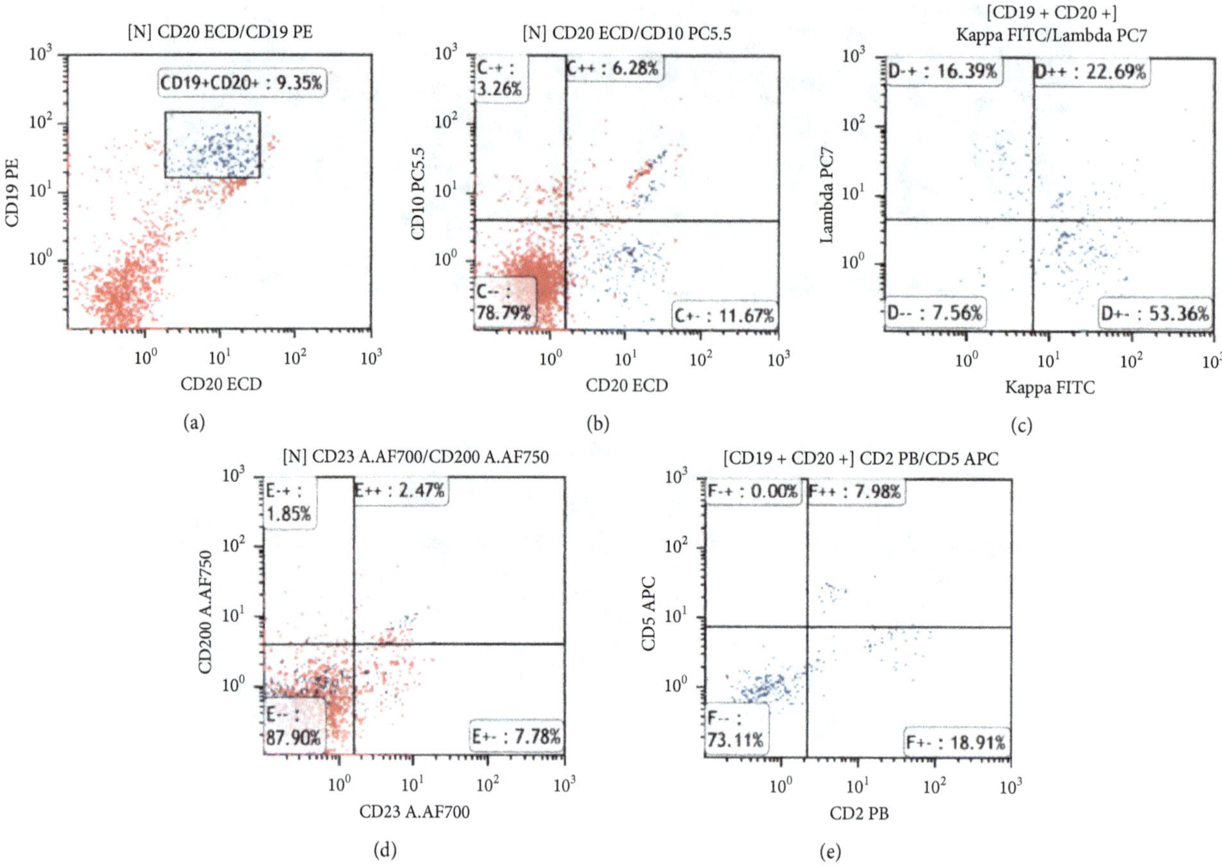

FIGURE 5: Flow cytometry results. We performed flow cytometry using 2 endoscopically biopsied fragments. The κ/λ ratio of CD19+/CD20+ cells is 3.3 (53.36/16.39), indicating positive light chain restriction.

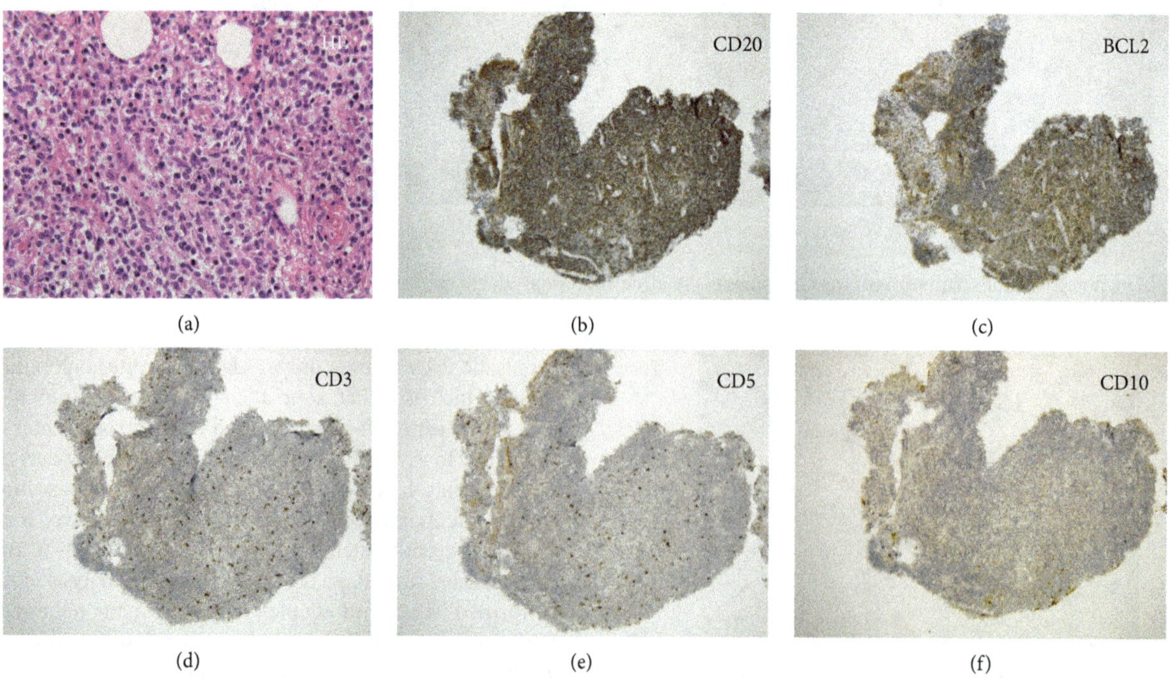

FIGURE 6: Continued.

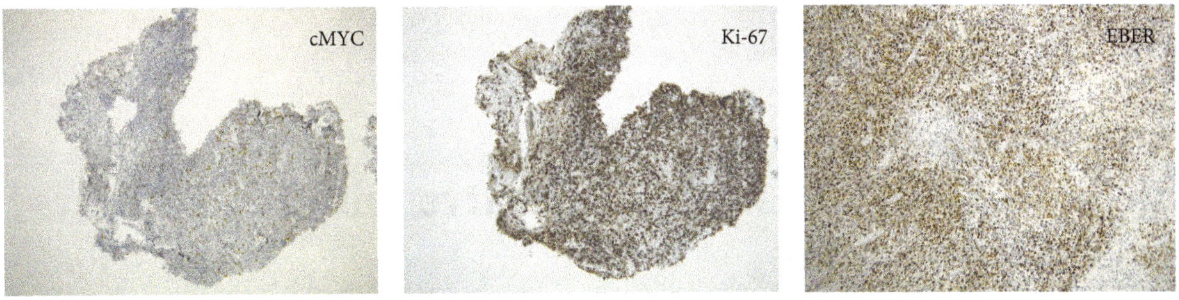

Figure 6: Pathological images. Infiltration of atypical, large lymphoid cells is seen in the endoscopic biopsy specimens (a): Hematoxylin-eosin stain. Lymphoma cells are positive for CD20 (b) and BCL2 (c), while they are negative for CD3 (d), CD5 (e), CD10 (f), and cMYC (g). The cells are diffusely positive for Ki-67 (h). The results of in situ hybridization for Epstein–Barr virus-encoded small RNA-1 (EBER) are also positive (i).

hours are required to obtain the results of flow cytometric analysis, and histological analysis with immunostaining generally takes days to weeks. Based on the flow cytometry results of our patient, we consulted with hematologists on the following day and performed bone marrow aspiration and biopsy 2 days after the endoscopy, resulting in timely preoperative diagnosis.

In conclusion, we encountered an SLE patient with diffuse large B-cell lymphoma in the jejunum. This case reinforces that lymphoma should be considered in the differential diagnosis of neoplastic lesions emerging in SLE patients. Moreover, flow cytometry analysis is useful in making a timely diagnosis of gastrointestinal lymphoma.

References

[1] C.-K. Lee, M. S. Ahn, E. Y. Lee et al., "Acute abdominal pain in systemic lupus erythematosus: focus on lupus enteritis (gastrointestinal vasculitis)," *Annals of the Rheumatic Diseases*, vol. 61, no. 6, pp. 547–550, 2002.

[2] D.-K. Chang, D.-H. Yoo, T.-H. Kim et al., "Burkitt's lymphoma presenting as ileocaecal intussusception in systemic lupus erythematosus," *Clinical Rheumatology*, vol. 18, no. 3, pp. 253–256, 1999.

[3] L. Song, Y. Wang, J. Zhang, N. Song, X. Xu, and Y. Lu, "The risks of cancer development in systemic lupus erythematosus (SLE) patients: a systematic review and meta-analysis," *Arthritis Research & Therapy*, vol. 20, no. 1, p. 270, 2018.

[4] M. Abu-Shakra, D. D. Gladman, and M. B. Urowitz, "Malignancy in systemic lupus erythematosus," *Arthritis & Rheumatism*, vol. 39, no. 6, pp. 1050–1054, 1996.

[5] L. Mellemkjaer, V. Andersen, M. S. Linet, G. Gridley, R. Hoover, and J. H. Olsen, "Non-Hodgkin's lymphoma and other cancers among a cohort of patients with systemic lupus erythematosus," *Arthritis & Rheumatology*, vol. 40, no. 4, pp. 761–768, 1997.

[6] K. Matsueda, M. Iwamuro, T. Takahashi et al., "Feasibility of flow cytometric analysis of restricted light chain in endoscopic biopsy specimens from patients with gastrointestinal tract B cell lymphoma: a pilot study," *BMC Research Notes*, vol. 12, no. 1, p. 571, 2019.

[7] A. Klein, A. Polliack, and A. Gafter-Gvili, "Systemic lupus erythematosus and lymphoma: incidence, pathogenesis and biology," *Leukemia Research*, vol. 75, pp. 45–49, 2018.

[8] S. Bernatsky, J. F. Boivin, L. Joseph et al., "An international cohort study of cancer in systemic lupus erythematosus," *Arthritis & Rheumatism*, vol. 52, no. 5, pp. 1481–1490, 2005.

[9] L. Cao, H. Tong, G. Xu et al., "Systemic lupus erythematous and malignancy risk: a meta-analysis," *PLoS One*, vol. 10, no. 4, Article ID e0122964, 2015.

[10] L.-H. Wang, W.-M. Wang, S.-H. Lin, and C.-C. Shieh, "Bidirectional relationship between systemic lupus erythematosus and non-Hodgkin's lymphoma: a nationwide population-based study," *Rheumatology*, vol. 58, no. 7, pp. 1245–1249, 2019.

[11] K. Ekström Smedby, C. M. Vajdic, M. Falster et al., "Autoimmune disorders and risk of non-Hodgkin lymphoma subtypes: a pooled analysis within the InterLymph Consortium," *Blood*, vol. 111, no. 8, pp. 4029–4038, 2008.

[12] J. K. King and K. H. Costenbader, "Characteristics of patients with systemic lupus erythematosus (SLE) and non-Hodgkin's lymphoma (NHL)," *Clinical Rheumatology*, vol. 26, no. 9, pp. 1491–1494, 2007.

[13] S. Bernatsky, R. Ramsey-Goldman, R. Rajan et al., "Non-Hodgkin's lymphoma in systemic lupus erythematosus," *Annals of the Rheumatic Diseases*, vol. 64, no. 10, pp. 1507–1509, 2005.

[14] O. Sela and Y. Shoenfeld, "Cancer in autoimmune diseases," *Seminars in Arthritis and Rheumatism*, vol. 18, no. 2, pp. 77–87, 1988.

[15] L. J. Kinlen, "Malignancy in autoimmune diseases," *Journal of Autoimmunity*, vol. 5, no. A, pp. 363–371, 1992.

[16] B. Tessier-Cloutier, D. D. Twa, E. Baecklund et al., "Cell of origin in diffuse large B-cell lymphoma in systemic lupus erythematosus: molecular and clinical factors associated with survival," *Lupus Science & Medicine*, vol. 6, no. 1, Article ID e000324, 2019.

[17] A. H. Draborg, K. Duus, and G. Houen, "Epstein-Barr virus in systemic autoimmune diseases," *Clinical and Developmental Immunology*, vol. 2013, pp. 535738–9, 2013.

[18] B. D. Poole, R. H. Scofield, J. B. Harley, and J. A. James, "Epstein-Barr virus and molecular mimicry in systemic lupus erythematosus," *Autoimmunity*, vol. 39, no. 1, pp. 63–70, 2006.

[19] C. Shannon-Lowe, A. B. Rickinson, and A. I. Bell, "Epstein-Barr virus-associated lymphomas," *Philosophical Transactions of the Royal Society B: Biological Sciences*, vol. 372, no. 1732, p. 20160271, 2017.

CholedochoClip: A Case of Obstructive Jaundice 14 Years after Cholecystectomy

Grace E. Kim[1] **John D. Morris,**[1,2] **and Peter E. Darwin**[1,2]

[1]*Department of Internal Medicine, University of Maryland Medical Center, Baltimore, MD 21201, USA*
[2]*Division of Gastroenterology and Hepatology, University of Maryland Medical Center, Baltimore, MD 21201, USA*

Correspondence should be addressed to Grace E. Kim; grace.kim@som.umaryland.edu

Academic Editor: I. Michael Leitman

Gallstone disease is a common gastrointestinal pathology that may result in surgical intervention. While cholecystectomy has relatively minimal risks, surgical clip migration is a rare complication that can cause severe morbidity and mortality. This report describes a rare phenomenon of a biliary stone forming onto a migrated surgical clip 14 years after cholecystectomy causing an obstructive jaundice. This case illustrates the importance of keeping a migrated surgical clip on the differential when encountering patients with symptoms of cholangitis after cholecystectomy.

1. Introduction

Gallstone disease is one of the most common gastrointestinal pathologies in the USA, and cholecystectomy remains the standard procedure for symptomatic stones. In this procedure, several surgical clips are placed to occlude cystic duct after gallbladder is removed to prevent biliary leaks. Laparoscopic cholecystectomy is the gold standard, embodying many advantages compared to open cholecystectomy including lower rates of complications, decreased length of hospitalization, and overall cost-effectiveness [1]. There still are risks including duct injury, bleeding, ventral hernia, bile leakage, and surgical site infection [2]. This case report delineates one of the rarer complications from a new stone formation on a surgical clip placed 14 years prior that migrated distally into the biliary duct causing obstructive jaundice.

2. Case Report

A 74-year-old female with history of hypertension and hyperlipidemia presented with a postprandial, nonradiating epigastric abdominal pain for several days. The pain came intermittently and lasted for hours at a time with spontaneous resolution. She denied fevers or chills but did endorse nausea and emesis. Her surgical history included a remote history of appendectomy decades ago and cholecystectomy 14 years ago. Patient is a never-smoker and denied drinking alcohol.

On presentation, she had scleral icterus with maximum total bilirubin of 3.9 mg/dL (reference range 0.1-1.4 mg/dL), alkaline phosphatase of 218 IU/L (reference range 30-140 IU/L), and aspartate aminotransferase (AST) and alanine aminotransferase (ALT) of 410 IU/L and 225 IU/L (reference range 7-40 IU/L and 10-65 IU/L). She had normal lipase of 23 U/L (reference range 10-51 U/L) and amylase of 60 U/L (reference range 25-115 U/L). White blood cells were also within normal limits at $6.4\ x10^9/L$ (reference range $4.0 - 10.8\ x10^9/L$)

She was initially started on ampicillin-sulbactam. Computed tomography (CT) of abdomen and pelvis with contrast read "marked intra- and extrahepatic biliary dilatation down to the level of the ampulla. Radiopaque foreign bodies are seen within the duodenum adjacent to the ampulla which could be obstructing." Liver and pancreas were both normal appearing with no masses. Gastroenterology service was consulted who recommended magnetic resonance cholangiopancreatography (MRCP) given lab findings suggestive of biliary obstruction, concerning for a stone or stricture. MRCP read that "there are 2 linear metallic (and less likely calcific) densities within the duodenum at the ampulla of Vater. These appear to represent metallic surgical clips rather than stones. Unfortunately, there is magnetic susceptibility artifact off

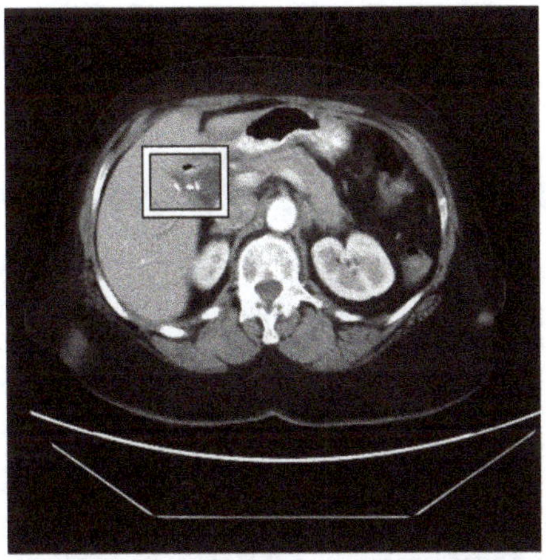

FIGURE 1: Abdominal CT showing the surgical clips by the cystic duct from the patient's prior cholecystectomy in 2004 (boxed).

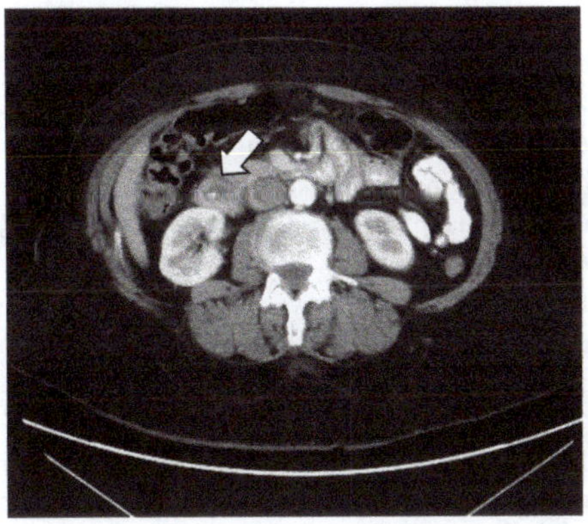

FIGURE 2: Abdominal CT showing a radiodense foreign body by the ampulla of Vater, most likely a migrated surgical clip from the prior cholecystectomy (arrow).

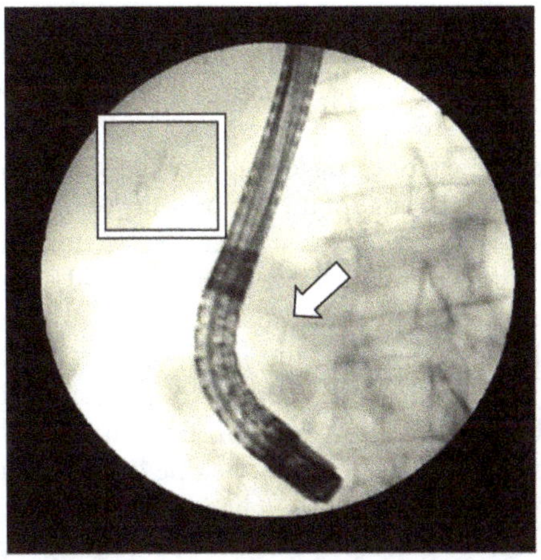

FIGURE 3: ERCP showing both the surgical clips by the cystic duct (boxed) as well as a foreign body that looks like a clip by the ampulla of Vater (arrow).

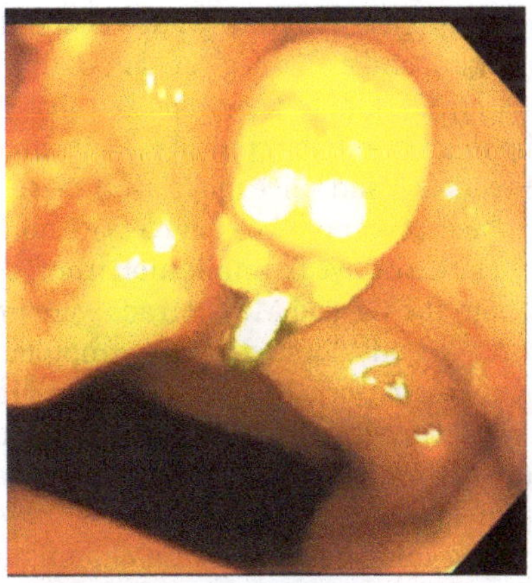

FIGURE 4: Image taken from ERCP showing a clip with stone attached, coming out of the ampulla of Vater.

of these obscuring adjacent structures, including the distal common bile duct. There is dilatation of the more proximal common bile duct measuring approximately 12 mm. There is mild-moderate intrahepatic ductal dilatation." Figures 1 and 2 show images from the CT surgical clips from cholecystectomy by the cystic duct (Figure 1) as well as common bile duct dilation with a hyperdense foreign body by the ampulla of Vater, most likely a migrated surgical clip (Figure 2). Endoscopic retrograde cholangiopancreatography (ERCP) was then performed, which located the surgical clip that migrated distally (Figure 3). The clip with a stone attached was then removed via balloon sweep (Figure 4), resulting in subsequent resolution of abdominal pain and normalization of the liver function tests.

3. Discussion

Cholecystectomy is a relatively benign procedure that is widely used. However, it does carry some risks of complications including biliary leakage and surgical clip migration. Gallstones forming on foreign bodies such as silk sutures have been reported as early as 1897 [3], with the first case of biliary stone formation from a migrated surgical clip reported in 1979 [4]. Surgical clip migration after laparoscopic cholecystectomy has been reported since 1992 [5], however the absolute number of this complication is low, accounting for less than 100 cases worldwide despite the increasing number of laparoscopic cholecystectomy procedures [6, 7]. While some clip migrations occur spontaneously without any symptoms, many of them result in biliary stricture, cholangitis, acute pancreatitis, choledochoduodenal fistula, and other severe, potentially fatal complications if not discovered in a timely manner [6, 8]. The most optimal approach to a migrated surgical clip causing obstruction is early detection and ERCP with sphincterotomy and clip removal, which provides both diagnostic and therapeutic measures to relieve the obstruction [6, 9].

Moreover, another rarer phenomenon depicted in this case is that the stone had formed onto the clip which potentiated the clinical presentation of obstructive jaundice. The stone seen on ERCP (Figure 4) had the clip almost embedded in the stone, suggesting that the stone had formed de novo around the edge of the clip over the years after the clip was placed. While the exact mechanism of stone formation after cholecystectomy is not well-understood, it is a complex, multifactorial process most likely due to the resultant stagnant biliary flow from the insertion of surgical clip in the setting of local inflammation and necrosis that initially prompted cholecystectomy [7, 10]. This in turn allows the clip to serve as a nidus for biliary stone development. Other factors include the number of clips used intraoperatively as well as incorrect placements of the clip causing incomplete occlusion of the cystic duct causing biliary leakage or partial occlusion of the common bile duct. These can further induce chronic inflammation around the biliary tree, enabling the clip to erode and migrate into the cystic and common bile ducts.

Albeit postsurgical clip migration has been well-published in the surgical literature [2, 10–12], it is nonetheless a rare complication and easily neglected in both medical and surgical fields [2, 13]. One review reported that the median time for a clip migration to be clinical evident after cholecystectomy is 2 years [6]; and since majority of these migrations occur within the first year or two of cholecystectomy [7, 10], it is even rarer to find a delayed complication from it. This could explain why both the CT and MRCP reads were rather vague about the foreign body located by the ampulla. Although there are some case reports of surgical clip migration years after cholecystectomy [14, 15], this is the first case of such finding reported from USA with such a complication from cholecystectomy performed over a decade ago.

Novel ways to mitigate postsurgical clip migration complications after cholecystectomy have been proposed in the surgical literature, including a total clipless cholecystectomy via harmonic sealing or ultrasound dissection of the cystic duct and artery [16, 17]. These approaches are still under active investigation and in the meantime, laparoscopic cholecystectomy remains the preferred procedure.

This case aims to raise awareness that the history of cholecystectomy does not rule out a biliary etiology when a patient presents with obstructive jaundice or biliary colic. This case also illustrates the importance of keeping a migrated surgical clip as well as a possible stone formation on the differential when encountering patients with cholangitis symptoms after a history of cholecystectomy.

References

[1] R. Fajardo, J. I. Valenzuela, S. C. Olaya et al., "Cost-effectiveness of laparoscopic versus open cholecystectomy," *Biomédica*, vol. 31, no. 4, pp. 514–524, 2011.

[2] L. Pang, J. Yuan, Y. Zhang, Y. Wang, and J. Kong, "Clip-stone and T clip-sinus: a clinical analysis of six cases on migration of clips and literature review from 1997 to 2017," *Journal of Minimal Access Surgery*, 2018.

[3] J. Homans, "Gall-stones formed around silk sutures twenty months after recovery from cholecystotomy," *Annals of Surgery*, vol. 26, no. 1, pp. 114–116, 1897.

[4] W. E. Walker, G. R. Avant, and V. H. Reynolds, "Cholangitis with a silver lining," *JAMA Surgery*, vol. 114, no. 2, pp. 214-215, 1979.

[5] J. L. Raoul, J. F. Bretagne, L. Siproudhis, D. Heresbach, J. P. Campion, and M. Gosselin, "Cystic duct clip migration into the common bile duct: a complication of laparoscopic cholecystectomy treated by endoscopic biliary sphincterotomy," *Gastrointestinal Endoscopy*, vol. 38, no. 5, pp. 608–611, 1992.

[6] V. H. Chong and C. F. Chong, "Biliary complications secondary to post-cholecystectomy clip migration: a review of 69 cases," *Journal of Gastrointestinal Surgery*, vol. 14, no. 4, pp. 688–696, 2010.

[7] K. K. Rawal, "Migration of surgical clips into the common bile duct after laparoscopic cholecystectomy," *Case Reports in Gastroenterology*, vol. 10, no. 3, pp. 787–792, 2016.

[8] T. Hong, X.-Q. Xu, X.-D. He, Q. Qu, B.-L. Li, and C.-J. Zheng, "Choledochoduodenal fistula caused by migration of endoclip after laparoscopic cholecystectomy," *World Journal of Gastroenterology*, vol. 20, no. 16, pp. 4827–4829, 2014.

[9] J. Martinez, W. Combs, and P. G. Brady, "Surgical clips as a nidus for biliary stone formation: diagnosis and therapy," *American Journal of Gastroenterology*, vol. 90, no. 9, pp. 1521–1524, 1995.

[10] J.-W. Qu, G.-Y. Wang, Z.-Q. Yuan, and K.-W. Li, "Hem-o-lok clips migration: an easily neglected complication after laparoscopic biliary surgery," *Case Reports in Surgery*, vol. 2017, Article ID 7279129, 4 pages, 2017.

[11] S. Ray and S. P. Bhattacharya, "Endoclip migration into the common bile duct with stone formation: a rare complication after laparoscopic cholecystectomy," *Journal of the Society of Laparoendoscopic Surgeons*, vol. 17, no. 2, pp. 330–332, 2013.

[12] E. S. Photi, G. Partridge, M. Rhodes, and M. P. N. Lewis, "Surgical clip migration following laparoscopic cholecystectomy as a cause of cholangitis," *Journal of Surgical Case Reports*, vol. 2014, no. 4, Article ID rju026, 2014.

[13] Y. Zheng, Y. Wang, X. Bai, D. Liu, and F. Li, "Nonmetal clip migration after laparoscopic cholecystectomy and bile duct exploration: is it rare?" *Asian Journal of Surgery*, 2018.

[14] A. G. Antunes, B. Peixe, and H. Guerreiro, "Pancreatitis and cholangitis following intraductal migration of a metal clip 5 years after laparoscopic cholecystectomy," *Gastroenterología y Hepatología*, vol. 40, no. 9, pp. 615–617, 2017.

[15] N. E. Cookson, R. Mirnezami, and P. Ziprin, "Acute cholangitis following intraductal migration of surgical clips 10 years after laparoscopic cholecystectomy," *Case Reports in Gastrointestinal Medicine*, vol. 2015, Article ID 504295, 3 pages, 2015.

[16] E. Sanawan, A. U. Qureshi, S. S. Qureshi, K. M. Cheema, and M. A. Cheema, "Effectiveness of ultrasound shear for clipless laparoscopic cholecystectomy versus conventional unipolar electrocautery in patients with cholelithiasis," *Journal of the College of Physicians and Surgeons Pakistan*, vol. 27, no. 10, pp. 611–615, 2017.

[17] A. C. Ramos, M. G. Ramos, M. Galvão-Neto et al., "Total clipless cholecystectomy by means of harmonic sealing," *Arquivos Brasileiros de Cirurgia Digestiva*, vol. 28, no. 1, pp. 53–56, 2015.

32

Extensive Superior Vena Caval Territory Thrombosis and Pulmonary Embolism: A Rare Clinical Entity of Haemorrhagic Pancreatitis

P. Thineskaran, K. Abiramy, T. Kumanan, V. Sujanitha, N. Suganthan, and G. Selvaratnam

University Medical Unit, Teaching Hospital, Jaffna, Sri Lanka

Correspondence should be addressed to P. Thineskaran; pthinafm069@gmail.com

Academic Editor: Gregory Kouraklis

Acute haemorrhagic pancreatitis is a severe form of pancreatitis often encountered in ethanol abuse. Extensive venous thrombosis resulting in pulmonary embolism is a rare presenting clinical entity of acute haemorrhagic pancreatitis. Here, we report a young male with an extensive deep vein thrombosis involving superior vena caval territory associated with haemorrhagic pancreatitis presented with pulmonary embolism managed supportively. Prompt recognition and appropriate intervention of this rare complication would improve the outcome in patients with acute pancreatitis.

1. Introduction

Acute pancreatitis is defined as "an acute inflammation of the pancreas, characterized by local inflammation that can trigger a systemic inflammatory response and it mostly occurs due to alcohol." Extensive deep venous thrombosis and pulmonary embolism are rare but life-threatening complications of acute pancreatitis. Hypercoagulable state in acute pancreatitis is due to release of pancreatic proteolytic enzymes that cause proteolytic damage and inflammation of the vessels. Here we report a case of severe haemorrhagic pancreatitis complicated with extensive deep vein thrombosis and pulmonary embolism in a young male.

2. Case Presentation

A 25-year-old previously healthy Sri Lankan male presented to the emergency department with a history of painful swelling of the left side on the neck and odynophagia of four days duration. He denied a history of fever and had no symptoms suggestive of upper airway obstruction. He had no significant past medical history to note, except he experienced an episode of severe epigastric pain which was treated as gastritis a year ago. He was an ethanol user, consuming 15 units per week. On examination, he was neither pale nor icteric. His pulse rate was 140 bpm, and blood pressure was 120/70 mmHg. He had tachypnea at rest with a respiratory rate of 32 per minute. Abdominal examination revealed mild tenderness over epigastric region though he denied any history of abdominal pain on admission. A swollen tender area, not moving with swallowing was noted in the lateral aspect of the neck without any palpable cervical lymphadenopathy. Examination of the thyroid gland and oral cavity showed no abnormality except poor oral hygiene. Rest of the systemic examination was unremarkable.

The initial full blood count showed white cell count of 12,580/mm^3 with predominant neutrophils, haemoglobin of 13.5 g/dL with a haematocrit of 44, and platelets of 206,000/mm^3. Initial inflammatory markers ESR and C-reactive protein (CRP) were 97 mm/1st hour and 26 mg/L, respectively. Serum amylase was 2180 IU/L, and corrected calcium was 2.21 mmol/L. Random blood glucose on admission was 122 mg/dL, and an ABG showed hypoxemia. Ultrasound scan with Doppler study of his neck showed extensive deep vein thrombosis involving internal jugular veins, subclavian veins, axillary veins, basilic veins, and upper part of superior vena cava. Ultrasound scan of abdomen revealed mixed echogenic area seen below the spleen suspicious for haematoma or haemorrhage into the cyst. At this point, he was diagnosed with an acute pancreatitis complicated with extensive deep vein thrombosis, and he was initiated with enoxaparin along with warfarin targeting an INR of 2.5 in addition to other supportive measures for acute pancreatitis.

Subsequent contrast enhanced-computed tomography of chest, abdomen, and pelvis with venogram showed extensive venous thrombosis involving in both internal jugular veins, subclavian veins, bracheocephalic vein, and superior vena cava up to the right atrium (Figure 1) and pulmonary arterial thromboembolism. It also revealed moderate right-sided pleural effusion and gross ascites and features of acute-on-chronic pancreatitis with two cystic collections suggestive of pseudo cyst formation (Figure 2).

The 2D echocardiography showed normal cardiac function with an ejection fraction of 55%. Extensive investigations done on him to identify an alternative cause for his deep vein thrombosis failed to show any positive results. Anticardiolipin antibody, protein C, S, Factor V Leiden mutation, hams test, and urine for haemosiderin were negative. Markers of autoimmune pancreatitis and pancreatic malignancy were normal.

On day 10 of admission, he developed a bout of severe abdominal pain associated with haemodynamic instability. An urgent ultrasonography of abdomen showed bleeding into the cyst, and it was managed with therapeutic aspiration of 2000 ml of haemorrhagic fluid and transfusion of packed cells while withholding the anticoagulant. Analysis of aspirate showed an exudative fluid with an amylase level of 10435 U/L and LDH of 6060 U/L, suggestive of haemorrhagic pancreatitis. Cytological analysis did not reveal evidence of a malignancy. Parenteral antibiotics and other supportive therapies were continued. Anticoagulant was reinstituted after few days. He made a gradual recovery and discharged from hospital on day 24.

On review at a month later, he showed significant clinical improvement with an evidence of resolving deep vein thrombosis.

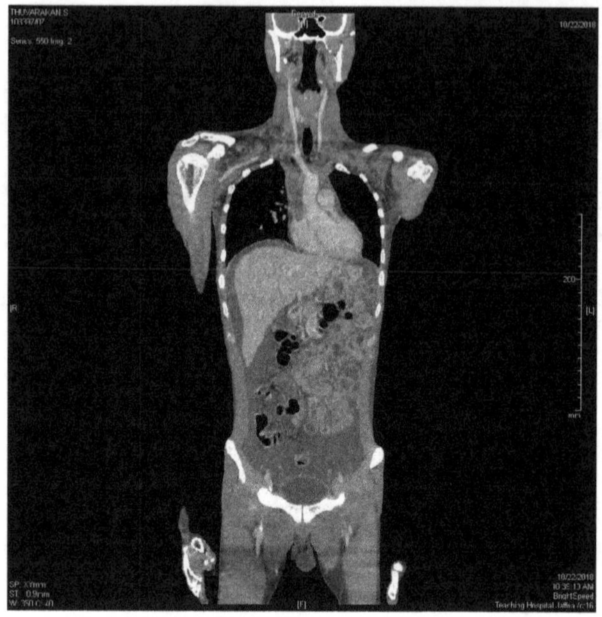

Figure 1: The contrast-enhanced computed tomography of neck, chest, abdomen, and pelvis showed extensive venous thrombosis involving in internal jugular veins, subclavian veins, brachiocephalic vein, and superior vena cava up to the right atrium.

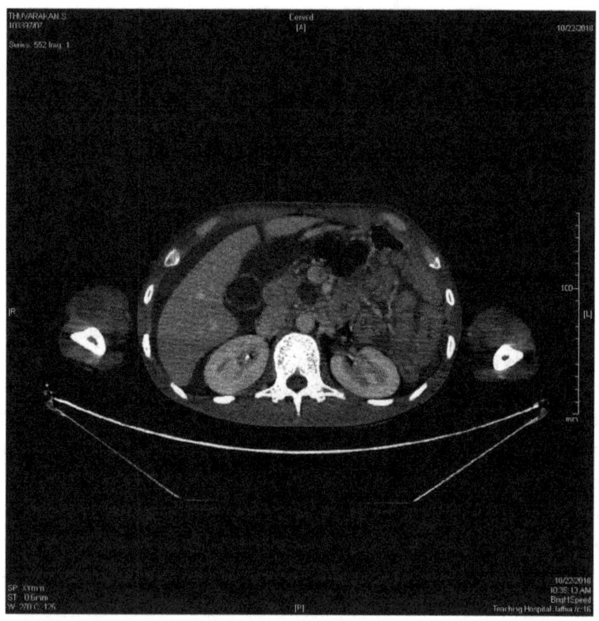

Figure 2: The contrast-enhanced computed tomography of abdomen shows two cystic collections suggestive of pseudo cysts in pancreas.

3. Discussion

Acute pancreatitis is an acute inflammatory process of the pancreas that presents with severe abdominal pain with elevated levels of pancreatic enzymes in the blood. Serum amylase and lipase are the important sensitive biochemical markers used to diagnose and monitor acute pancreatitis in clinical practice. The contrast-enhanced computed tomography of the pancreatic system is the widely used preferred diagnostic imaging and used in prognostic assessment of pancreatitis as well.

According to the revised Atlanta classification system, this patient had moderately severe acute pancreatitis. His Balthazar grade was D with a moderate severity. His Acute Physiology and Chronic Health Evaluation II score was 8 points with 8.7% estimated nonoperative mortality. An inherited or acquired thrombophilic state can leads to venous thrombosis. However, this patient had negative test results for any inherited or acquired prothrombotic conditions. Therefore, in this context, it is assumed that his extensive thrombosis involved in deep veins of neck and pulmonary regions were secondary to severe recurrent acute pancreatitis.

The vascular complications are the major cause of morbidity and mortality of acute pancreatitis that are related to haemorrhage resulting from arterial erosion or pseudoaneurysms, ischaemic complications, and venous or arterial complications—specifically splanchnic thrombosis and associated varices [1]. Extensive deep vein thrombosis involving the pulmonary, neck, and calf veins are a rare complication of acute pancreatitis that has been described in few case reports in the literature to date [2]. A case has been reported with acute pancreatitis with ischaemic cerebrovascular accident and pulmonary embolism which was successfully managed with anticoagulation [3]. Hypercoagulable state said to occur due to release of proteolytic enzyme in pancreatic juice in a cyst communicating with the pancreatic duct penetrates into the vascular system that causes proteolytic damage and inflammation of the vessels [4]. The pancreatic elastase is a major role in the development of pulmonary vascular injury after acute pancreatitis. The combination of hepatic dysfunction and hypertrypsinemia (resulting in raised fibrinogen and factor VIII concentrations) and cachexia, immobility also cause hypercoaguable state of acute pancreatitis. Furthermore, the sub sensitivity of contractile response to phenylephrine in both mesenteric and pulmonary rings might be due to the complications of this pathological condition in the early stage of pancreatitis [5].

Prompt investigations and clinical vigilance should be emphasized among clinically suspected acute pancreatitis because accurate diagnosis and timely radiological intervention procedures could reduce mortality. Early institution of intravenous heparin or thrombolysis is recommended to prevent further complications of acute pancreatitis once a diagnosis was confirmed.

4. Conclusion

Extensive venous thrombosis is a rare presentation of acute haemorrhagic pancreatitis. Anticipation of this rare complication would aid in early diagnosis, specific therapy, and to prevent fatal pulmonary embolism, a rare but catastrophic phenomenon of thrombosis in patients with acute haemorrhagic pancreatitis.

References

[1] R. M. Mendelson, J. Anderson, M. Marshall, and D. Ramsay, "Vascular complications of pancreatitis," *ANZ Journal of Surgery*, vol. 75, no. 12, pp. 1073–1079, 2005.

[2] R. L. Kistner, J. J. Ball, R. A. Nordyke, and G. C. Freeman, "Incidence of pulmonary embolism in the course of thrombophlebitis of the lower extremities," *The American Journal of Surgery*, vol. 124, no. 2, pp. 169–176, 1972.

[3] P. Alavinejad, E. Hajiani, and A. Parsi, "Acute pancreatitis complicated by vascular emboli," *Govaresh*, vol. 20, pp. 205–207, 2015.

[4] G. Lungarella, C. Gardi, M. Margherita de Santi, and P. Luzi, "Pulmonary vascular injury in pancreatitis: evidence for a major role played by pancreatic elastase," *Experimental and Molecular Pathology*, vol. 42, no. 1, pp. 44–59, 1985.

[5] P. A. Banks, M. L. Freeman, and The Practice Parameters Committee of the American College of Gastroenterology, "Practice parameters committee of the American college of gastroenterology practice guidelines in acute pancreatitis," *The American Journal of Gastroenterology*, vol. 101, no. 10, pp. 2379–2400, 2006.

33

Pancreatic Solid Pseudopapillary Tumor Associated with Elevated DHEA and Testosterone

Elias Estifan,[1] **Yana Cavanagh**,[2] **Ashima Kapoor**,[1] **and Matthew Grossman**[2]

[1]*Department of Internal Medicine, St. Joseph's University Medical Center-New York Medical College, USA*
[2]*Department of Gastroenterology, St. Joseph's University Medical Center-New York Medical College, USA*

Correspondence should be addressed to Elias Estifan; egestifan@gmail.com

Academic Editor: I. Michael Leitman

Solid pseudopapillary neoplasms (SPN) of the pancreas are extremely rare epithelial tumors with low malignant potential. They account for only 1-2% of pancreatic lesions. These masses often go unnoticed and when they become symptomatic it is often due to mass effect on neighboring structures. We encountered an unusual presentation in a healthy 34-year-old female who was found to have elevated dehydroepiandrosterone (DHEA) and testosterone levels during the evaluation of irregular menses. Subsequent abdominal imaging revealed an enhancing 2.7 cm pancreatic tail mass that was concerning for a pancreatic neoplasm. The patient underwent endoscopic ultrasound which confirmed the presence of a hypoechoic, 2.3 x 1.7 cm mass in the pancreatic tail. An intact interface was seen between the mass and adjacent structures, suggesting the absence of local invasion. Fine needle biopsy was performed and cytology was consistent with SPN. The patient later underwent curative distal pancreatectomy, with subsequent normalization of her menses. SPN are generally inactive on laboratory screening modalities (i.e., AFP, CEA, CA 19-9, and CA 125) and our patient showed no evidence of pancreatic insufficiency, pancreatic parenchymal injury, abnormal liver function, or cholestasis. Similarly to our patient, most SPN are asymptomatic. One retrospective study (spanning 15 years) reported vague abdominal pain in ~70% of patients, on initial presentation. Symptoms of tumor mass effect were the second most common. To our knowledge, this is the first reported presentation of elevated DHEA and testosterone levels associated with a solid pseudopapillary tumor in the absence of an underlying adrenal lesion or dysfunction. Despite extensive workup, no alternate etiology or correlatable medical condition could be elucidated for our patient's hormonal dysregulation. We, therefore, recommend further review and investigation into this potential correlative relationship in an effort to guide the future diagnosis and management of this unusual neoplasm.

1. Introduction

Solid pseudopapillary neoplasms (SPN) of the pancreas are an extremely rare epithelial tumor with low malignant potential. SPN was first described by Dr. Virginia Kneeland Frantz in 1959. It was initially known as Frantz's tumor until 1996 when the World Health Organization redefined this lesion as a "solid pseudopapillary tumor." SPN have solid as well as papillary histological features and account for 1-2% of exocrine pancreatic tumors [1–3]. They have an overwhelming predilection for adolescent girls and young women but have rarely been reported in older females, males, and children [1, 2].

SPN generally present with nonspecific clinical pictures which can include abdominal or back pain, distension, and a palpable mass [3, 4]. Up to 39.2% of tumors are discovered incidentally on imaging and are asymptomatic [5]. SPN predominantly occur in the pancreas but can occur at extrapancreatic sites, such as the ovary, testis, and mesentery [6–8]. In one study on 97 patients, pancreatic SPN tumors were localized to the pancreatic head in 38.1%, pancreatic neck in 12.4%, and pancreatic body/tail in 49.5% [5]. The prognosis is generally good. Wang et al. reported that surgical resection carries low morbidity and mortality and is effective even in the presence of local invasion and metastases [5]. A recent review reported the 5-year and 10-year recurrence-free survival as 89.5% and 86.3%, respectively [9].

2. Case Presentation

A 34-year-old female with no notable past medical history or manifestations of hyperandrogenism underwent evaluation

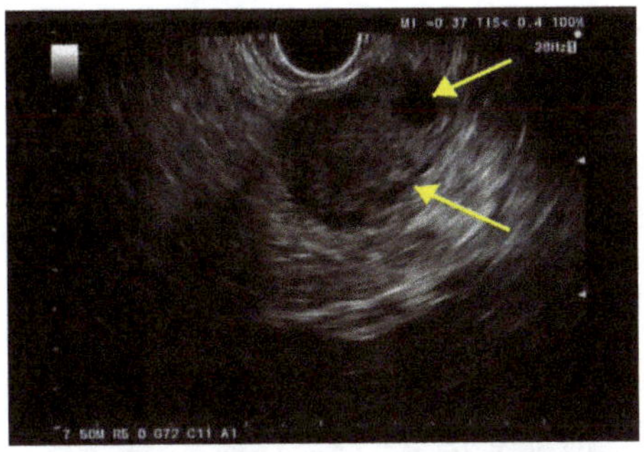

FIGURE 1: Solid mass with cystic component during an endoscopic ultrasound.

by her gynecologist for abnormal menstrual cycles. She described her menstrual cycle as regularly occurring every 40 to 35 days and reported it as heavy. She was found to have elevated dehydroepiandrosterone (DHEA) of 336 mcg/dL (23-266 mcg/dL), as well as borderline total testosterone of 45 ng/dL (2-45 ng/dL) and free testosterone level of 6.5 pg/mL (0.1-6.4 pg/mL), with no reported intake of exogenous androgens, hormonal birth control modalities, or glucocorticoids. Also, the patient had no known heart disease, osteoporosis, or anorexia nervosa. Endocrinology consultation and additional hormonal evaluation were unremarkable, with estradiol of 24 pg/mL (19-144 pg/mL), 17-hydroxyprogesterone of 42 ng/dL (23-102 ng/dL), FSH of 7.2 mIU/mL (2.5-10.2 mIU/mL), LH of 4.5 mIU/mL (1.9-12.5 mIU/mL), and TSH of 1.74 mIU/L (0.4-4.5 mIU/L). She subsequently underwent an abdominal computed tomography (CT) scan due to concern for an underlying adrenal adenoma. No ovarian or adrenal abnormalities were noted in imaging; however an indeterminate pancreatic tail mass measuring 2.7 x 1.3 x 2.0 cm was seen. Subsequent MRI of the abdomen further characterized the lesion as an enhancing pancreatic tail mass, concerning for pancreatic neoplasm.

The patient then underwent endoscopic ultrasound (EUS) for further evaluation and biopsy. EUS confirmed a hypoechoic mass in the pancreatic tail, measuring 2.3 x 1.7 cm (Figure 1). An intact interface was seen between the mass and adjacent structures suggesting an absence of invasion and cytology revealed SPN (Figures 2, 3, and 4). The patient was advised to undergo distal pancreatectomy and splenectomy, which she tolerated well, without any complication. Immunohistochemical staining of the resected specimen was positive for beta-catenin, CD10, and nuclear progesterone receptors (Figures 5, 6, and 7). Estrogen receptors were predominantly negative. Chromogranin and synaptophysin were negative.

Postsurgically, laboratory testing revealed normalized total testosterone of 33 ng/dL (2-45 ng/dL) and free testosterone level of 2.6 pg/mL (0.2-5.0 pg/mL); however dehydroepiandrosterone (DHEA) remained elevated at 351 mcg/dL (23-266 mcg/dL). The remaining hormonal workup was unremarkable, with estradiol of 162 pg/mL (56-214 pg/mL), 17-hydroxyprogesterone of 134 ng/dL (129-431 ng/dL), FSH of 1.7 mIU/mL (1.5-9.1 mIU/mL), LH of 3.4 mIU/mL (0.5-16.9 mIU/mL), and TSH of 1.98 mIU/L (0.4-4.5 mIU/L).

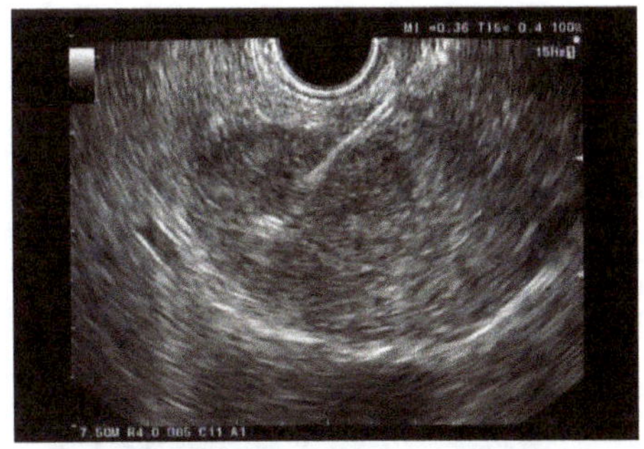

FIGURE 2: Fine needle aspiration during endoscopic ultrasound.

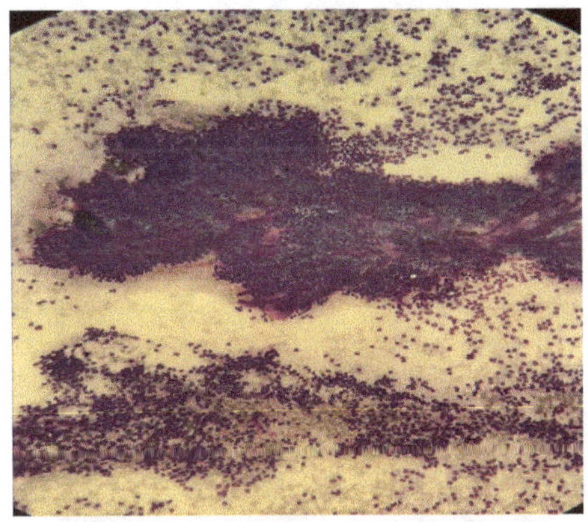

FIGURE 3: Cellular neoplasm showing papillary architecture (top) and numerous single cells also present (bottom).

3. Discussion

Solid pseudopapillary tumors are often asymptomatic but may manifest vague abdominal pain or mass effect on neighboring abdominal structures. One retrospective study (conducted between 1998 and 2013) noted the most frequent presenting complaints to be vague abdominal pain in 70% of their patient base. The remaining 30% displayed signs of compression by a tumor or were asymptomatic [10]. There was no reported evidence of pancreatic insufficiency, abnormal liver function test, cholestasis, elevated pancreatic enzyme, or elevation of tumor markers in their cohort [10].

Interestingly, there is a female predilection of SPN. Multiple studies described the female predominance and female-to-male ratio of nearly 5:1 [1, 5, 9–13]. Chhabra et al. attributed the underlying female predominance to a relationship with sex hormones (i.e., estrogen and progesterone); however, their role in neoplasm growth and histogenesis remains debated [14]. Similarly to our case, progesterone receptors are identified on most SPN tumors, while estrogen receptors are rarely present [15]. Furthermore, there are no significant qualitative differences in sex hormone–receptor status between SPN obtained from male and female patients [12, 14, 15]. Interestingly, however, the rate of SPN growth is accelerated in pregnancy suggesting a hormonal basis [15].

One common cause of hyperandrogenism is polycystic ovary syndrome (PCOS) [16]. In women with PCOS ovarian androgens increase and up to 50% also have elevated DHEA

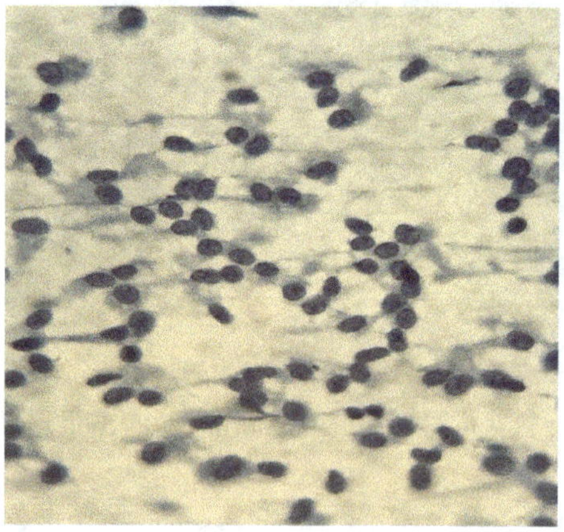

FIGURE 4: High power image shows cells with round to oval nuclei with fine chromatin and inconspicuous nucleoli and some with characteristic nuclear grooves.

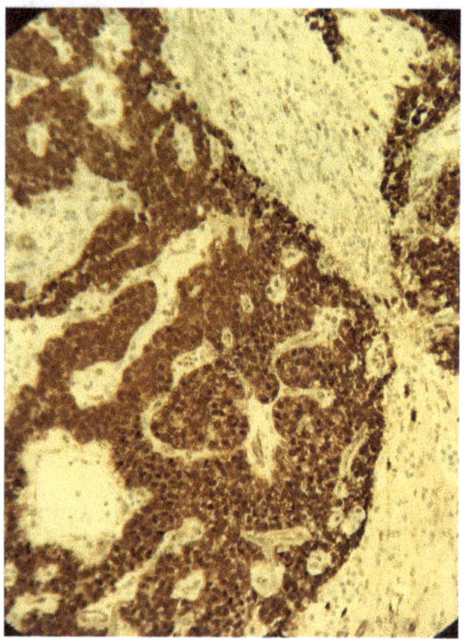

FIGURE 5: Immunohistochemical staining shows nuclear positivity for beta-catenin in the tumor cells, which is characteristic of SPN.

levels. Another study of 611 women aged 25-50 years explored the association between testosterone concentrations and body composition and found an interesting positive dose-response relationship. As such, increased testosterone has been associated with obesity and PCOS. Although testosterone and sex hormone bending globulin (SHBG) may play an important role in the development of menstrual irregularities in obese women, our patient's BMI was only 24 [16, 17]. High blood glucose is an alternate risk factor for hypogonadism as it is associated with reduced LH states, in which testosterone levels are reduced [18]; however, this is in contrast to our patient who had elevated testosterone levels. Androstenedione is normally produced by the adrenals and to a lesser extent by the testis. Androstenedione can be interconverted to testosterone by an enzyme present in the pancreas based on a canine model. Interestingly, one study reported that androstenedione was significantly higher

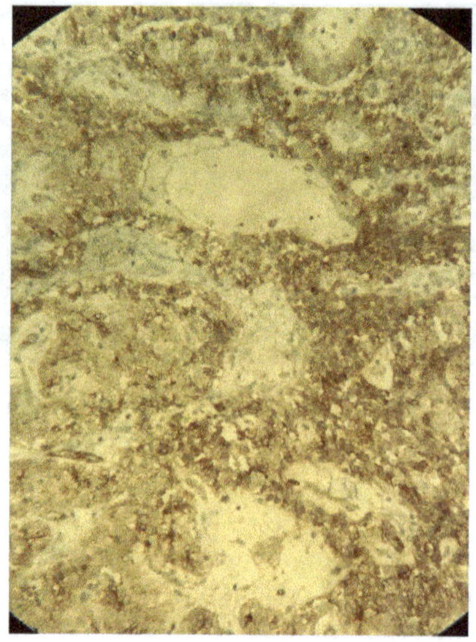

FIGURE 6: Immunohistochemical staining for CD10, showing membranous staining in the tumor cells.

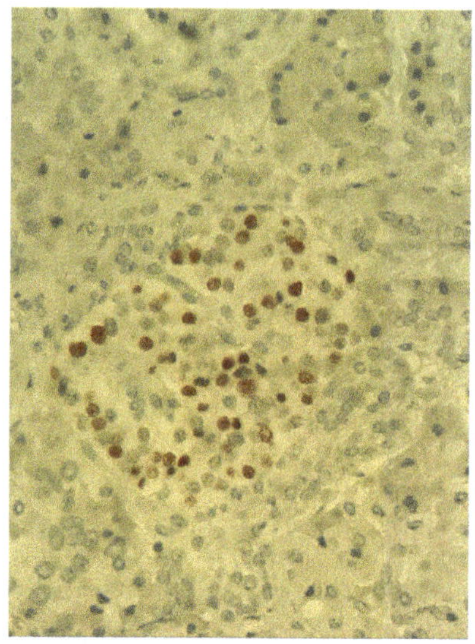

FIGURE 7: Immunohistochemical staining shows positive nuclear positivity for progesterone receptors.

in patients with pancreatic cancer, while testosterone levels were significantly lower in their examined population. The increased androstenedione was associated with pancreatic cancer and may have been produced by the pancreatic tumors in their examined population [19]. However, this is, again, in contrast to our patient who had elevated testosterone.

This case appears to be the first documented presentation of SPN in concomitance with elevated DHEA and testosterone level, in an otherwise asymptomatic female. Our patient was not on hormonal birth control and endocrine evaluation revealed no alternate etiology to explain her hormonal dysregulation. The patient remains asymptomatic at one-year follow-up with mitigation of functional endogenous androgen effect and normalization of her menstrual cycle. Although there is a reported female predominance of SPN, the underlying role of sex hormones (i.e., estrogen and progesterone) in SPN growth and histogenesis remains theoretical. We recommend further review and investigation into this interesting potential correlative relationship in an effort to guide future diagnosis and management of this unusual neoplasm.

Disclosure

The abstract was presented in the ACG 2018 Annual Scientific Meeting on 08/10/2018.

References

[1] D. Li, H. Li, Y. Xu, Q. Wang, R. Chen, and F. Zhou, "Solid pseudopapillary tumor of the pancreas: clinical features and imaging findings," *Clinical Imaging*, vol. 48, pp. 113–121, 2018.

[2] F. Limaiem, H. Mestiri, S. Mejri, A. Lahmar, and S. Mzabi, "Solid pseudopapillary neoplasm of the pancreas in two male patients: gender does not matter," *Pan African Medical Journal*, vol. 27, 2017.

[3] F. Yang, C. Jin, J. Long et al., "Solid pseudopapillary tumor of the pancreas: a case series of 26 consecutive patients," *The American Journal of Surgery*, vol. 198, no. 2, pp. 210–215, 2009.

[4] W. P. Beach, *Surgial Management of Solid-Pseudopapillary Neoplasms of the Pancreas (Franz or Hamoudi Tumors) A Large Single-Institutional Series*, vol. 208, 2009.

[5] P. Wang, J. Wei, J. Wu et al., "Diagnosis and treatment of solid-pseudopapillary tumors of the pancreas: A single institution experience with 97 cases," *Pancreatology*, vol. 18, no. 4, pp. 415–419, 2018.

[6] H. Wu, Y. Huang, X. Liu, and M. Xu, "Extrapancreatic solid pseudopapillary neoplasm followed by multiple metastases: Case report," *World Journal of Gastrointestinal Oncology*, vol. 9, no. 12, pp. 497–501, 2017.

[7] W. Cheuk, I. Beavon, D. T. Y. Chui, and J. K. C. Chan, "Extrapancreatic solid pseudopapillary neoplasm: report of a case of primary ovarian origin and review of the literature," *International Journal of Gynecological Pathology*, vol. 30, no. 6, pp. 539–543, 2011.

[8] K. Michalova, M. Michal, M. Sedivcova et al., "Solid pseudopapillary neoplasm (SPN) of the testis: Comprehensive mutational analysis of 6 testicular and 8 pancreatic SPNs," *Annals of Diagnostic Pathology*, vol. 35, pp. 42–47, 2018.

[9] F. Yang, X. Yu, Y. Bao, Z. Du, C. Jin, and D. Fu, "Prognostic value of Ki-67 in solid pseudopapillary tumor of the pancreas: Huashan experience and systematic review of the literature," *Surgery*, vol. 159, no. 4, pp. 1023–1031, 2016.

[10] A. Yagcı, S. Yakan, A. Coskun et al., "Diagnosis and treatment of solid pseudopapillary tumor of the pancreas: experience of one single institution from Turkey," *World Journal of Surgical Oncology*, vol. 11, article 308, 2013.

[11] Y.-Q. Cai, S.-M. Xie, X. Ran, X. Wang, G. Mai, and X.-B. Liu, "Solid pseudopapillary tumor of the pancreas in male patients: report of 16 cases," *World Journal of Gastroenterology*, vol. 20, no. 22, pp. 6939–6945, 2014.

[12] M. C. C. Machado, M. A. C. Machado, T. Bacchella, J. Jukemura, J. L. Almeida, and J. E. M. Cunha, "Solid pseudopapillary neoplasm of the pancreas: distinct patterns of onset, diagnosis, and prognosis for male versus female patients," *Surgery*, vol. 143, no. 1, pp. 29–34, 2008.

[13] M. Jiménez-Fuertes, J. R. Ramírez-García, J. Ruiz-Tovar, G. Díaz García, and M. Durán-Poveda, "Solid Pseudopapillary Neoplasm of the Pancreas," *Cirugía Española (English Edition)*, vol. 94, no. 2, pp. e31–e33, 2016.

[14] C. Author, "Solid pseudopapillary epithelial neoplasm of pancreas in pregnancy: Case Report of a Rare Co-Occurrence," *journal of medical science and clinical research*, vol. 5, no. 8, pp. 26978–26983, 2017.

[15] Y.-W. Tien, K.-H. Ser, R.-H. Hu, C.-Y. Lee, Y.-M. Jeng, and P.-H. Lee, "Solid pseudopapillary neoplasms of the pancreas: is there a pathologic basis for the observed gender differences in incidence?" *Surgery*, vol. 137, no. 6, pp. 591–596, 2005.

[16] N. Güdücü, S. S. Kutay, U. Görmüş, Z. N. Kavak, and İ. Dünder, "High DHEAS/free testosterone ratio is related to better metabolic parameters in women with PCOS," *Gynecological Endocrinology*, vol. 31, no. 6, pp. 495–500, 2015.

[17] S. Wei, M. D. Schmidt, T. Dwyer, R. J. Norman, and A. J. Venn, "Obesity and menstrual irregularity: associations with shbg, testosterone, and insulin," *Obesity*, vol. 17, no. 5, pp. 1070–1076, 2009.

[18] P. Dandona, S. Dhindsa, A. Chandel, and A. Chaudhuri, "Hypogonadotropic hypogonadism in men with type 2 diabetes," *Postgraduate Medical Journal*, vol. 121, no. 3, pp. 45–51, 2015.

[19] C. Fernández-del Castillo, G. Robles-Díaz, V. Díaz-Sánchez, and A. Altamirano, "Pancreatic cancer and androgen metabolism," *Pancreas*, vol. 5, no. 5, pp. 515–518, 1990.

34

Prolonged Hypercupremia after Laparoscopic Vertical Sleeve Gastrectomy Successfully Treated with Oral Zinc

Timothy R. Koch[1] **Elizabeth A. Zubowicz,**[1] **and John B. Gross Jr.**[2]

[1]*Center for Advanced Laparoscopic General & Bariatric Surgery, MedStar Washington Hospital Center and Georgetown University School of Medicine, Washington, DC 20010, USA*
[2]*Division of Gastroenterology and Hepatology, Mayo Clinic, 200 First Street S.W., Rochester, MN 55905, USA*

Correspondence should be addressed to Timothy R. Koch; timothy.r.koch@medstar.net

Academic Editor: I. Michael Leitman

A 30-year-old female underwent vertical sleeve gastrectomy. Postoperatively, hypercupremia and elevated ceruloplasmin were identified. Further testing revealed normal blood levels of transaminases, alkaline phosphatase, and albumin. She stopped ingestion of multivitamins, began a copper-free multivitamin, and then began a low copper diet, but with no improvement in hypercupremia. Protein electrophoresis was normal with no M-spike. Urinary copper excretion was normal at 0.24 micromol/24 hours (normal: < 0.55), and there were no Kayser-Fleischer rings on slit lamp examination. Two years postoperatively, she lost 44% of excess preoperative weight and she began zinc sulfate before meals twice daily (115 mg elemental Zinc/day). At 2 months and 8 months later, plasma copper and ceruloplasmin had essentially normalized. Increased production of ceruloplasmin could have been a response to significant weight loss or the presence of nonalcoholic steatohepatitis. The mechanism of zinc's beneficial effect is uncertain but may be related to suppressing hepatic synthesis of or secretion of ceruloplasmin.

1. Introduction

The global epidemic of obesity continues to be a major health risk factor. The prevalence of obesity was found to have doubled since 1980 in more than 70 countries in a recent international study of 195 countries [1]. The vertical sleeve gastrectomy has become the most common operation for the surgical management of medically complicated obesity, and in 2016 a vertical sleeve gastrectomy was performed for 53.6% of 609,987 global bariatric surgical procedures [2].

Disorders of copper metabolism appear to be common after bariatric surgery [3]. In a report describing hypocupremia in individuals who had undergone Roux-en-Y gastric bypass (RYGB) surgery, Gletsu-Miller and associates also included identification of hypercupremia in 10 of 136 subjects (for a prevalence of 7.4%) [3]. In a retrospective review of 54 subjects after RYGB, we identified hypercupremia in 19% of individuals at 18 months or longer after RYGB surgery, but in only 8% of individuals at less than 18 months after RYGB surgery [4]. At that time we speculated that the likely origin for identification of hypercupremia after RYGB was the result of joint national practice guidelines recommending two multivitamins with minerals daily for postbariatric surgery patients [5], which would supply 4 mg of copper daily. We report herein a case of a woman after laparoscopic vertical sleeve gastrectomy whose hypercupremia did not improve by conversion to a copper-free multivitamin and the addition of a low copper diet.

2. Case Presentation

This study was reviewed and approved on December 10, 2017, by the Human Studies Subcommittee of the MedStar Research Institute, Hyattsville, MD, USA.

Micronutrient levels were measured by a commercially available private laboratory. Serum iron was determined by a colorimetric method, serum ceruloplasmin was determined by an immunological method, and plasma copper

Table 1: Summary of biochemical findings.

Months after surgery	Copper	Ceruloplasmin	Zinc	Iron
5 months	45	4.9	14	10
12 months*	41		12	
14 months†	41	4.8		
17 months‡	36			
24 months	39			16
27 months¥	28	2.9	12	
33 months**	28	2.9	15	
	(Normal range: 11-26 μmol/L)	(Normal range: 1.4-2.9 μmol/L)	(Normal range: 8.6-21 μmol/L)	(Normal range: 4.8-28 μmol/L)

*Multivitamin had been stopped.
†Taking a copper-free multivitamin containing 15 mg/day zinc.
‡Using a low copper diet and taking a copper-free multivitamin with 15 mg/day zinc.
¥Two months after starting 115 mg/day zinc; **eight months after starting 115 mg/day zinc.

and zinc were separately determined by inductively coupled plasma/mass spectrometry.

A 30-year-old female (preoperative body mass index: 49 kg/m^2) underwent a laparoscopic vertical sleeve gastrectomy with no immediate postoperative complication. When she was seen 5 months after surgery, she was taking two daily chewable multivitamins with minerals (containing 4 mg elemental copper and 24 mg elemental zinc). Hypercupremia was present, in association with elevated ceruloplasmin, noted in retrospect (see Table 1). Follow-up testing demonstrated persistently normal blood levels of aspartate aminotransferase, alanine transaminase, alkaline phosphatase, glucose, creatinine, free thyroxine, and albumin. She was not taking an estrogen-containing medication and she had not had placement of a copper-intrauterine device.

At 11 months after surgery, she discontinued oral intake of multivitamins. At 12 months postoperatively, when hypercupremia persisted, she began oral intake of one copper-free multivitamin daily containing 15 mg of zinc. Despite this change in her multivitamin supplementation, high levels of plasma copper persisted at her 14-month postoperative visit. A search for underlying causes showed normal protein electrophoresis (no M-spike was identified), negative celiac disease markers, and negative anti-nuclear antibody. Of note, urinary copper excretion was normal at 0.24 μmol/24 hours (normal: < 0.55 μmol/24 hours), which did not support the diagnosis of a copper overload disorder. She was instructed on a low-copper diet, which she then began.

At the 2-year postoperative visit, she had obtained loss of 44% of her excess preoperative weight (body mass index: 34 kg/m^2). Hypercupremia was still present. Slit lamp examination revealed no Kayser-Fleischer rings. She then began oral zinc sulfate 220 mg taken fifteen minutes before meals twice daily (100 mg elemental Zn), with one daily copper-free multivitamin containing 15 mg zinc. At her follow-up visit 2 months later, plasma copper and serum ceruloplasmin levels had essentially normalized, and at her follow-up visit 8 months later these improvements in plasma copper and serum ceruloplasmin were reconfirmed (see Table 1).

Table 2: Differential diagnosis of hypercupremia.

PBC*	PSC**
Cirrhosis	Hemochromatosis
Pregnancy	Oral contraceptive/estrogen use
Thyrotoxicosis	Diabetes mellitus
Hypertension	Infections
Chronic renal failure	
Lung & breast cancer	Leukemia
Monoclonal gammopathy	

*PBC: primary biliary cholangitis; **PSC: primary sclerosing cholangitis.

3. Discussion

The differential diagnosis of hypercupremia is complex (see Table 2) and includes the following: liver disorders, gynecologic origins, endocrine origins, infections, hypertension, chronic renal failure, and neoplasia [6]. In this case report, careful examination did not identify a disorder associated with the development of hypercupremia. Individuals with persistently high blood levels of copper-binding proteins may deposit copper in Descemet's membrane and lens capsule [7]. Slit-lamp examination was however unremarkable in this patient.

Table 1 demonstrates that the high levels of plasma copper correlated with high levels of serum ceruloplasmin. At the same time, a normal urinary copper excretion and absence of Kayser-Fleischer rings excluded a more generalized copper overload syndrome. Our initial speculation was that the likely origin for the common identification of hypercupremia after bariatric surgery was the result of joint national practice guidelines recommending two multivitamins with minerals daily for postbariatric surgery patients [5]. Two daily multivitamins with minerals would supply 4 mg of copper daily. However, in our patient's case, there was no significant improvement in her hypercupremia after stopping standard multivitamin supplementation, switching to a copper-free multivitamin containing 15 mg/day zinc, or adopting a low copper diet. As seen in Table 1, hypercupremia persisted

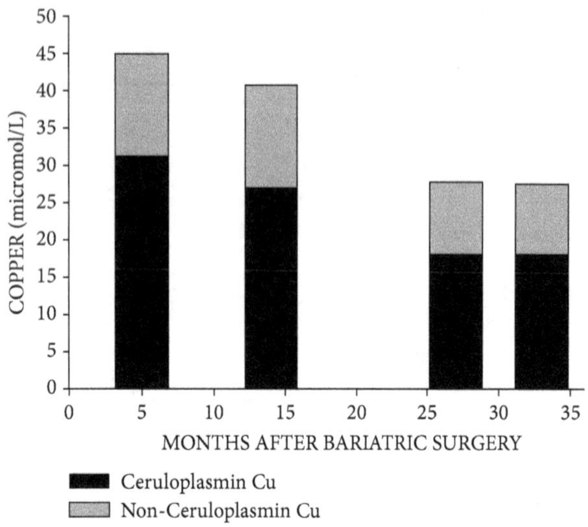

FIGURE 1: Concentrations of plasma copper (Cu) are shown at postoperative visits. The black bars demonstrate the contributions of ceruloplasmin copper to the plasma copper concentrations while the gray bars demonstrate the contributions of non-ceruloplasmin copper to the plasma copper concentrations. Note that there was a 38% decline in plasma copper between the 5-month postoperative visit and the postoperative visit after initiation of therapy with oral zinc.

one year after stopping multivitamin supplements containing copper. In previously reported studies of patients with Wilson's disease, a low copper diet may improve clinical outcomes [8]. For these reasons, we believe that it is unlikely that the increased production of ceruloplasmin in this case was simply a reflection of an excess of available copper.

Oral zinc therapy (as zinc acetate) has been approved by the United States Food and Drug Administration for maintenance treatment of individuals with Wilson's disease who have received treatment with a chelating agent. In patients with Wilson's disease who have received chelation therapy, studies from both Europe [9] and the United States [10] have revealed that treatment with oral zinc results in identification of increased liver copper concentrations at follow-up liver biopsies.

One possible interpretation of these results is that oral zinc suppresses hepatic synthesis of or secretion of ceruloplasmin. To examine this possible mechanism, in Figure 1, we depict postoperative copper levels related to ceruloplasmin copper and non-ceruloplasmin copper. In examination of hypercupremia at the 5-month postoperative visit compared to the plasma copper concentration after initiation of oral zinc, Figure 1 demonstrates the 38% decline in plasma copper. Within this decline, there was a 42% decline in ceruloplasmin copper, but a 29% decline in non-ceruloplasmin copper. This finding could support the notion that oral zinc suppresses hepatic synthesis of or secretion of ceruloplasmin. Additional studies utilizing serial liver biopsies for determination of liver copper and ceruloplasmin concentrations are required to examine this potential mechanism.

Increased production of ceruloplasmin in this patient could have been a response to significant weight loss or to the presence of nonalcoholic fatty liver disease, since her body mass index was still 34 kg/m^2 in follow-up after bariatric surgery. An initial report described an association between nonalcoholic fatty liver disease and low liver copper concentrations [11]. In that report, lower liver copper was reported in those individuals with more severe hepatic steatosis [11], which raises the question of whether the finding of low liver copper was a "dilution" effect due to the presence of extensive steatosis. A recent review of the potential role of copper in nonalcoholic fatty liver disease suggested that serum copper levels rise in the progression from nonalcoholic fatty liver disease to nonalcoholic steatohepatitis and that antioxidant food agents that bind copper may be useful in the treatment of nonalcoholic fatty liver disease [12]. Since serum ceruloplasmin may be a reactive inflammatory marker, a cautious interpretation of the reported rise in serum copper levels [12] may be justified.

In conclusion, hypercupremia may occur after vertical sleeve gastrectomy and after RYGB. This finding stands in contrast to reports of hypocupremia after RYGB [3, 4]. Use of a daily copper-free multivitamin with mineral supplement and instruction on a low copper diet are reasonable initial approaches for the treatment of hypercupremia. In individuals with persistent hypercupremia, an evaluation for conditions associated with hypercupremia is important and should include testing for monoclonal gammopathy and slit lamp examination. This report suggests that oral zinc may be effective in decreasing the concentrations of serum ceruloplasmin and plasma copper in patients with hypercupremia following vertical sleeve gastrectomy.

Disclosure

T. R. Koch is a consultant for Goldberg Segalla LLP. This article has been published previously only in abstract form as part of the American College of Gastroenterology National Meeting in Philadelphia, PA in October 2018.

Authors' Contributions

Timothy R. Koch participated in literature review, in evaluation of clinical data, and in preparation of the manuscript. Elizabeth A. Zubowicz participated in evaluation of clinical data and in preparation of the manuscript. John B. Gross, Jr. participated in literature review and in preparation of the manuscript. All authors read and approved the final paper.

Acknowledgments

None of the authors was supported by funding for this case report. The authors wish to thank Anyea S. Lovette, M.S., R.D. for her discussions regarding this manuscript.

References

[1] The GBD 2015 Obesity Collaborators, "Health effects of overweight and obesity in 195 countries over 25 years," *The New England Journal of Medicine*, vol. 377, no. 1, pp. 13–27, 2017.

[2] L. Angrisani, A. Santonicola, P. Iovino et al., "IFSO worldwide survey 2016: primary, endoluminal, and revisional procedures," *Obesity Surgery*, vol. 28, no. 12, pp. 3783–3794, 2018.

[3] N. Gletsu-Miller, M. Broderius, J. K. Frediani et al., "Incidence and prevalence of copper deficiency following roux-en-y gastric bypass surgery," *International Journal of Obesity*, vol. 36, no. 3, pp. 328–335, 2012.

[4] J. Lee, E. Oweis, T. R. Shope, F. C. Finelli, and T. R. Koch, "Mechanisms involved in the alteration of serum copper levels after Roux-en-Y gastric bypass surgery (RYGB)," *American Journal of Gastroenterology*, vol. 107, no. 1, p. S130, 2012.

[5] J. I. Mechanick, A. Youdim, D. B. Jones et al., "Clinical practice guidelines for the perioperative nutritional, metabolic, and nonsurgical support of the bariatric surgery patient-2013 update: cosponsored by American Association of Clinical Endocrinologists, the Obesity Society, and American Society for Metabolic & Bariatric Surgery," *Endocrine Practice*, vol. 19, no. 2, pp. 337–372, 2013.

[6] C. C. Pfeiffer and R. Mailloux, "Excess copper as a factor in human diseases," *Journal of Orthomolecular Medicine*, vol. 2, no. 3, pp. 171–182, 1987.

[7] S. Shah, E. M. Espana, and C. E. Margo, "Ocular manifestations of monoclonal copper-binding immunoglobulin," *Survey of Ophthalmology*, vol. 59, no. 1, pp. 115–123, 2014.

[8] G. J. Brewer, V. Yuzbasiyan-Gurkan, R. Dick, Y. Wang, and V. Johnson, "Does a vegetarian diet control Wilson's disease?" *Journal of the American College of Nutrition*, vol. 12, no. 5, pp. 527–530, 1993.

[9] T. U. Hoogenraad, J. Van Hattum, and C. J. A. Van den Hamer, "Management of Wilson's disease with zinc sulphate: experience in a series of 27 patients," *Journal of the Neurological Sciences*, vol. 77, no. 2-3, pp. 137–146, 1987.

[10] G. J. Brewer, V. Yuzbasiyan-Gurkan, D. Y. Lee, and H. Appelman, "Treatment of Wilson's disease with zinc. VI. Initial treatment studies," *Journal of Laboratory and Clinical Medicine*, vol. 114, no. 6, pp. 633–638, 1989.

[11] E. Aigner, M. Strasser, H. Haufe et al., "A role for low hepatic copper concentrations in nonalcoholic fatty liver disease," *American Journal of Gastroenterology*, vol. 105, no. 9, pp. 1978–1985, 2010.

[12] L. Antonucci, C. Porcu, G. Iannucci, C. Balsano, and B. Barbaro, "Non-alcoholic fatty liver disease and nutritional implications: special focus on copper," *Nutrients*, vol. 9, no. 10, p. 1137, 2017.

35

A Rare Case of Splenic *Pneumocystis jirovecii* in a HIV-Positive Patient

Hafsa Abbas ,[1,2] Harish Patel,[1,2] Ahmed Baiomi,[1,2] Masooma Niazi,[3] Trupti Vakde,[2,4] and Sridhar Chilimuri[2]

[1]*Division of Gastroenterology, BronxCare Hospital Center, Bronx, NY 10457, USA*
[2]*Department of Medicine, BronxCare Hospital Center, Bronx, NY 10457, USA*
[3]*Department of Pathology, BronxCare Hospital Center, Bronx, NY 10457, USA*
[4]*Division of Pulmonary and Critical Care, Department of Medicine, BronxCare Hospital Center, Bronx, NY 10457, USA*

Correspondence should be addressed to Hafsa Abbas; hafsaabbas20@gmail.com

Academic Editor: Yoshihiro Moriwaki

Introduction. Human immunodeficiency virus (HIV) positive individuals with the CD4 count less than 200 cells/mm^3 are at risk for opportunistic infections. *Pneumocystis jirovecii,* a fungal pathogen, is a common cause of opportunistic infections with predominantly pulmonary involvement. Disseminated *P. jiroveciii* infection presenting with hepatosplenic lesion is extremely rare. *Case Summary.* A 31-year-old male with HIV with and acquired immunodeficiency syndrome (AIDS) presented with diarrhea for 3 weeks. He had splenomegaly and inguinal lymphadenopathy on physical examination. Laboratory parameters revealed anemia and hypoalbuminemia, while stool studies for infectious etiology and fecal leucocyte were negative. Computed tomography (CT) of the chest and abdomen depicted consolidation of the lungs and a large splenic mass. He underwent fiberoptic bronchoscopy with transbronchial biopsy which was consistent with *P. jirovecii* pneumonia. He also had a ultrasound-guided core biopsy of the splenic mass which revealed necrotizing granulomas with *Pneumocystis jirovecii* infection on Grocott-Gomori's methenamine silver (GMS) stain and was initiated on treatment for *P. jirovecii* with sulfamethoxazole with trimethoprim. *Conclusion.* Malignancy and atypical infection are key differentials in patients presenting with hepatosplenic lesions. HIV positive patients are at increased risk of AIDS-related lymphoma. Tissue diagnosis is often required for further evaluation. Disseminated *P. jirovecii* presenting with splenic mass and liver lesion is extremely rare.

1. Introduction

An opportunistic infection is defined as an infection affecting individuals with weakened immune system. Human immunodeficiency virus (HIV) positive patients with CD4 count below 200/mm^3 are at high risk of the opportunistic infection [1]. Patients with HIV are at increased risk of lymphoma and often present with the extranodal disease with tumor burden [2]. Acquired immune deficiency syndrome (AIDS) related lymphoma is common in HIV-positive patients, especially in those with lower CD4 count [3].

Pneumocystis jirovecii, previously known as *Pneumocystis carinii,* is a common opportunistic fungal pathogen mostly affecting immunocompromised individuals [4, 5]. Pulmonary infection is the most common presentation for *P. jirovecii* infection and is often life-threatening [5–7]. Pharmacological prophylaxis is recommended in patients with CD4 count below 200/mm^3. However, patients with a high HIV viral load in the absence of antimicrobial prophylaxis can present with a disseminated extrapulmonary infection [4, 8]. Extrapulmonary manifestation is exceedingly rare and requires a thorough evaluation to exclude other etiologies such as lymphoma or other malignancies.

We report a case of disseminated pneumocystis in a patient with AIDS presenting with splenic mass and liver nodules along with concurrent *P. jirovecii* pneumonitis. On our review of literature, splenic involvement of pneumocystis is very rare, and only a few cases have been reported so far [4, 9–12].

2. Case Summary

A 31-year-old man was evaluated in the emergency room (ER) of our institution for persistent diarrhea of 3 weeks duration. He also reported abdominal pain along with lightheadedness. He described the abdominal pain as vague, diffuse, nonradiating, and mild in intensity without any precipitating or relieving factors. He reported up to 10 episodes of watery diarrhea which did not contain any blood. He also complained of fever and dysuria. About 3 weeks before the current presentation, the patient had presented to the ER with dysuria, abdominal pain, and intermittent diarrhea. At that time he was admitted and treated for a urinary tract infection (UTI) with ciprofloxacin and later discharged home. As per patient, his diarrhea had worsened after taking the antibiotics and had presented with the current symptoms. There was no nausea, vomiting, constipation, fever, and early satiety or appetite changes. He had a prior history of HIV/AIDS, had not been adherent to antiretroviral therapy or PCP prophylaxis. He had a high viral load and low CD4 count.

He was a current smoker and admitted smoking 4 or more cigarettes per day but denied using alcohol except on social occasions or illicit drugs. He did not have a family history of liver, stomach, or colon cancer. His medications included acetaminophen and ciprofloxacin.

On examination, he was found to have a temperature of 39.1°C, blood pressure of 108/52 mmHg, a pulse rate of 99 beats per minute, and a respiratory rate of 16 breaths per minute. The patient was alert, fully oriented, and communicative. The abdomen was scaphoid, nontender, and nondistended with normal bowel sounds. There was no palpable hepatomegaly; however, the spleen was palpable. Shotty cervical and inguinal lymph nodes were palpated. The rest of the physical examination was unremarkable.

Routine laboratory tests showed a hemoglobin level of 8 g/dL, white blood cell count of 3.7 k/uL, serum potassium level of 3.4 mEq/L, and albumin level of 1.7 g/dL. Stool studies including *Clostridium difficile* cytotoxin, fecal leucocyte stain, and fecal fat were negative. His blood and stool cultures were negative for the growth of *Mycobacterium avium* complex. A chest X-ray revealed a right lower lobe consolidation and bilateral pleural effusions. The patient was initiated on broad spectrum antibiotics for hospital-acquired infection. A CT of the chest was done as a part of workup revealed moderate right and small left pleural effusions, consolidation in the dependent lung bases, nodular opacities in both lungs, some cavitary in nature, and patchy ground glass opacity in both lungs (Figure 1). Sputum for acid-fast bacilli (AFB) was negative, ruling out pulmonary tuberculosis. CT abdomen and pelvis done for chronic diarrhea and abdominal pain revealed a hypodense lesion within the cephalad aspect of the spleen, a 6.7 cm splenic mass with adjacent small nodule, multiple hypodense hepatic lesions, measuring up to 12 mm in diameter, and mild ascites in the upper abdomen (Figure 2). Magnetic resonance imaging (MRI) abdomen showed a heterogeneous lesion within the upper pole of the spleen measuring 5.2 × 4.3 cm in size with absent enhancement centrally, with some enhancement along the peripheral aspect of the lesion, suggesting central necrosis (Figure 3). He underwent an ultrasound-guided core biopsy with an 18-gauge (18G) needle. Two core biopsies were obtained for histologic analysis of the splenic mass. The histopathology revealed necrotizing granulomas on hematoxylin and eosin stain (Figures 4 and 5) with *Pneumocystis jirovecii* infection on Grocott-Gomori's methenamine silver (GMS) stain (Figures 6(a) and 6(b)). A fiberoptic bronchoscopy with transbronchial biopsy was also done revealing *P. jirovecii* pneumonia, while bronchoalveolar lavage was negative for malignant cells. His alpha fetoprotein (AFP) level was 3.2 ng/ml. Results of the rest of the laboratory parameters are given in Table 1. The patient was started on sulfamethoxazole with trimethoprim, and no steroids were given. Antiretroviral therapy was not started at the time of discharge due to concerns over IRS (immune reconstitution syndrome). He continued to follow-up at our hospital as an outpatient.

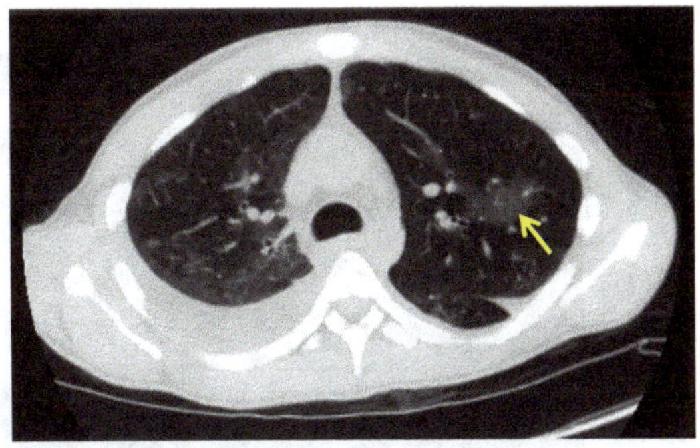

FIGURE 1: Cross-sectional computerized scan of the chest revealing nodular opacities and ground glass opacities (GGOs) with cavitation in lung field.

3. Discussion

There are a wide array of differentials for a patient presenting with splenic lesion [13]. Angiosarcoma, lymphoma, hemangioendothelioma, and metastasis are the common malignant etiologies of the splenic lesion. MRI of the splenic lesion with and without gadolinium enhancement can assist in further characterization, but is not diagnostic [14]. Image-guided percutaneous biopsy of the spleen with 18G needle is safe and is a favorable alternative to diagnostic splenectomy [15]. It is essential to characterize the vascular pattern of splenic lesion prior to biopsy. Given the risk of malignancy, our patient required splenic biopsy.

Before AIDS pandemic, there were sporadic cases of *P. jirovecii* pneumonia in individuals with immunosuppression due to corticosteroids or chemotherapy [4, 16]. Now, it is the most common respiratory opportunistic infection in AIDS patients. Pneumonia or interstitial pneumonitis is the most common presentation of *P. jirovecii* in HIV/AIDS patients [12]. The first case of fatal extrapulmonary pneumocystis was

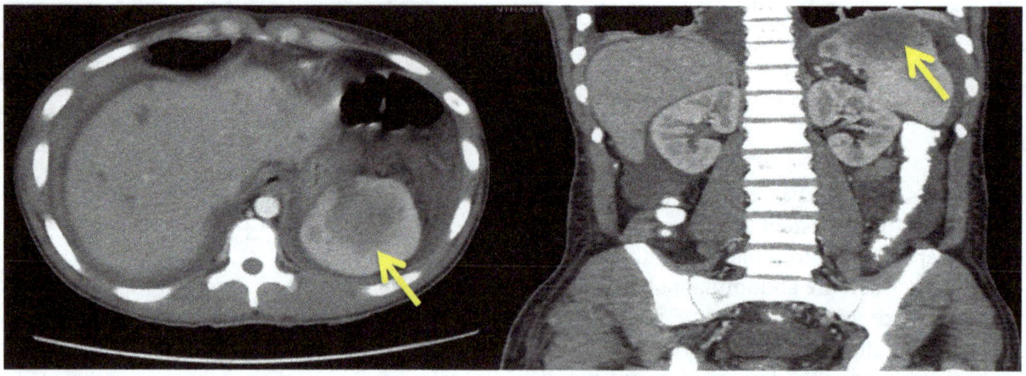

Figure 2: Cross-sectional and coronal computerized tomogram of abdomen with intravenous contrast revealing a hypodense lesion of 6.7 cm in the cephalad aspect of the spleen with adjacent small nodule, multiple liver lesion, and ascites.

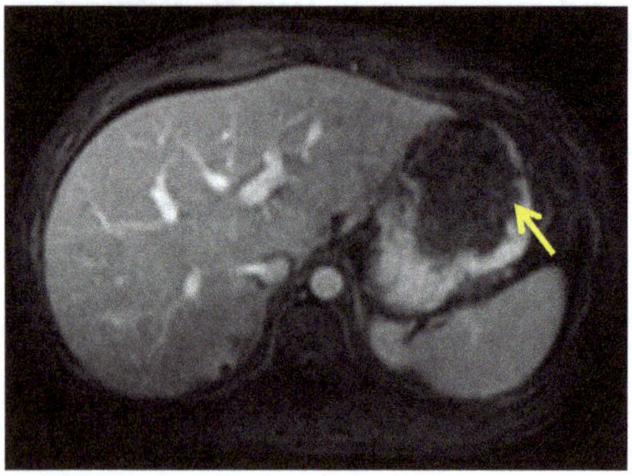

Figure 3: Magnetic resonance imaging of abdomen with gadolinium revealing a heterogeneous lesion in upper pole of the spleen measuring approximately 5.2 × 4.3 cm in size.

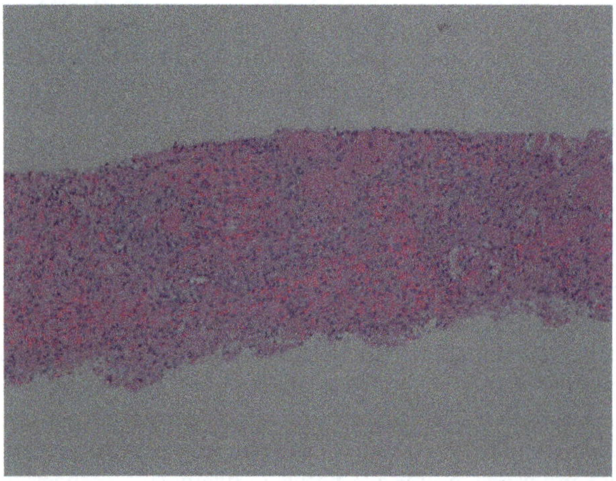

Figure 4: Splenic biopsy with *Pneumocystis jirovecii* infection showing necrotizing granulomatous inflammation/frothy exudate (hematoxylin and eosin stain, magnification ×100 low power).

reported in 1960 [17]. Extrapulmonary or disseminated pneumocystis infection is uncommon, about 0.5% to 2.5% in patients with AIDS [18, 19] but has been described and well documented [8, 20–27].

Disseminated pneumocystis has a highly variable pattern of tissue involvement. It can involve the spleen, liver,

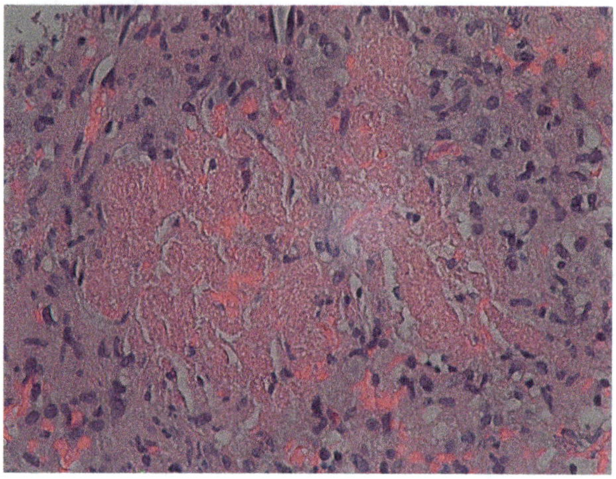

Figure 5: Splenic biopsy with *Pneumocystis jirovecii* infection showing necrotizing granuloma and frothy exudate surrounded by epitheloid cells (hematoxylin and eosin, magnification ×400).

gastrointestinal tract [22], skin [28], heart, bone marrow with lymph nodes [8], kidneys, thyroid, and skeletal muscle [24]. The clinical presentation has a wide array of symptoms. Diffuse organ involvement can result in systemic symptoms, whereas local involvement can produce local symptoms, such as isolated involvement of the small intestine [29] causing acute abdomen and thyroid disease, causing left-sided neck swelling and dysphagia [30]. Pneumocystis of the liver has been reported to be associated with hypoalbuminemia, ascites, and anasarca [9, 31, 32].

Splenic involvement of pneumocystis can present with left upper quadrant pain, splenic mass, thrombocytopenia, and splenomegaly [33]. Typical features of splenic pneumocystis on CT abdomen are multiple hypodense lesions with punctate or rim-like calcifications [9, 34].

Our patient with AIDS had presented with abdominal pain, and imaging revealed hypodense lesions in both spleen and liver. Splenic biopsy and transbronchial biopsy revealed pneumocystis consistent with disseminated pneumocystis. Disseminated *P. jirovecii* was diagnosed with splenic and transbronchial lung biopsy, and hence, hepatic biopsy was not required. Although the liver lesions were not biopsied but the clinical presentation of our patient including ascites,

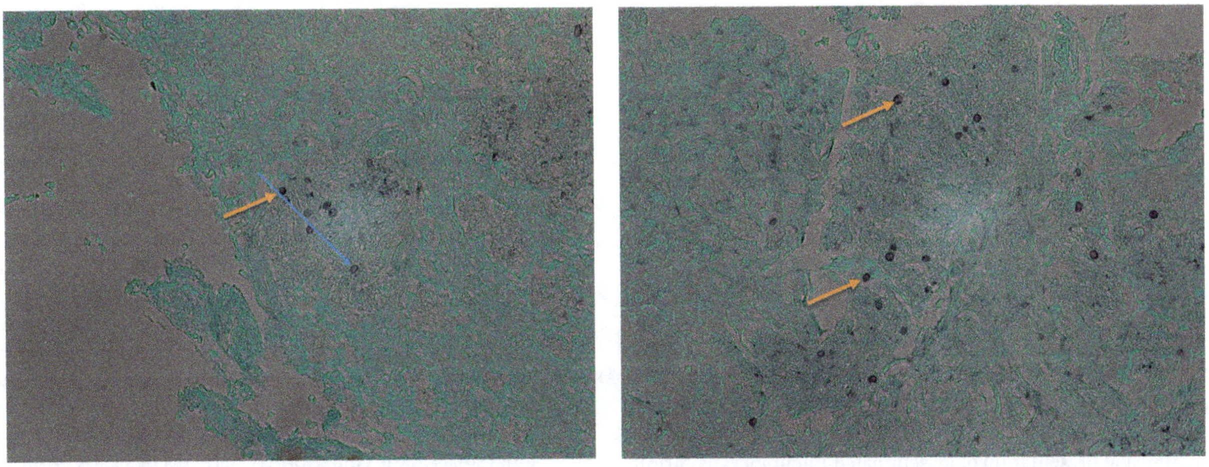

(a) (b)

FIGURE 6: Splenic biopsy on Grocott-Gomori methenamine silver (GMS) stain with 400 times magnification showing the necrotic and frothy infiltrate containing multiple *Pneumocystis jirovecii* organisms (arrow indicates *P. jirovecii*).

TABLE 1: Initial laboratory work up.

Parameter	Initial laboratory results	Reference range
Hemoglobin (g/dL)	8.7	12–16
Hematocrit (%)	26.6	42–51
White blood cell count (per mm^3)	3.7	4.8–10.8
Platelet count (k/μL)	344	150–400
Sodium (mEq/L)	135	135–145
Potassium (mEq/L)	3.4	3.5–5.0
HCO_3 (mEq/L)	19	24–30
BUN (mg/dl)	6	6–20
Creatinine (mg/dL)	1	0.5–1.5
Glucose (mg/dL)	67	70–120
Lactic acid (mmol/L)	1.5	0.5–1.6
AST (mg/dL)	74	9–48
ALT (mg/dL)	63	5–40
Total bilirubin/direct (mg/dL)	0.2	0.2–1.2
Alkaline phosphatase (U/L)	83	53–141
Albumin (g/dL)	1.8	3.2–4.8
Alpha fetoprotein (AFP) (ng/mL)	3.2	<10
Hepatitis A IgM	Negative	Negative
Hepatitis B core total antibody	Negative	Negative
Hepatitis B surface antibody	Positive	Negative
Hepatitis B surface antigen	Negative	Negative
Hepatitis C antibody	Negative	Negative
HIV RNA PCR (copies/mL)	206,000	Not detectable
Absolute CD4 cells	<20	490–1740

hypoalbuminemia and hypodense liver lesions on CT is similar to prior cases reporting hepatic pneumocystis.

4. Conclusion

Patients with HIV and AIDS presenting with hepatosplenic mass have a wide array of differentials with opportunistic infection and the malignancy being the most common etiology. Image-guided splenic tissue aspiration is required for the diagnosis. As presented in the index case, disseminated *P. jirovecii* infection can be a possible etiology for the splenic mass.

References

[1] B. C. Zanoni and R. T. Gandhi, "Update on opportunistic infections in the era of effective antiretroviral therapy," *Infectious Disease Clinics of North America*, vol. 28, no. 3, pp. 501–518, 2014.

[2] K. L. Grogg, R. F. Miller, and A. Dogan, "HIV infection and lymphoma," *Journal of Clinical Pathology*, vol. 60, no. 12, pp. 1365–1372, 2007.

[3] A. Levine, "Acquired immunodeficiency syndrome-related lymphoma," *Blood*, vol. 80, no. 1, pp. 8–20, 1992.

[4] C. B. O'Neal and S. C. Ball, "Splenic pneumocystosis: an a typical presentation of extrapulmonary Pneumocystis infection," *AIDS Read*, vol. 18, no. 10, pp. 503–508, 2008.

[5] J. Truong and J. V. Ashurst, *Pneumocystis (Carinii) Jirovecii Pneumonia*, StatPearls, Treasure Island, FL, USA, 2019.

[6] C. A. Mecoli, D. Saylor, A. C. Gelber, and L. Christopher-Stine, "*Pneumocystis jirovecii* pneumonia in rheumatic disease: a 20-year single-centre experience," *Clinical and Experimental Rheumatology*, vol. 35, no. 4, pp. 671-673, 2019.

[7] A. Ricciardi, E. Gentilotti, L. Coppola et al., "Infectious disease ward admission positively influences *P. jirovecii* pneumonia (PjP) outcome: a retrospective analysis of 116 HIV-positive and HIV-negative immunocompromised patients," *PLoS One*, vol. 12, no. 5, Article ID e0176881, 2017.

[8] A. J. Kallen and M. R. Wallace, "A typical Pneumocystis carinii infection in AIDS," *Southern Medical Journal*, vol. 91, no. 8, pp. 759-760, 1998.

[9] P. F. Rockley, C. M. Wilcox, M. Moynihan, K. Hewan-Lowe, and D. A. Schwartz, "Splenic infection simulating lymphoma: an unusual presentation of disseminated Pneumocystis carinii infection," *Southern Medical Journal*, vol. 87, no. 4, pp. 530–536, 1994.

[10] A. Galimberti, E. Morandi, G. Giani et al., "Pneumocystosis of splenic localization in the course of HIV infection: a new indication for splenectomy: description of a case," *Annali Italian di Chirugia*, vol. 68, no. 4, pp. 559–562, 1997.

[11] A. Grasland, J. Pouchot, C. Michon, A. Hertig, A. Simonpoli, and P. Vinceneux, "Splenic pneumocystosis disclosing extrapulmonary pneumocystosis of fatal outcome," *Annales de Medecine Interne (Paris)*, vol. 148, no. 2, pp. 184-185, 1997.

[12] C. J. Harvey, A. G. Rockall, W. R. Lees, and R. F. Miller, "Splenic pneumocystosis in AIDS: unusual ultrasound appearances," *International Journal of STD & AIDS*, vol. 8, no. 5, pp. 342–344, 1997.

[13] H.-J. Lee, J. W. Kim, J. H. Hong et al., "Cross-sectional imaging of splenic lesions: RadioGraphics fundamentals | online presentation," *RadioGraphics*, vol. 38, no. 2, pp. 435-436, 2018.

[14] A. Luna, R. Ribes, P. Caro, L. Luna, E. Aumente, and P. R. Ros, "MRI of focal splenic lesions without and with dynamic gadolinium enhancement," *American Journal of Roentgenology*, vol. 186, no. 6, pp. 1533–1547, 2006.

[15] M. D. F. McInnes, A. Z. Kielar, and D. B. Macdonald, "Percutaneous image-guided biopsy of the spleen: systematic review and meta-analysis of the complication rate and diagnostic accuracy," *Radiology*, vol. 260, no. 3, pp. 699–708, 2011.

[16] P. D. Walzer, D. P. Perl, D. J. Krogstad, P. G. Rawson, and M. G. Schultz, "Pneumocystis cariniiPneumonia in the United States," *Annals of Internal Medicine*, vol. 80, no. 1, pp. 83–93, 1974.

[17] C. D. Anderson and H. J. Barrie, "Fatal pneumocystis pneumonia in an adult: report of a case," *American Journal of Clinical Pathology*, vol. 34, no. 4, pp. 365–370, 1960.

[18] M. C. Raviglione, "Extrapulmonary pneumocystosis: the first 50 cases," *Clinical Infectious Diseases*, vol. 12, no. 6, pp. 1127–1138, 1990.

[19] E. E. Telzak, R. J. Cote, J. W. M. Gold, S. W. Campbell, and D. Armstrong, "Extrapulmonary Pneumocystis carinii infections," *Clinical Infectious Diseases*, vol. 12, no. 3, pp. 380–386, 1990.

[20] A. D. Abati, L. Opitz, C. Brones, D. E. Burstein, and L. Gallo, "Cytology of extrapulmonary Pneumocystis carinii infection in the acquired immunodeficiency syndrome," *Acta Cytologica*, vol. 36, no. 3, pp. 440–444, 1992.

[21] C. Bazin, P. Hazera, A. Greder et al., "Extrapulmonary and disseminated pneumocystosis in HIV infection," *Presse Medicale*, vol. 22, no. 4, pp. 161–165, 1993.

[22] E. Bierhoff, A. Tran, E. Pakos, J. Rockstroh, and U. Pfeifer, "Perforation of the small intestine in a patient with disseminated Pneumocystis carinii infection in AIDS," *General & Diagnostic Pathology*, vol. 141, no. 3-4, pp. 255–260, 1996.

[23] O. J. Cohen and M. Y. Stoeckle, "Extrapulmonary Pneumocystis carinii infections in the acquired immunodeficiency syndrome," *Archives of Internal Medicine*, vol. 151, no. 6, pp. 1205–1214, 1991.

[24] G. Z. Panos, I. Karydis, S. E. Velakoulis, and M. E. Falagas, "Multi-skeletal Pneumocystis jiroveci (carinii) in an HIV-seropositive patient," *International Journal of STD & AIDS*, vol. 18, no. 2, pp. 134–137, 2007.

[25] B. Terris, C. Marche, and F. Potet, "Extra-pulmonary pneumocystosis in the course of AIDS: report of a case," *Annales de Pathologie*, vol. 16, no. 1, pp. 41–44, 1996.

[26] E. Valdes, F. Borzoni, D. Onnis, S. Piras, A. Vespa, and C. Varsi, "Disseminated Pneumocystis carinii infection: clinico-pathologic findings in an AIDS patient," *Pathologica*, vol. 86, no. 6, pp. 659–664, 1994.

[27] T. Wakabayashi, S. Oka, K. Shimada, I. Nakano, T. Iwatsubo, and S. Mori, "Disseminated Pneumocystis carinii infection in a hemophiliac patient with acquired immunodeficiency syndrome," *Virchows Archiv A Pathological Anatomy and Histopathology*, vol. 42, no. 4, pp. 262–266, 1994.

[28] D. L. Bundow and D. M. Aboulafia, "Skin involvement with Pneumocystis despite dapsone prophylaxis: a rare cause of skin nodules in a patient with AIDS," *The American Journal of the Medical Sciences*, vol. 313, no. 3, pp. 182–186, 1992.

[29] T. R. Carter, P. H. Cooper, W. A. Petri, C. K. Kim, P. D. Walzer, and R. L. Guerrant, "Pneumocystis carinii infection of the small intestine in a patient with acquired immune deficiency syndrome," *American Journal of Clinical Pathology*, vol. 89, no. 5, pp. 679–683, 1988.

[30] J. E. Gallant, R. E. Enriquez, K. L. Cohen, and L. W. Hammers, "Pneumocystis carinii thyroiditis," *The American Journal of Medicine*, vol. 84, no. 2, pp. 303–306, 1988.

[31] R. B. Poblete, K. Rodriguez, R. T. Foust, K. R. Reddy, and M. J. Saldana, "Pneumocystis carinii hepatitis in the acquired immunodeficiency syndrome (AIDS)," *Annals of Internal Medicine*, vol. 110, no. 9, pp. 737-738, 1989.

[32] W. A. Hagopian and J. S. Huseby, "Pneumocystis hepatitis and choroiditis despite successful aerosolized pentamidine pulmonary prophylaxis," *Chest*, vol. 96, no. 4, pp. 949-951, 1989.

[33] V. A. Pilon, R. M. Echols, J. S. Celo, and S. L. Elmendorf, "Disseminated Pneumocystis carinii infection in AIDS," *The New England Journal of Medicine*, vol. 316, no. 22, pp. 1410-1411, 1987.

[34] E. K. Fishman, D. Magid, and J. E. Kuhlman, "Pneumocystis carinii involvement of the liver and spleen," *Journal of Computer Assisted Tomography*, vol. 14, no. 1, pp. 146–148, 1990.

36

Long-Term Survival in Locally Advanced *KRAS* Wild-Type Pancreatic Adenocarcinoma

Marion Alhenc-Gelas,[1] Romain Cohen,[1] Pascale Cervera,[2] Jean-Christophe Vaillant,[3] and Thierry André[1]

[1] *Sorbonne Université, Department of Medical Oncology, AP-HP, Hôpital Saint-Antoine, F-75012 Paris, France*
[2] *Sorbonne Université, Department of Pathology, AP-HP, Hôpital Saint-Antoine, F-75012 Paris, France*
[3] *Sorbonne Université, Department of Digestive and Hepatobiliary Surgery, AP-HP, Pitié-Salpêtrière Hospital, F-75013 Paris, France*

Correspondence should be addressed to Romain Cohen; romain.cohen@aphp.fr

Academic Editor: Chia-Tung Shun

Pancreatic adenocarcinoma remains a cancer associated with a poor prognosis. For locally advanced pancreatic cancer (LAPC), median overall survival is approximately 16 months. Here we report the case of a 52-year-old LAPC patient treated with chemotherapy followed by chemoradiotherapy that was associated with a 14-year complete remission. A peritoneal relapse was then observed and chemotherapy was undergone until the patient died of infectious complications, 17 years after his diagnosis. The tumor was found *KRAS*, *TP53*, *BRCA1*, and *BRCA2* wild-type. This *KRAS* wild-type LAPC-long survivor case report emphasizes the need to develop molecular approaches to predict LAPC patients' prognosis.

1. Introduction

Pancreatic adenocarcinoma (PC) is the fifth leading cause of cancer death and the second leading digestive cancer in incidence in Western countries, with a 5-year survival rate of less than 5% [1, 2]. For locally advanced PC (LAPC), median overall survival (OS) is approximately 16 months [3]. Here we report the case of long survivor of *KRAS* wild-type LAPC who benefited from a therapeutic strategy combining cytotoxic agents and radiotherapy.

2. Case Report

On July 2000, a 52-year-old man presented a loss of weight associated with dyspepsia. Ultrasonography showed a 4 cm mass in the head of the pancreas infiltrating biliary ducts, portal vein and an involvement of superior mesenteric artery greater than 180°. No metastatic dissemination was found. Pathological examination of the tumor revealed a moderately differentiated tubular pancreatic adenocarcinoma showing eosinophilic abundant cytoplasm and vesicular nucleus with a clear nucleolus. The patient previously received 10 cycles of a regimen combining gemcitabine 1,000 mg/m(2) as a 10-mg/m^2/min infusion on day 1 and oxaliplatin 100 mg/m(2) as a 2-hour infusion on day 2 every 2 weeks [4]. Tumor stability was observed while CA19.9 level decreased from 147 U/mL to 47 U/mL. In March 2001, chemoradiotherapy was performed (45 Gy with a 10 Gy boost associated with 5-fluorouracil) and resulted in a radiological tumoral stability, with a normalized CA19.9 level.

Between April 2001 and May 2015, no tumor recurrence was detected. During this period, the patient presented several episodes of hematemesis, attributed to severe ulcerated bulbitis. The bulbitis was likely a side-effect of radiotherapy.

In May 2015, a disease recurrence was observed with jaundice due to an extrinsic obstruction of the common bill duct. Endoscopic biliary catheterism failed and eventually a surgical biliojejunal derivation was performed; peritoneal involvement was observed during the procedure. Chemotherapy was initiated in September 2015, with 5FU and oxaliplatin (FOLFOX regimen). Oxaliplatin was stopped after 7 cycles because of neuropathy and irinotecan was introduced after normalization of bilirubin for 5 more cycles until January 2016, followed with maintenance treatment by capecitabine until June 2016. At this time, disease remained stable with peritoneal diffuse infiltration and biliary duct dilatation.

Then, the patient benefited from a 12-month therapeutic-free interval. A diffuse lymph node tumor progression was detected in July 2017. A combination of capecitabine and oxaliplatin was initiated. Confirmed stable disease was observed and the treatment was withheld in December 2017 because of infectious complications. From January to March 2018, the patient presented several episodes of angiocholitis related to an anastomotic hepaticojejunal stenosis. A percutaneous biliary derivation was successfully performed with adapted antibiotherapy. Nevertheless the patient presented a new septic episode which revealed the appearance of multiples intrahepatic abscesses. CT-scans conducted at this period did not reveal any tumoral progression, but a neoplastic cholangitis could not be excluded from the causes of the biliary obstruction. Unfortunately in March 2018 the patient finally died of this medically challenging infectious complication.

An exploratory molecular analysis was performed on patient's tumor sample. No mutation was detected in *PIK3CA, BRAF, BRCA1,* and *BRCA 2* genes, neither in *KRAS* and *TP53* genes. No loss of MMR protein expression was observed (i.e., mismatch repair proficiency).

3. Discussion

Here we report the case of a very long survivor of LAPC with *KRAS* wild-type mutational status. Long-term PC survivors are poorly characterized, with few described prognostic clinical, biological, or molecular parameters [5].

The patient was treated with chemoradiotherapy after induction chemotherapy. This strategy has not been demonstrated to improve neither OS (15.2 *versus* 16.5 months, hazard ratio (HR) 1.03, p=0.83) nor progression-free survival (HR 0.78, p=0.06) in the LAP07 phase III study but it enhances median delay to treatment reintroduction (6.1 *versus* 3.7 months, 95% confidence interval (95%CI) 4.8 - 7.0 months, p=0.02) [3]. Based on this trial, a prognostic nomogram for LAPC patients with 5 independent prognostic factors of OS has been designed: age, pain, tumor size, albumin, and CA19-9. The PROLAP score dichotomizes LAPC patients into three prognosis groups with median OS of 15.4, 11.7, and 8.5 months (p<0.0001) [6]. According to the nomogram, the predicted median survival time of our 17-year LAPC survivor would have been about 14 months (95%CI 11.75-15.5) and the 4-year survival probability about 4% (95%CI 2-9). Nevertheless LAP07 study brought out the existence of long survivors after chemoradiotherapy who experience long remission periods without antitumor treatments.

Several genetic features have also been identified as prognosis biomarkers of PC patients. In 2012, an association was suggested between the number of mutated oncogenes and survival [7]. Focusing on the 4 main oncogenic drivers in PC (*KRAS, CDKN2A, SMAD4,* and *TP53*), a statistically significant association was found between the number of altered genes (1 or 2 *versus* 3 or 4) and OS (p=0.041) in a cohort of 79 patients. It is worth noting that these genetic alterations are harbored by the vast majority of PC (> 90% for *KRAS* and *CDKN2A,* 75% for *TP53* and 55% for *SMAD4)* [8, 9]. Nevertheless the prognostic impact of *KRAS* mutation remains a matter of debate. Recently, Bournet and colleagues did not find *KRAS* mutational status as an OS prognostic factor, even if *KRAS* codon 12 mutation was significantly associated with a worse prognosis [10]. Similarly, *KRAS* mutation was not associated with OS in another cohort of 178 PC patients [11].

Interestingly *KRAS* wild-type status might be a predictive factor of response to EGFR inhibitors. In a phase IIb randomized trial evaluating first-line gemcitabine with or without nimotuzumab (a humanized monoclonal antibody acting like an *EGFR* inhibitor), 12-month OS rate was 53.8% versus 15.8% in the *KRAS* wild-type population (HR 0.32, 95%CI 0.13-0.84, p=0.026). It is worth noting that the proportion of *KRAS* wild-type patients in this study was surprisingly much higher than that usually described in literature (26.5% in the combination arm and 41.7% in the gemcitabine arm) [12]. This result suggests that *EGFR* inhibitors might be efficient in first-line treatment for *KRAS* wild-type advanced PC patients.

4. Conclusion

Our case report emphasizes the need to develop molecular approaches in the field of PC to predict the patients' prognosis with more accuracy and to promote personalized therapeutic strategies.

Authors' Contributions

All authors contributed equally to the manuscript. Romain Cohen is the article guarantor.

References

[1] A. Jemal, R. Siegel, J. Xu, and E. Ward, "Cancer statistics, 2010," *CA: A Cancer Journal for Clinicians*, vol. 60, no. 5, pp. 277–300, 2010.

[2] J. Ferlay, I. Soerjomataram, R. Dikshit et al., "Cancer incidence and mortality worldwide: sources, methods and major patterns in GLOBOCAN 2012," *International Journal of Cancer*, vol. 136, no. 5, pp. E359–E386, 2015.

[3] P. Hammel, F. Huguet, J.-L. Van Laethem et al., "Effect of chemoradiotherapy vs chemotherapy on survival in patients with locally advanced pancreatic cancer controlled after 4 months of gemcitabine with or without erlotinib the LAP07 randomized clinical trial," *Journal of the American Medical Association*, vol. 315, no. 17, pp. 1844–1853, 2016.

[4] C. Louvet, T. André, G. Lledo, P. Hammel, H. Bleiberg, C. Bouleuc et al., "Gemcitabine combined with oxaliplatin in advanced pancreatic adenocarcinoma: final results of a GERCOR multicenter phase II study," *Journal of Clinical Oncology*, vol. 20, no. 6, pp. 1512–1518, 2002.

[5] J. H. Jo, M. J. Chung, J. Y. Park et al., "Clinical characteristics of long-term survivors of inoperable pancreatic cancer," *Pancreas*, vol. 43, no. 7, pp. 1022–1031, 2014.

[6] D. Vernerey, F. Huguet, A. Vienot et al., "Prognostic nomogram and score to predict overall survival in locally advanced untreated pancreatic cancer (PROLAP)," *British Journal of Cancer*, vol. 115, no. 3, pp. 281–289, 2016.

[7] S. Yachida, C. M. White, Y. Naito et al., "Clinical significance of the genetic landscape of pancreatic cancer and implications for identification of potential long-term survivors," *Clinical Cancer Research*, vol. 18, no. 22, pp. 6339–6347, 2012.

[8] A. F. Hezel, A. C. Kimmelman, B. Z. Stanger, N. Bardeesy, and R. A. Depinho, "Genetics and biology of pancreatic ductal adenocarcinoma," *Genes & Development*, vol. 20, no. 10, pp. 1218–1249, 2006.

[9] T. Tatarian and J. M. Winter, "Genetics of pancreatic cancer and its implications on therapy," *Surgical Clinics of North America*, vol. 96, no. 6, pp. 1207–1221, 2016.

[10] B. Bournet, F. Muscari, C. Buscail et al., "*KRAS* G12D mutation subtype is a prognostic factor for advanced pancreatic adenocarcinoma," *Clinical and Translational Gastroenterology*, vol. 7, article e157, 2016.

[11] M. Haas, S. Ormanns, S. Baechmann et al., "Extended RAS analysis and correlation with overall survival in advanced pancreatic cancer," *British Journal of Cancer*, vol. 116, no. 11, pp. 1462–1469, 2017.

[12] B. Schultheis, D. Reuter, M. P. Ebert et al., "Gemcitabine combined with the monoclonal antibody nimotuzumab is an active first-line regimen in KRAS wildtype patients with locally advanced or metastatic pancreatic cancer: a multicenter, randomized phase IIb study," *Annals of Oncology*, vol. 28, no. 10, pp. 2429–2435, 2017.

37

Cholecystomegaly: A Case Report and Review of the Literature

Mohammad Bagher Jahantab, Vahid Salehi, Saadat Mehrabi, Lotfolah Abedini, and Mohammad Javad Yavari Barhaghtalab

General Surgery Department, Shahid Beheshti Hospital, Yasuj University of Medical Sciences, Yasuj, Iran

Correspondence should be addressed to Mohammad Javad Yavari Barhaghtalab; mj.yavari.barhaghtalab@yums.ac.ir

Academic Editor: Yoshifumi Nakayama

Chronic cholecystitis or symptomatic gallbladder is a prolonged mechanical or functional disorder of abnormal gallbladder emptying. Most of the patients have recurrent pain attacks (acute biliary colic), but when pain lasts more than 24 hours, it requires urgent surgical intervention (acute cholecystitis). The length of a fully distended gallbladder is about 7 to 10 cm. We report a case of a huge and severely inflamed gallbladder, as we have just found only a few previous case reports of the huge gallbladder in the literature. This case report and review may help to find a mechanism for the development of a giant gallbladder. The patient was a 36-year-old woman, who had been known to have a symptomatic gallstone for at least three years. The patient underwent laparotomy, and a giant 22 cm roundish severely inflamed and overdistended gallbladder with wall thickening and tight adhesion to adjacent organs was found under the right liver lobe. Femininity and diabetes seem to be risk factors for developing a huge gallbladder, and several hypotheses are encountered: (1) a long-lasting obstructed cystic duct or biliary tree, and accumulation of mucosal secretion from the gallbladder epithelium, (2) an obstructed hepatic/cystic duct junction with a stone acting like a check valve and bile trapping mechanism, and (3) gallbladder dysfunction and cholecystoparesis affecting through reduced cholecystokinin and celiac parasympathetic nerve disturbance in diabetes and diabetic autonomic neuropathy. Open cholecystectomy is the technique of choice in surgical excision of a huge gallbladder; however, laparoscopy could be performed by expert hands.

1. Background

Cholecystitis is the inflammation of the gallbladder. Symptoms include postprandial right upper quadrant or epigastric abdominal pain, and it is often called biliary colic. If biliary colic is left untreated, then most of the patients will develop chronic noninfectious inflammation of the gallbladder wall (chronic cholecystitis) [1]. When the pain lasts more than 24 hours without resolving, it can progress to a more severe form of cholecystitis (acute cholecystitis), so then requiring an urgent intervention [1, 2]. Contrary to the biliary colic, the pain of acute cholecystitis does not decrease [1].

In the etiology of cholecystitis, obstruction of the cystic duct by a gallstone or rarely an obstructive tumor is the initiating event that leads to distention, inflammation, edema, and mechanical dysfunction of the gallbladder. In this regard, the gallbladder wall becomes grossly thickened and reddish with subserosal hemorrhages and pericholecystic fluid. The mucosa may show hyperemia and patchy necrosis. Hypokinetic functioning of the gallbladder can also lead to a static state of gallbladder bile and is a precipitating factor for sludge and gallstone formation [1, 2]. Mucosal toxin lysolecithin (a product of lecithin), bile salts, platelet-activating factor, and an increase in prostaglandin synthesis may be associated with the inflammatory process in acute cholecystitis [1].

Cholecystectomy is the most common abdominal surgery in Western countries. Before the adventure of laparoscopic cholecystectomy by Philippe Mouret in 1987, an open technique was the standard procedure for cholecystectomy for more than 100 years (Carl Langenbuch made the first successful cholecystectomy in 1882). Now, the laparoscopic technique is the preferred method for the treatment of cholecystitis [2, 3].

The gallbladder is a pear-shaped sac that measures around 7 to 10 cm long and 4 cm wide, with an average capacity of 30 to 50 mL. When obstructed, the gallbladder can distend markedly and contain up to 300 mL of fluid [1, 4, 5]. We report a case with a huge and severely inflamed gallbladder, as we have just found only a few earlier case reports with a huge gallbladder in the literature [6–18]. This case report and review may help to find the mechanism for the development of a giant gallbladder or cholecystomegaly.

2. Case Presentation

The patient was a 36-year-old woman, a known case of symptomatic gallstone for at least three years. She was admitted to the emergency department at Yasuj Shahid Beheshti Hospital in April 2019, with a 2-day history of progressive increasing abdominal pain in the right upper quadrant with the radiation of pain to the epigastric area. The patient also had nausea, vomiting, and anorexia. She had 3 times previous admissions for the same problem last year, in which she did not give consent for operation and she did not use any medications.

On examination, she was hemodynamically stable and was not febrile. She had no jaundice, and the patient had abdominal tenderness in the right upper quadrant, and the gallbladder was palpable, with a positive Murphy's sign.

Laboratory tests showed a white blood cell (WBC) count of 9300 mm^3, mild increase in total bilirubin, direct bilirubin, and aspartate aminotransferase (AST) (1.24 mg/dl, 0.68 mg/dl, and 36 u/l, retrospectively), a erythrocyte sedimentation rate (ESR) of 58.4 mm in one hour, and a C-reactive protein (CRP) of 58.4 mg/dL. Serum amylase, lipase, alanine transaminase (ALT), and alkaline phosphatase were all at normal levels. Urine analysis was normal.

Abdominal sonography showed a dilated edematous gallbladder with a thickened wall more than 10 mm (the gallbladder size and dimensions were not included in the ultrasound report), with many small stones and sludge in which the largest one was about 25 mm and was indicative of acute cholecystitis. The common bile duct and hepatic ducts had normal caliber without any pathology. As the diagnosis was exact and there was no clinical suspicion for the complications of acute cholecystitis such as cholangitis or gallbladder perforation according to the ultrasound report, other diagnostic modalities such as computed tomography (CT) scan was not performed. The patient underwent open cholecystectomy through midline laparotomy on the day of admission. The findings of abdominal sonography were compatible with what we saw during laparotomy. A giant roundish severely inflamed and overdistended gallbladder with wall thickening and with tight adhesion to adjacent organs was found under the right liver lobe. Decompression of the gallbladder with needle aspiration was performed to decrease the size and make the cholecystectomy easier. After the decompression, a large impacted stone in the neck of the gallbladder was palpated. Cholecystectomy was performed successfully, and the exact size of the gallbladder was about 22 cm length, 6 cm width, and 1 cm thickness for the gallbladder wall. Figure 1 shows the gross pathology of the specimen after fixation in formalin (the difference between the real postoperation and the gross pathology gallbladder size was due to the formalin shrinking effect).

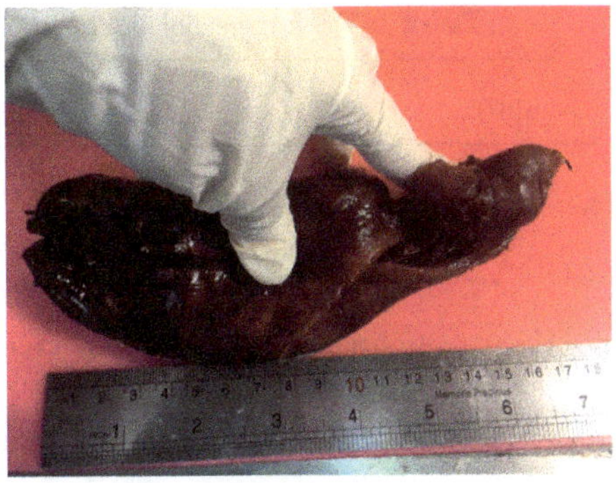

FIGURE 1: The huge gallbladder after fixation in formalin.

The patient got well after the operation and was discharged in good condition on the fourth day of admission. Histopathological evaluation revealed chronic gangrenous cholecystitis, with no sign of malignant change. The patient was followed up in the next 4 weeks after the operation without any complications.

3. Discussion

Grosberg [6] reported the first published giant gallbladder in the literature. Bloom and Stachenfeld [7] discussed the diabetic cholecystomegaly observed in three cases for the first time. Cohen et al. [8] presented a case with acromegalic cholecystomegaly. Maeda et al. [9] resected a congenital form of the giant gallbladder. Tessier et al. [10] removed a huge gallbladder by laparoscopic surgery. Hsu et al. [11] reported the first and the only huge cancerous gallbladder in the literature. Panaro et al. [12] presented the largest gallbladder even reported in the world in a patient with Byler's disease (a group of diseases known as progressive familial intrahepatic cholestasis). The patient had chronic diarrhea and severe pruritus and was referred for liver transplantation. Taj [13] was issued in the Guinness Book of World Records as the first surgeon who operated the world's longest gallbladder through laparoscopic cholecystectomy at Capital Development Authority (CDA) hospital. Zong et al. [14] presented a huge congenital form of the gallbladder, which was marked as a giant celiac cyst before the operation. Kuznetsov et al. [15] reported the only huge gallbladder found in the literature without any evidence of acquired, congenital, and obstructive cause for the enlargement of the gallbladder. Edlin et al. [16] presented a patient with chronic cholecystitis who underwent cholecystostomy and then laparoscopic cholecystectomy. Kankaria et al. operated a huge gallbladder mucocele, belonged to Suman from Jaipur, India, through a laparoscopic approach, and the Guinness Book of World Records accepted it for the longest gallbladder in the world till now [17, 18]. Table 1 shows the huge gallbladders reported in the literature in the order of published year till now.

Our case study was comparable with the earlier studies according to size, procedure method, and pathology. All the patients were female except two diabetic cholecystomegaly patients who were male and in one whom sex identity was not mentioned. It shows that men develop less likely to have

Table 1: The huge gallbladders reported in the literature in the order of published year till now.

	Year	Country	Author	Age (years)	Sex	Gallbladder size	Kind of operation	Pathology
1	1962	USA	Grosberg [6]	95	Female	14 cm	Open cholecystectomy	Acute gangrenous cholecystitis
2	1969	USA	Bloom and Stachenfeld [7]	61/66/70	Female/male/male	3 to 9 times normal size	Nonoperative management	Three cases of diabetic cholecystomegaly
3	1974	USA	Cohen et al. [8]	65	Female	18 cm	Nonoperative management	Visceromegaly as a feature of acromegaly
4	1979	Japan	Maeda et al. [9]	36	Female	18 cm	Open cholecystectomy	Neither inflammatory nor obstructive marked as a congenital giant gallbladder
5	2005	USA	Tessier et al. [10]	78	Female	17 cm	Laparoscopic cholecystectomy after needle decompression	Stone impaction and dilatation in the neck of the gallbladder, acute and chronic cholecystitis
6	2011	Taiwan	Hsu et al. [11]	87	Female	16.4 cm	Emergency laparotomy with extended cholecystectomy	Acute suppurative cholecystitis with a fungating tumor showing poorly differentiated adenocarcinoma
7	2012	France	Panaro et al. [12]	17	Not available (N/A)	43 cm	Open cholecystectomy at the time of liver transplantation	Byler's (intrahepatic cholestasis), no pathologic change in the gallbladder
8	2012	Pakistan	Taj [13]	70	Female	25.5 cm	Laparoscopic cholecystectomy	N/A
9	2013	China	Zong et al. [14]	55	Female	30 cm	Open cholecystectomy	No obstructive cause, so congenital giant gallbladder considered
10	2014	Russia	Kuznetsov et al. [15]	77	Female	24 cm	Open cholecystectomy	No acquired, congenital and obstructive cause
11	2015	United Kingdom	Edlin et al. [16]	88	Female	12 cm	Cholecystostomy and then laparoscopic cholecystectomy 6 weeks later	Chronic cholecystitis
12	2017	India	Kankaria et al. [17, 18]	46	Female	30 cm	Laparoscopic cholecystectomy	Chronic cholecystitis, cholelithiasis, gallbladder mucocele with a large impacted stone
13	2019	Iran	Jahantab (current report)	36	Female	22 cm	Open cholecystectomy	Chronic gangrenous cholecystitis

huge gallbladders except in diabetic patients. The patients' ages were from 17 to 95 years. According to the size, in Panaro's case report, the largest gallbladder even seen in the world till now was about 43 cm. However, the gallbladder size in our case was about 22 cm, and it was smaller than five previous reported studies [12–18]; it is large enough to be presented as a case report, as there are no defined borders proposed to distinguish between simply enlarged and giant gallbladders [15].

According to the procedure method used, Tessier et al. [10, 13, 16–18] performed laparoscopic cholecystectomy. In our study, classic open cholecystectomy was preferred as like as some other studies [6, 9, 11, 12, 14, 15]. In giant gall stones, it is much difficult to do laparoscopic cholecystectomy, so conversion from laparoscopic to open cholecystectomy is often performed because the giant stones are associated with more inflammation and thickening of the gallbladder wall and could make it much more difficult to hold the gallbladder with a grasper and expose Calot's triangle anatomy and retrieve such a large gallstone [19, 20]. Because of these whys and wherefores, open cholecystectomy is the ideal procedure in such cases [19]. However, this procedure is much difficult in these instances, but it is not an absolute indication for open cholecystectomy, and laparoscopy could be performed by an expert laparoscopic surgeon [20].

In the earlier case reports and our study, the dominant pathologies for giant gallbladders were as follows: chronic inflammation (cholecystitis), congenital, diabetes, visceromegaly due to acromegaly, inappropriate accumulation of mucus (mucocele), malignancy (adenocarcinoma), cholelithiasis, and cholestatic liver disease (Byler's disease). In our study, chronic inflammation (gangrenous cholecystitis) and an obstructive stone were the dominant pathologies. According to the existence of an obstructive stone in the gallbladder, our results were as same as Grosberg, Kankaria, and Tessier's studies [6, 10, 17, 18] in which a large impacted stone at the gallbladder neck was found. In the other studies, there was no obstructive etiology [8, 10–12, 14, 15]. In Bloom and Stachenfeld [7] and Zong's [14] case reports, as there was no inflammation and obstruction, it was considered to be a congenital etiology.

For the establishment of an overdistended huge gallbladder, several hypotheses could be identified: (1) The first process could be the hydrops of the gallbladder, in which an impacted stone without cholecystitis is present. Bile could not enter the gallbladder due to the long-lasting obstructed cystic duct or biliary tree, but the gallbladder epithelium will continue to secrete mucus and the gallbladder will become distended with clear-white mucinous material leading in the gallbladder wall edema, dilatation, inflammation, infection, and maybe perforation [1, 21, 22]. (2) The second hypothesis could be that the stones may move down and obstruct the hepatic/cystic duct junction acutely. One huge stone or multiple large stones act like a check valve allowing bile to enter but not exit (bile trapping) and impair drainage, and this leads to the slow resorption of the bile, distension, and enlargement of the gallbladder. When the disease progresses, the giant gallbladder became filled with bile, which leads to swelling and inflammation and targets the contractile ability of the gallbladder and can cause the gallbladder to grow large [14, 22]. (3) Another hypothesis is associated with physiological gallbladder contraction and relaxation which are regulated by both the endocrine and autonomic nervous system. Cholecystokinin (CCK) stimulates the gallbladder to contract and release stored bile into the intestine, and the parasympathetic nerve evokes gallbladder evacuating [23]. It has been shown that postprandial plasma cholecystokinin secretion and maximal gallbladder emptying after feeding were much reduced during hyperglycemia [24]. In patients with diabetic autonomic neuropathy, cholinergic action would be diminished by disturbance of the celiac parasympathetic nerve, resulting in gallbladder dysfunction and cholecystoparesis [23], so we could hypothesize that cholecystomegaly could occur in conjunction with diabetes and diabetic autonomic neuropathy through gallbladder dysfunction and cholecystoparesis.

The strength of this study is its comprehensive literature review, and its limitation is that we just check English literature for this review. Femininity and diabetes seem to be risk factors for developing a huge gallbladder. Conditions in which gallbladder increases in size are inflammation, acromegaly, diabetes, congenital, mucocele, malignancy, cholelithiasis, and intrahepatic cholestasis. Large or giant gallbladders need special surgical intervention. Open cholecystectomy is the technique of choice in surgical excision of a huge gallbladder, but laparoscopy could be performed, too by expert hands. The primary take away lesson of this report is to take enough time for our patients and give enough information to convince them to operate in a proper time to prevent a difficult, time-consuming, and high-risk operation instead of an easy, rapid, and low-risk surgery.

Abbreviations

WBC: White blood cell
CT: Computed tomography
AST: Aspartate aminotransferase
CRP: C-reactive protein
ALT: Alanine transaminase
CDA: Capital Development Authority hospital
N/A: Not available
CCK: Cholecystokinin.

Authors' Contributions

MBJ evaluated the patient clinically and operated the patient (main surgeon) and revised the manuscript. VS, SM, and HA revised the manuscript. MJYB evaluated the patient clinically and helped to operate the patient (cosurgeon), reviewed the literature, and prepared the manuscript. All authors read and approved the final manuscript.

Acknowledgments

The authors express their gratitude to the patient who kindly gave consent for this case to be presented in this paper. The authors also wish to thank Dr. Aida Iraji at the Central Research Laboratory of Shiraz University of Medical Sciences for her assistance in editing this manuscript.

References

[1] K. R. Haisley and J. G. Hunter, "Gallbladder and the extrahepatic biliary system: Chapter 32,""Gallbladder and the extrahepatic biliary system: Chapter 32," in *Schwartz's Principles of Surgery*, F. Brunicardi, D. K. Andersen, T. R. Billiar et al., Eds., McGraw-Hill, New York, NY, USA, 11th edition, 2019.

[2] M. W. Jones and T. Ferguson, *Chronic Cholecystitis*, StatPearls Publishing, Treasure Island, FL, USA, 2020.

[3] M. W. Jones and J. G. Deppen, *Open Cholecystectomy*, StatPearls Publishing, Treasure Island, FL, USA, 2020.

[4] J. W. Meilstrup, *Imaging Atlas of the Normal Gallbladder and its Variants*p. 4, 1st edition, CRC Press, Boca Raton, FL, USA, 1994.

[5] C. D. Clemente, *Gray's Anatomy of the Human Body: Hardcover*p. 132, 30th edition, Lippincott Williams & Wilkins, Philadelphia, PA, USA, 1985.

[6] S. J. Grosberg, "Giant gallbladder," *The American Journal of Digestive Diseases*, vol. 7, no. 11, pp. 1039-1040, 1962.

[7] A. A. Bloom and R. Stachenfeld, "Diabetic cholecystomegaly," *JAMA: The Journal of the American Medical Association*, vol. 208, no. 2, pp. 357–359, 1969.

[8] G. A. Cohen, W. M. Smoak, and L. D. Goldberg, "Acromegalic cholecystomegaly," *Journal of Nuclear Medicine: Official Publication, Society of Nuclear Medicine*, vol. 15, no. 8, pp. 720-721, 1974.

[9] Y. Maeda, T. Setoguchi, T. Yoshida, and T. Katsuki, "A giant gallbladder," *Gastroenterologia Japonica*, vol. 14, no. 6, pp. 621–624, 1979.

[10] D. J. Tessier, L. McMahon, and K. L. Harold, "Cholecystomegaly: laparoscopic treatment," *Journal of Minimal Access Surgery*, vol. 1, no. 2, pp. 82-83, 2005.

[11] K.-F. Hsu, C.-L. Yeh, M.-L. Shih, C.-B. Hsieh, and H.-M. Hsu, "Giant gallbladder: adenocarcinoma complicated with empyema," *The Journal of Trauma: Injury, Infection, and Critical Care*, vol. 70, no. 1, p. 261, 2011.

[12] F. Panaro, L. Chastaing, and F. Navarro, "Hepatobiliary and Pancreatic: giant gallbladder associated with Byler's disease," *Journal of Gastroenterology and Hepatology*, vol. 27, no. 3, p. 620, 2012.

[13] N. Taj, World's biggest gall bladder: doctor's Guinness book entry honoured. The Express Tribune, Pakistan January 10, 2012. https://tribune.com.pk/story/319049/worlds-biggest-gall-bladder-doctors-guinness-book-entry-honoured/.

[14] L. Zong, P. Chen, L. Wang et al., "A case of congenital giant gallbladder with massive hydrops mimicking celiac cyst," *Oncology Letters*, vol. 5, no. 1, pp. 226–228, 2013.

[15] A. V. Kuznetsov, A. V. Borodach, E. N. Fedin, and A. D. Khromova, "Giant gallbladder: a case report and review of literature," *International Journal of Surgery Case Reports*, vol. 5, no. 10, pp. 673–676, 2014.

[16] J. C. Edlin, M. Alfa-Wali, and A. Bond, "A mass more ordinary," *BMJ Case Reports*, vol. 2015, 2015.

[17] R. Yadav and J. Kankaria, "Longest gallbladder: a case report," *International Journal of Surgery Case Reports*, vol. 33, pp. 127–129, 2017.

[18] B. Kuchay. Doctors remove world's longest gallbladder through laparoscopic surgery. Story Trender, Powered by Caters Media Group. 2011; http://www.storytrender.com/9423/doctors-remove-worlds-longest-gallbladder-through-laparoscopic-surgery/.

[19] S. Dalal, S. B. Pankaj, R. Pankaj, S. Bhoriwal, R. Kumar, and Sujata, "Giant gallstone: a rare indication of open cholecystectomy," *Journal of Case Reports*, vol. 4, no. 1, pp. 17–19, 2014.

[20] P. O. Igwe and O. N. Diri, "Laparoscopic cholecystectomy for giant gall stone: report of two cases," *International Journal of Surgery Case Reports*, vol. 67, pp. 207–210, 2020.

[21] R. R. Khothsymuong and J. Kaminski, "Gallbladder hydrops," *Journal of Diagnostic Medical Sonography*, vol. 20, no. 4, pp. 256–259, 2004.

[22] S. Amarnath, A. D. Polavarapu, and V. Gumaste, "Spontaneous perforation of an acalculous hydropic gallbladder in a diabetic patient with neuropathy: an underdiagnosed entity," *Gastroenterology Research*, vol. 12, no. 6, pp. 315–319, 2019.

[23] H. Itoh, T. Matsumoto, N. Tanimoto et al., "Cholecystoparesis with diabetic autonomic neuropathy," *Internal Medicine*, vol. 36, no. 9, pp. 624–627, 1997.

[24] S. Y. De Boer, A. A. M. Masclee, W. F. Lam, J. Schipper, J. B. M. J. Jansen, and C. B. H. W. Lamers, "Hyperglycemia reduces gallbladder emptying and plasma hormone secretion to modified sham feeding and regular feeding," *Hepatology*, vol. 17, no. 6, pp. 1022–1027, 1993.

38

A Rare Complication of Noncompliance Status Post-Transhiatal Esophagectomy and Esophago-Gastroanastomosis

Daniel Ramirez,[1] **Graham Appelbe**,[1] **Venkatramana Vattipally**,[2] **and Justin Miller**[3]

[1]*Department of Internal Medicine, Ascension Genesys Medical Center, Grand Blanc, MI, USA*
[2]*Department of Radiology, Ascension Genesys Medical Center, Grand Blanc, MI, USA*
[3]*Department of Gastroenterology, Ascension Genesys Medical Center, Grand Blanc, MI, USA*

Correspondence should be addressed to Daniel Ramirez; djramirez10@gmail.com

Academic Editor: Shiro Kikuchi

Gastropleural fistulas are a complication of peptic ulcers in hiatal hernias, trauma, infections, surgical complications, and malignancy. Presenting symptoms may include gastric and chest pain with respiratory failure in the setting of pneumonitis, hydropneumothorax, or tension pneumothorax. We describe a 57-year-old male with a history of transhiatal esophagectomy and esophago-gastroanastomosis who presented in the setting of dyspnea and dark orogastric tube output. Upper endoscopy revealed multiple gastric ulcers with a dominant ulceration communicating with an adjacent space, and a fistulous tract was demonstrated on computed tomography chest, confirming a gastropleural fistula, a rare life-threatening condition.

1. Introduction

Gastropleural fistulas (GPFs) are a rare and dangerous complication of different pathologies including peptic ulcer disease, trauma, infections, surgical complications, and malignancy [1]. Presentation is typically insidious, and symptoms may include abdominal and chest pain, respiratory failure, and signs of septic shock [1–7]. Treating physicians should have a high index of suspicion with high-risk patients, as prompt diagnosis is essential to decrease mortality in this life-threatening diagnosis. We describe a 57-year-old male with a history of transhiatal esophagectomy and esophago-gastroanastomosis secondary to high-grade dysplasia who presented in the setting of dyspnea and dark orogastric tube (OGT) suction. Respiratory distress worsened, and the patient was emergently intubated in the Emergency Room. Bronchoscopy revealed clear airways; however, esophagogastroduodenoscopy (EGD) revealed multiple gastric ulcers with a dominant ulceration communicating with an adjacent space. Computed tomography (CT) of the chest confirmed suspicion of fistulous tract, and this patient was diagnosed with the rare condition of GPF requiring urgent correction with endoscopic suture placement.

2. Case Report

The patient was a 57-year-old male with a history of COPD and transhiatal esophagectomy with esophago-gastro-anastomosis and J-tube placement (2005) secondary to high-grade dysplasia within a segment of Barrett's esophagus. Since 2005, he had numerous hospitalizations for dysphagia, regurgitation, and aspiration with subsequent balloon dilation without significant relief. Several records indicate a significant history of leaving against medical advice (AMA) and noncompliance with tobacco abuse and eating solid foods leading to multiple EGD with subsequent removal of retained food products. Also noted on previous endoscopies were findings suggesting functional gastric outlet obstruction and multiple Forrest class III gastric ulcers thought to be from ischemia and stasis.

Prior to this admission, the patient ingested solid food which induced abdominal pain, nausea and nonbloody,

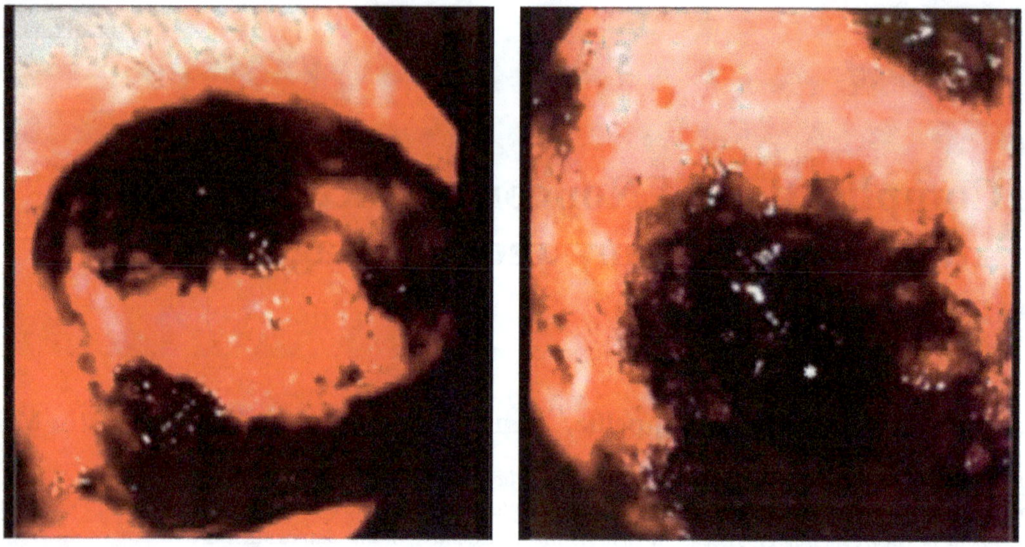

(a) (b)

FIGURE 1: (a) Dominant ulceration along the greater curvature. (b) Image within ulceration revealing fistula opening leading to pleural space marked by the asterisk.

nonbilious emesis. In the ER, the patient became dyspneic requiring intubation for airway protection. OGT suctioned approximately 1200 cc of dark-colored fluid. Pertinent physical findings included cachectic appearance with right-sided coarse lung sounds. The abdomen was nondistended, soft, and nontender, and without organomegaly or masses. The J-tube was in place without discharge or erythema.

Chest X-ray showed right middle and lower lobe infiltrate. Labs were significant for leukocytosis (WBC 22.9 K/cmm), anemia (hemoglobin of 8.8 g/dL), thrombocytosis (platelets greater than 1000 K/cmm), and lactic acid of 9.92 mmol/L. Electrolyte abnormalities included sodium of 129 mmol/L, chloride of 75 mmol/L, and hyperglycemia with glucose at 248 mg/dL. Arterial blood gas showed hypercapnia without significant hypoxia, and EKG showed sinus tachycardia without ischemic changes. He received a 30 mL/kg bolus of intravenous fluids, antibiotics including vancomycin/cefepime with the addition of clindamycin for aspiration coverage, and 80 mg IV pantoprazole and was admitted to the Intensive Care Unit (ICU). Due to worsening hypoxia and the suspicion of aspiration, Critical Care performed bronchoscopy which showed a normal-appearing trachea as well as clear bilateral lung lobes. Secretions were suctioned and the right lung wash-out specimens were sent for pathology; however, there were no reported findings of food material or bleeding. Gastroenterology was consulted for concern of upper GI bleed with dark liquid from OGT and a decrease in Hgb from 8.8 to 6.2 g/dL requiring 2 units of packed red blood cells (pRBCs).

EGD discovered 1.5 L of dark gastric content that was suctioned revealing 5 clean-based gastric ulcers. One such ulcer measured approximately 2×2.5 cm in diameter and approximately 1 cm deep at 44 cm from the incisors, along the greater curvature. At the base of this ulcer appeared an external communication with a questionable fistula (Figure 1). Biopsies obtained revealed inflammatory granulation tissue without signs of malignancy. Subsequent insertion of the gastric tube after endoscopy was completed, and follow-up CT imaging (Figure 2) showed right-sided gastric pull-through with a concerning fistulous tract connecting to the underlying lung parenchyma, as the distal tip of the gastric feeding tube terminated within a focal air lucency within the lung parenchyma. A large consolidation with right-sided pleural effusion was also identified, likely contributing to this patient's worsening respiratory status. Due to these concerning findings, a decision was made to transfer this patient to a tertiary center where he was known to the cardiothoracic surgical group for further surgical management. The patient was subsequently treated with endoscopic suturing and continued on antibiotic therapy; however, despite treatments, he succumbed to his illness several months later.

3. Discussion

First described in 1960 by Markowtts and Herter, GPF can be an acquired complication from peptic ulcerations via hiatal hernia, trauma, and perforation with abscess formation [1]. Case reports have described oral intake of steroids or anti-inflammatory drugs increasing the risk of gastric perforations, and several studies have demonstrated that GPF can also be a serious complication from surgical interventions and malignancy [2–6]. As the diaphragm acts as an effective barrier, communicating fistulas from the stomach and pleural space through the diaphragm are extremely rare. Diagnosis is normally via contrast radiology, upper endoscopy, and/or via open operation.

Prognosis of this rare complication depends on the time of diagnosis and intervention with prolonged use of antibiotics, acid-suppressing medications, and strict NPO with total parenteral nutrition which can result in successful outcomes. In the absence of universal guidelines, there are conflicting reports on the proper care of GPF. A majority of

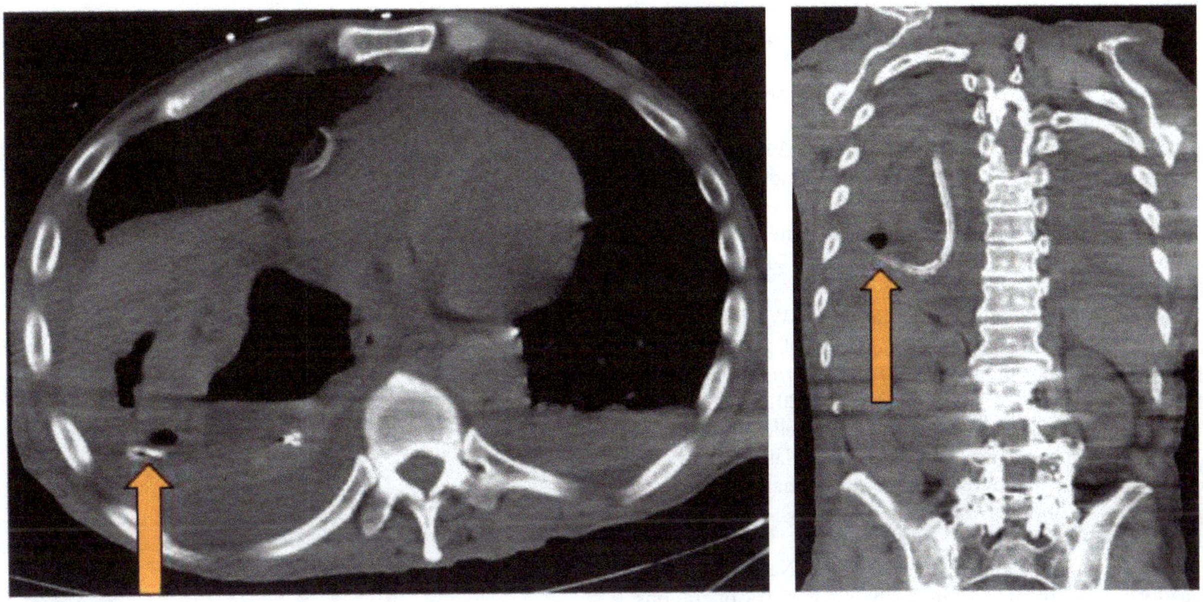

(a) (b)

FIGURE 2: The arrow in (a) and (b) demonstrate a catheter passing from the stomach into the pleural cavity consistent with gastropleural fistula.

reports agree that the laparoscopic approach and surgical interventions are definitive treatments as data indicate higher mortality with conservative management [7–9]. Meta-analysis of several case reports and retrospective studies has evaluated the outcomes of various surgical and endoscopic interventions. Stent placement, endoscopic clipping techniques, or surgical sealants have all shown high success rates of repair with decreased morbidity and mortality when compared to nonsurgical therapies [8, 9]. Contemporary studies have shown improving trends with fistula repairs with evidence implying that complex endoscopic surgical treatments or combined treatment with simultaneous or sequential endoscopic methods can optimize management [8]. While postoperative complication management is crucial, preoperative modifiable factors have also been investigated. Several reviews have implicated potential quality improvements to postsurgical patients and distinguished tobacco abuse and hyperobesity as modifiable risk factors and that as the quantity and chronicity of tobacco use rose, it showed positive correlation to postsurgical complications [10–12].

This case provides an excellent example of septic shock in the setting of an extremely rare surgical and traumatic complication. GPF are infrequent and life-threatening with insidious onset and nonspecific symptoms. This diagnosis has been historically difficult to establish and is often misdiagnosed, as is noted in several reviews and case reports [2, 5–7]. A high index of suspicion should be held in patients with significant risk factors including previous surgeries, malignancy, and gastric ulcerations. Providing awareness of this uncommon pathology may help eliminate delay of diagnosis, as rapid surgical or endoscopic correction appears to be the definitive form of treatment. In the case of our patient, the combination of esophago-gastroanastomosis with gastric pull-through and the chronic history of tobacco abuse and NPO noncompliance likely led to persistent inflammation at the numerous gastric ulcer sites eventually leading to this devastating complication.

Disclosure

J. Miller and is the article guarantor.

Authors' Contributions

D. Ramirez drafted the manuscript and reviewed the literature. G. Appelbe revised the manuscripts. V. Vattipally formatted and described the CT image. J. Miller reviewed and revised the manuscript.

References

[1] A. M. Markowttz and F. P. Herter, "Gastro-pleural fistula as a complication of esophageal hiatal hernia∗," *Annals of Surgery*, vol. 152, no. 1, pp. 129–134, 1960.

[2] P. A. O'keefe and P. Goldstraw, "Gastropleural fistula following pulmonary resection," *Thorax*, vol. 48, no. 12, pp. 1278-1279, 1993.

[3] C. J. Warburton and P. M. A. Calverley, "Gastropleural fistula due to gastric lymphoma presenting as tension pneumothorax and empyema," *European Respiratory Journal*, vol. 10, no. 7, pp. 1678-1679, 1997.

[4] M. A. Bozkurt, O. Köneş, İ. Başoğlu, and H. Alış, "Gastropleural fistula: a rare complication of ewing sarcoma," *The Korean Journal of Thoracic and Cardiovascular Surgery*, vol. 46, no. 4, pp. 293-294, 2013.

[5] R. L. Armstrong and P. B. Heyse, "Gastropleural fistula in metastatic ovarian cancer," *Journal of Surgical Case Reports*, vol. 2014, no. 5, p. rju033, 2014.
[6] S. M. Iqbal, C. Zhi, M. Masud, H. M. Aslam, and M. A. Qadir, "Gastropleural fistula: a rare complication of a common procedure," *Cureus*, vol. 11, no. 2, p. e413, 2019.
[7] F. Alghanim, A. Alkhaibary, A. Alzakari, and A. AlRumaih, "Gastropleural fistula as a rare complication of gastric sleeve surgery: a case report and comprehensive literature review," *Case Reports in Surgery*, vol. 2018, Article ID 2416915, 5 pages, 2018.
[8] P. Rogalski, J. Daniluk, A. Baniukiewicz, E. Wroblewski, and A. Dabrowski, "Endoscopic management of gastrointestinal perforations, leaks and fistulas," *World Journal of Gastroenterology*, vol. 21, no. 37, pp. 10542–10552, 2015.
[9] P. Rogalski, A. Swidnicka-Siergiejko, J. Wasielica-Berger et al., "Endoscopic management of leaks and fistulas after bariatric surgery: a systematic review and meta-analysis," *Surgical Endoscopy*, 2020, In press.
[10] E. H. Livingston, D. Arterburn, T. L. Schifftner, W. G. Henderson, and R. G. DePalma, "National surgical quality improvement program analysis of bariatric operations: modifiable risk factors contribute to bariatric surgical adverse outcomes," *Journal of the American College of Surgeons*, vol. 203, no. 5, pp. 625–633, 2006.
[11] M. Parthasarathy, M. Greensmith, D. Bowers, and T. Groot-Wassink, "Risk factors for anastomotic leakage after colorectal resection: a retrospective analysis of 17,518 patients," *Colorectal Disease*, vol. 19, no. 3, pp. 288–298, 2016.
[12] P. Agostini, H. Cieslik, S. Rathinam et al., "Postoperative pulmonary complications following thoracic surgery: are there any modifiable risk factors?" *Thorax*, vol. 65, no. 9, pp. 815–818, 2010.

39

Use of Argon Plasma Coagulation and Endoscopic Hemoclips for Postsurgical Gastrointestinal Fistula

Abdullah Sohail,[1] Ahmad Khan,[1] Hamza Shah,[2] and Ragheb Rezko[3]

[1]*West Virginia University Charleston Division, Charleston, West Virginia, USA*
[2]*Charleston Area Medical Center, Charleston, West Virginia, USA*
[3]*West Virginia University, Morgantown, West Virginia, USA*

Correspondence should be addressed to Abdullah Sohail; abdullah.sohail@camc.org

Academic Editor: Haruhiko Sugimura

A 72-year-old male was diagnosed with a duodenal mass and underwent extensive surgical resection. The patient's post-op course was complicated by an anastomotic leak that was first treated conservatively; however, his condition continued to deteriorate. An upper endoscopy was performed, which showed misplacement of drain forming a fistulous track through the lumen of the bowel. We removed the drain and used argon plasma coagulation to de-epithelize the lumen and closed the fistula with hemostasis clips. The patient's clinical status improved significantly. Our case emphasizes the success of endoscopic techniques as an alternative option in the management of postsurgical anastomotic leaks and fistulas in the right clinical setting and patient population.

1. Introduction

Postsurgical anastomotic leaks and fistulas are a serious complication after major abdominal surgery resulting in significant morbidity and mortality [1]. Its occurrences depend on surgical procedure type, technique, expertise, and anatomical location [2]. The estimated incidence is reported between 4% to 17% in surgical procedures involving the upper gastrointestinal (GI) tract and 2% to 7% in colorectal surgeries. Similarly, associated mortality is described 10% to 65% in the upper GI tract and 6% to 22% in lower GI tract surgeries [3, 4].

Historically, the mainstay of treatment has been either conservative management such as prolonged bowel rest with total parenteral nutrition (TPN) or surgical interventions. Lately, endoscopic treatments have emerged as an alternative option for the management of anastomotic leaks/fistulas with better clinical outcomes [5].

We present a case of a postsurgical anastomotic leak and enterocutaneous fistula formation after an extensive small bowel resection who deteriorated with conservative/surgical interventions and had successful outcomes with endoscopic treatment.

2. Case Report

A 72-year-old male presented to the emergency department with complaints of four-day history of epigastric abdominal pain, nausea, vomiting, constipation, and inability to tolerate oral diet. He reported early satiety and 24 pounds of unintentional weight loss in the last four months. He was hemodynamical stable on presentation. Abdominal examination revealed mild epigastric tenderness with moderate abdominal distention. The basic laboratory workup was within normal limits. However, computed tomography (CT) abdomen and pelvis with intravenous and oral contrast showed eccentric thickening of the third and fourth part of the duodenum (Figure 1). A magnetic resonance imaging showed a heterogeneous mass in the duodenum measuring $13.1 \times 5.9 \times 7.5$ cm (Figure 2). An esophagogastroduodenoscopy (EGD) was performed to obtain the biopsy of the mass which turned

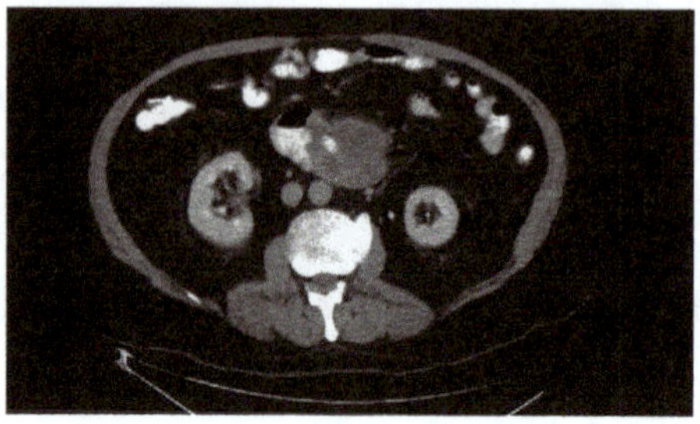

Figure 1: Initial CT scan showing mass in the duodenum.

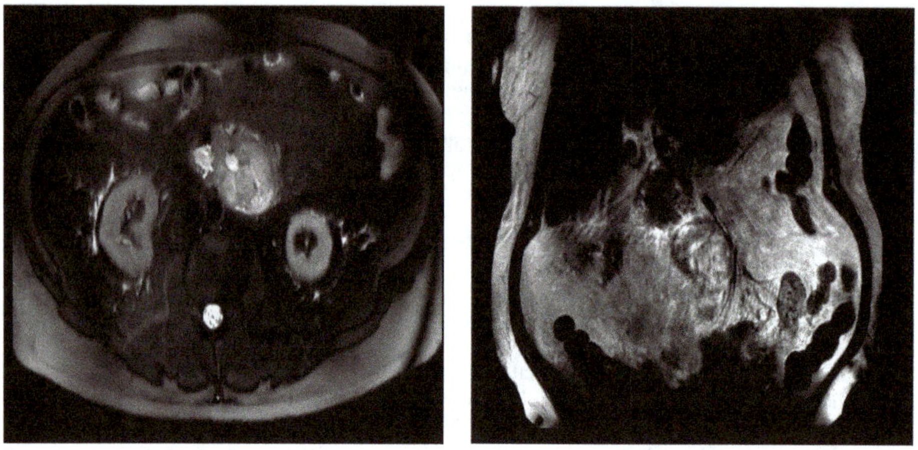

(a) (b)

Figure 2: MRI abdomen confirming duodenal mass in both (a) sagittal and (b) coronal sections.

out to be adenocarcinoma of the small bowel (Figures 3–5). He underwent open distal duodenectomy with extensive small bowel resection. His postoperative course was complicated by fever, hypotension, tachycardia, and persistent abdominal pain. A follow-up CT scan of the abdomen revealed an anastomotic leak at the surgical site (Figure 6). Although the patient was started on complete bowel rest, TPN, and broad-spectrum antibiotics, his clinical condition continued to deteriorate. Two 8 French pigtail drainage catheters were placed around the anastomosis leak which continued to have high output over the next few days (Figure 7). A follow-up CT revealed a persistent anastomotic leak with the formation of an enterocutaneous fistula involving the duodenum. A repeat EGD was performed, and the tip of one of the catheter was found in the lumen of the duodenum forming a fistulous tract (Figures 8–10). The catheter was removed, and we applied argon plasma coagulation (APC) through the fistulous tract and around the edges to allow de-epithelialization and granulation tissue formation. The closure of the tract was achieved by placing over the scope hemoclips (Figure 11). A follow-up CT scan of the abdomen and pelvis showed resolution of the anastomotic leak (Figure 12). The patient's clinical condition markedly improved and was transferred out of the ICU and later discharged home.

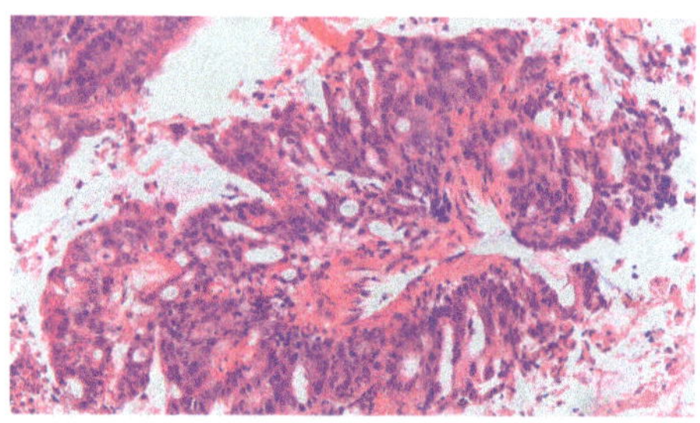

Figure 3: Invasive moderately differentiated adenocarcinoma with extracellular mucin production.

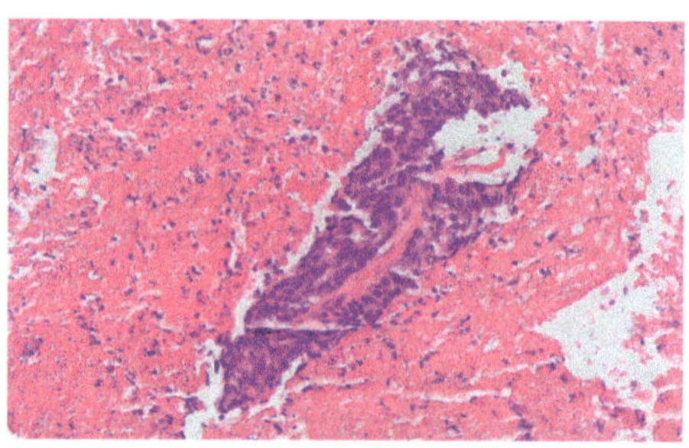

Figure 4: A group of malignant columnar shaped epithelioid cells in a background of abundant necroinflammatory debris.

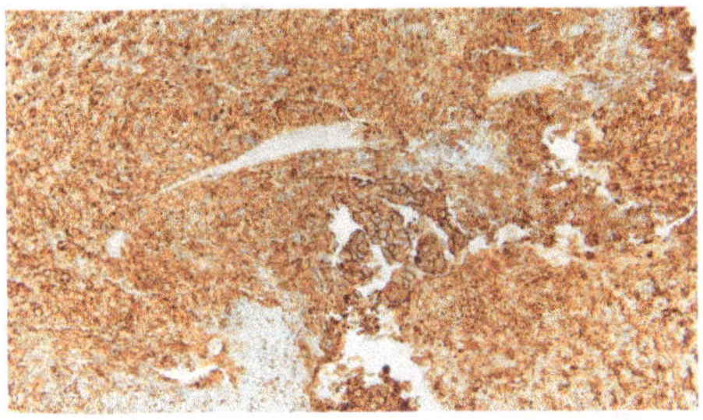

FIGURE 5: Malignant cells are positive for MOC-31 stain.

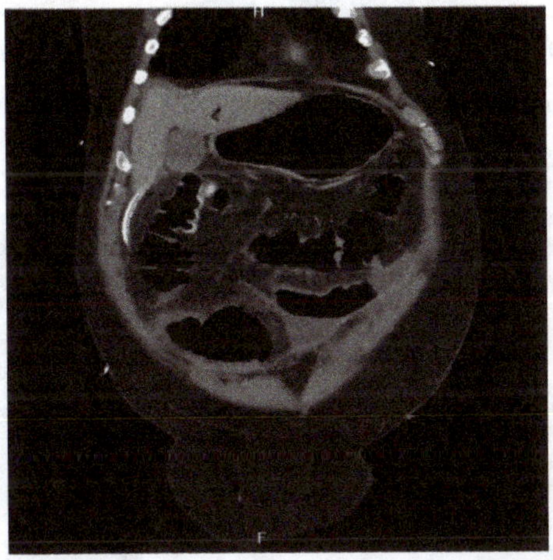

FIGURE 6: CT abdomen showing extravasation of contrast material.

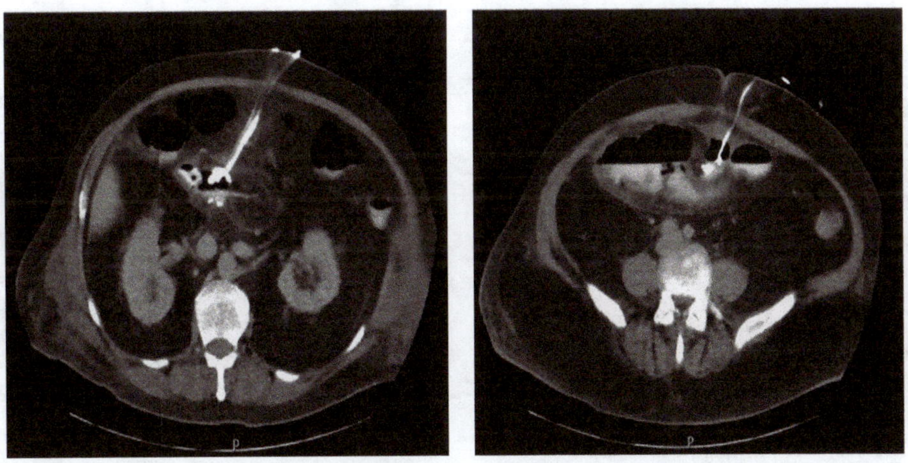

(a) (b)

FIGURE 7: CT showing drainage catheters at the anastomotic site.

3. Discussion

The endoscopic management of postsurgical intestinal anastomotic leaks and fistulas serves as an alternative to conservative and surgical treatment options. These techniques have the advantage of being minimally invasive that results in a shorter length of stay and antibiotic therapy. Different endoscopic modalities used have unique mechanisms and are used in combination or alone [6].

The use of self-expandable metal stents (SEMS) allows the diversion of the gastrointestinal contents away from the site of leakage to provide a stable environment for healing [7, 8]. Extraction of fully covered SEMS is easier than partially or uncovered SEMS which makes these preferred over the others. Also, the latter become rapidly embedded in

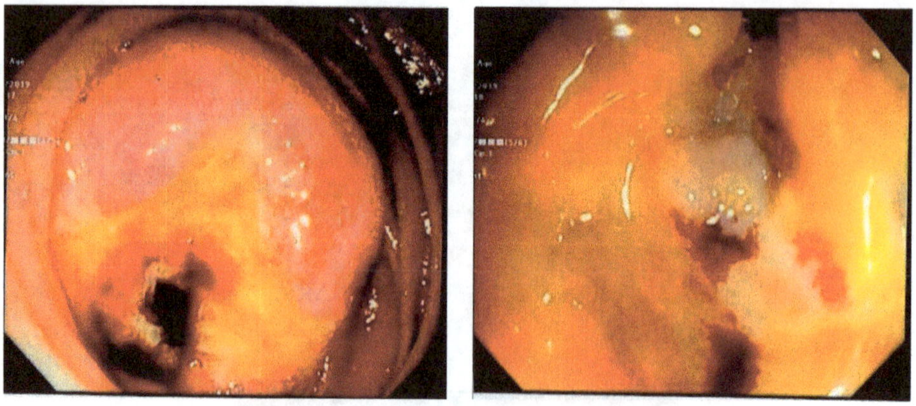

(a) (b)

Figure 8: Endoscopic images of misplaced drainage catheter in the lumen of the duodenum.

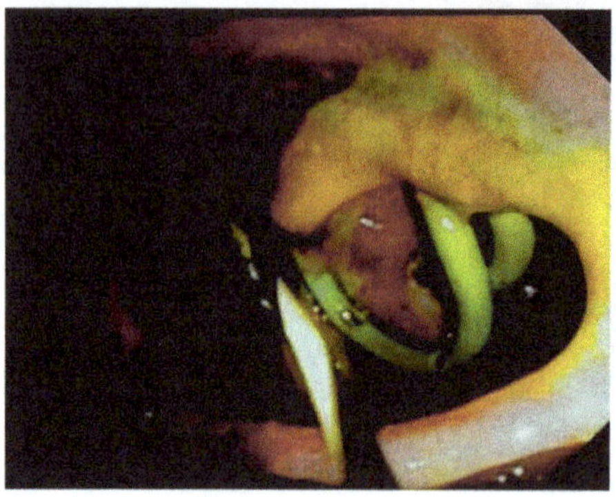

Figure 9: Drainage catheter in the lumen of the duodenum.

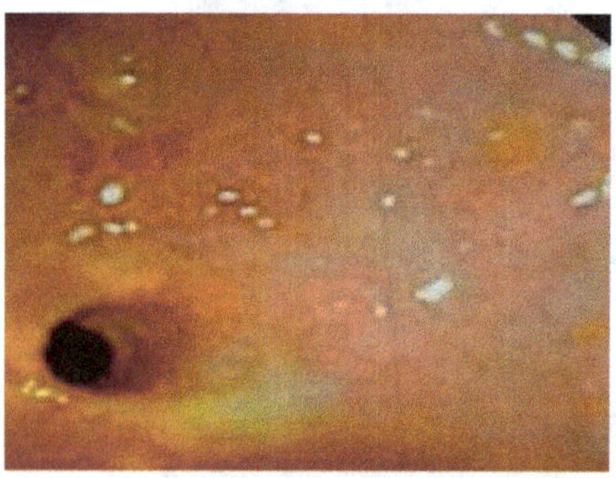

Figure 10: Fistulous tract opening in the lumen.

the mucosa due to tissue hyperplasia that makes them less favorable.

Hemostatic clips including through the scope (TTS) clips and over the scope (OTS) clips are used in closing the GI defects [9]. TTS clips have a disadvantage of a weak and superficial grasp and hence are less preferred and also OTS provides better pressure for tissue opposition. Haito-Chavez et al. reported a series of 188 patients who underwent management with OTS with an overall success rate of 90% and 73.3% for intestinal perforations and leaks, respectively [10].

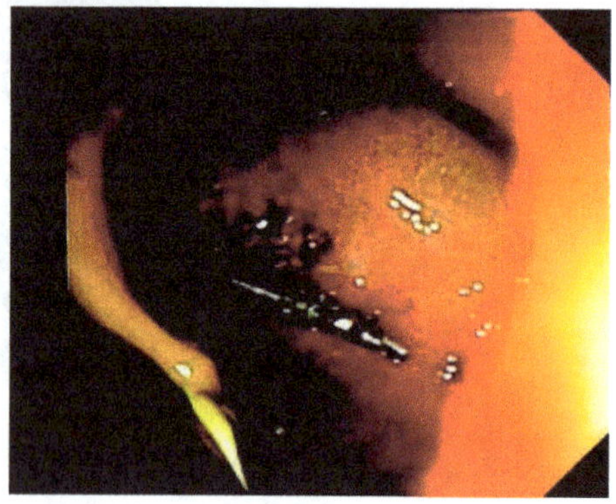

Figure 11: Closure of the tract by placing hemoclips.

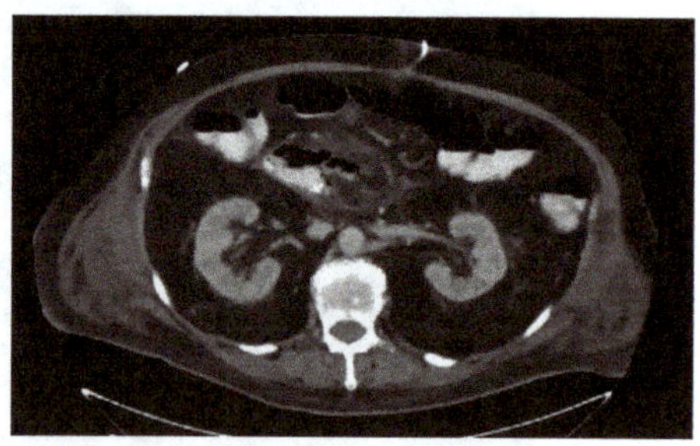

Figure 12: Follow-up CT scan showing resolution of anastomotic leakage.

Endoscopic suturing devices can also be used in the management of GI defects depending upon the location and type of the lesions. The Overstitch device (Apollo Endosurgery) is the most commonly used device that helps to apply sutures in a continuous or interrupted fashion. Sharaiha et al. reported the results from a large multicenter study for comprising of 122 patients who underwent endoscopic suturing to anchor stents ($n = 47$; 38.5%), fistulas ($n = 40$; 32.7%), leaks ($n = 15$; 12.3%), and perforations ($n = 20$; 16.4%). The immediate clinical success was ascertained in 79.5%, and long-term clinical success was noted in 78.8% after a mean follow-up of 68 days [11].

The vacuum-assisted closure (VAC) device is another promising option to be considered. In this technique, a vacuum-sealed sponge connected to a constant suction is inserted into the wound cavity. This helps in the removal of fluid and debris, promoting granulation tissue. Wedemeyer et al. successfully treated 8 patients with postesophagectomy leaks with VAC. The leak got healed in 7 out of 8 patients (88%) with a mean duration of 23 days [12].

One of the major issues in the postsurgical leak healing process is the epithelialization of the defect and subsequent tract formation which results in the formation of chronic draining fistulas. This usually slows down the healing process and limits the use of other endoscopic therapies. Therefore, de-epithelialization of the leak edges is vital in these cases and can be achieved by Argon Plasma coagulation (APC) as one of the preferred methods [13, 14]. The possible adverse effects of APC include perforation, pneumoperitoneum, and subcutaneous bubbling of gas [15, 16].

Postsurgical anastomotic leaks have serious complications with significant morbidity and mortality. As mentioned, there are several endoscopic techniques which have shown efficacy and promising outcomes with no single standard technique to manage individual defects, rather a combination of techniques, complementary to each other. The choice of the endoscopic technique depends on several factors including the site, size, duration of the leak, and operator experience with these techniques. In our patient, we used APC to de-epithelize or denude the luminal surface of the involved intestinal tract and later used hemostatic clips. The hemostatic clip was used since the size of the defect was small. Our case emphasizes the use of endoscopic techniques to treat postsurgical anastomotic leaks and fistulas early on in suitable patients as a successful alternative option to conventional therapies; however, future large case series or prospective studies are required to validate the efficacy and safety of endoscopic therapies.

Disclosure

The clinical vignette was presented in the West Virginia American College of Physician (ACP) Annual Conference on October 26, 2019.

Authors' Contributions

Abdullah Sohail, MD, wrote the manuscript and is the article guarantor. Ahmad Khan, MD, wrote and revised the manuscript. Ragheb Rezko, MD, helped with pathology images and description. Hamza Shah, DO, revised the manuscript and gave the final approval.

References

[1] M. Rutegård, P. Lagergren, I. Rouvelas, and J. Lagergren, "Intrathoracic anastomotic leakage and mortality after esophageal cancer resection: a population-based study," *Annals of Surgical Oncology*, vol. 19, no. 1, pp. 99–103, 2012.

[2] H. M. Shehab, S. M. Hakky, and K. A. Gawdat, "An endoscopic strategy combining mega stents and over-the-scope clips for the management of post-bariatric surgery leaks and fistulas (with video)," *Obesity Surgery*, vol. 26, no. 5, pp. 941–948, 2016.

[3] H. Lang, P. Piso, C. Stukenborg, R. Raab, and J. Jähne, "Management and results of proximal anastomotic leaks in a series of 1114 total gastrectomies for gastric carcinoma," *European Journal of Surgical Oncology (EJSO)*, vol. 26, no. 2, pp. 168–171, 2000.

[4] J. S. Marshall, A. Srivastava, S. K. Gupta, T. R. Rossi, and J. R. DeBord, "Roux-en-Y gastric bypass leak complications," *Archives of Surgery*, vol. 138, no. 5, pp. 520–523, 2003.

[5] K. Alanezi and J. D. Urschel, "Mortality secondary to esophageal anastomotic leak," *Annals of Thoracic and Cardiovascular Surgery: Official Journal of the Association of Thoracic and Cardiovascular Surgeons of Asia*, vol. 10, no. 2, pp. 71–75, 2004.

[6] Y. Sevim, S. U. Celik, H. Yavarifar, and C. Akyol, "Minimally invasive management of anastomotic leaks in colorectal surgery," *World Journal of Gastrointestinal Surgery*, vol. 8, no. 9, pp. 621–626, 2016.

[7] A. N. Holm, J. G. de la Mora Levy, C. J. Gostout, M. D. Topazian, and T. H. Baron, "Self-expanding plastic stents in treatment of benign esophageal conditions," *Gastrointestinal Endoscopy*, vol. 67, no. 1, pp. 20–25, 2008.

[8] S. Evrard, O. Le Moine, G. Lazaraki, A. Dormann, I. E. Nakadi, and J. Devière, "Self-expanding plastic stents for benign esophageal lesions," *Gastrointestinal Endoscopy*, vol. 60, no. 6, pp. 894–900, 2004.

[9] K. F. Binmoeller, H. Grimm, and N. Soehendra, "Endoscopic closure of a perforation using metallic clips after snare excision of a gastric leiomyoma," *Gastrointestinal Endoscopy*, vol. 39, no. 2, pp. 172–174, 1993.

[10] Y. Haito-Chavez, J. K. Law, T. Kratt et al., "International multicenter experience with an over-the-scope clipping device for endoscopic management of GI defects (with video)," *Gastrointestinal Endoscopy*, vol. 80, no. 4, pp. 610–622, 2014.

[11] R. Z. Sharaiha, N. A. Kumta, E. M. DeFilippis et al., "A large multicenter experience with endoscopic suturing for management of gastrointestinal defects and stent anchorage in 122 patients: a retrospective review," *Journal of Clinical Gastroenterology*, vol. 50, no. 5, pp. 388–392, 2016.

[12] J. Wedemeyer, M. Brangewitz, S. Kubicka et al., "Management of major postsurgical gastroesophageal intrathoracic leaks with an endoscopic vacuum-assisted closure system," *Gastrointestinal Endoscopy*, vol. 71, no. 2, pp. 382–386, 2010.

[13] A. A. Van Bodegraven, E. J. Kuipers, H. J. Bonenkamp, and S. G. M. Meuwissen, "Esophagopleural fistula treated endoscopically with argon beam electrocoagulation and clips," *Gastrointestinal Endoscopy*, vol. 50, no. 3, pp. 407–410, 1999.

[14] H. M. Shehab and H. M. Elasmar, "Combined endoscopic techniques for closure of a chronic post-surgical gastrocutaneous fistula: case report and review of the literature (with video)," *Surgical Endoscopy*, vol. 27, no. 8, pp. 2967–2970, 2013.

[15] A. C. Tan, P. P. Schellekens, P. Wahab, and C. J. Mulder, "Pneumatosis intestinalis, retroperitonealis, and thoracalis after argon plasma coagulation," *Endoscopy*, vol. 27, no. 09, pp. 698-699, 1995.

[16] N. Hoyer, R. Thouet, and U. Zellweger, "Massive pneumoperitoneum after endoscopic argon plasma coagulation," *Endoscopy*, vol. 30, p. S44, 1998.

Gastric Outlet Obstruction as the Initial Presentation of Upper Tract Urothelial Carcinoma

Karl Andersen,[1] Sarah Burroughs,[1] Assad Munis,[2] Ryan T. Hoff,[2] and Alan Shapiro[2]

[1]*Advocate Lutheran General Hospital, 1775 Dempster Street, Park Ridge, IL 60068, USA*
[2]*Department of Internal Medicine, Division of Gastroenterology, Advocate Lutheran General Hospital, 1775 Dempster Street, Park Ridge, IL 60068, USA*

Correspondence should be addressed to Sarah Burroughs; sarah.burroughs@aah.org

Academic Editor: Daniel C. Damin

GOO is often the first sign of advanced upper gastrointestinal neoplasms. The most common neoplasms associated with GOO include gastric, pancreatic, and biliary tract cancers. Urinary tract urothelial carcinoma has been a rarely documented cause of GOO.

1. Introduction

Gastric outlet obstruction (GOO) is a syndrome characterized by abdominal pain and vomiting secondary to mechanical obstruction. GOO is often the first sign of advanced upper gastrointestinal neoplasms, either as a result of direct invasion into the lumen of the digestive system or by external compression. Symptoms of obstruction are often vague and include early satiety, weight loss, gastroesophageal reflux disease (GERD), and abdominal pain [1]. Causes of GOO include peptic ulcer disease, gastric polyps, infiltrative disease, and malignancy. The most common neoplastic causes of GOO include gastric, pancreatic, and biliary tract cancers [2]. Locally invasive upper tract urothelial carcinoma (UTUC) is a rare cause of malignant GOO. This case report demonstrates the potential difficulty in diagnosing this disease and the need for a multidisciplinary approach.

2. Case Presentation

An 80-year-old female initially presented to her primary care physician's office with three weeks of right-sided flank pain. Her past medical history was notable for GERD, chronic constipation, and Barrett's esophagus. Her initial physical exam was significant for tenderness to palpation in the right lower quadrant of her abdomen, and was otherwise unremarkable. A computed tomography (CT) scan of her abdomen and pelvis showed dilatation of the renal pelvis, a thickened and dilated terminal ileum, and inflammatory changes with increased tissue around the right ureter. She was evaluated by urology and underwent a cystoscopy, which showed a ureteral stricture that was unable to be traversed. A ureteral stent was placed across the stricture. Urine cytology and ureteral brushings were negative for malignancy. Her symptoms modestly improved. Two months later, she continued to report right-sided flank pain despite stent placement. She underwent removal of right ureteral stent, ureteroscopy, and pyelogram which showed stable narrowing of the ureter in addition to dilatation of the upper and lower pole calices from prior evaluation. She was instructed to follow up in 6–8 weeks for diuretic renal scan.

Two weeks later, she presented with five days of diffuse abdominal pain and nonbloody, nonbilious emesis. She denied constipation or diarrhea but did report a lack of flatulence. Her physical exam was significant for diffuse, mild abdominal tenderness. Laboratory studies showed a serum white blood cell count of 11.7/mcL, and a urinalysis with moderate leukocyte esterase and moderate bacteria. Liver enzymes, lipase, and bilirubin were normal. A CT scan of the abdomen and pelvis with intravenous contrast showed an increase in the mass-like thickening of the right renal pelvis measuring 3.1 × 2.3 cm in size and partially encasing the renal artery and vein. It extended into the retroperitoneum resulting in compression of the duodenum. New gallbladder distention and biliary ductal dilatation was noted, with the common bile duct measuring 1.2 cm in diameter (Figures 1 and 2). A small bowel follow-through confirmed partial obstruction of the second portion of the duodenum (Figure 3). A CT-guided core and fine needle aspiration biopsy was then performed of the mass, revealing poorly differentiated upper tract urothelial carcinoma (UTUC) with immunohistochemical stains positive for CK-7, p63, and GATA3, and negative for PAX-8 and CK-20.

A gastrojejunostomy tube was inserted for nutrition and gastric decompression. She was evaluated by medical oncology and successfully completed four cycles of gemcitabine and cisplatin, which led to a decrease in mass size and resolution of the GOO, allowing for removal of the gastrojejunostomy tube. She then underwent a right nephroureterectomy followed by four more cycles of chemotherapy. Four months later, she was readmitted for small bowel obstruction secondary to peritoneal metastasis. A percutaneous endoscopic gastrostomy tube was inserted for decompression; however, the patient continued to decline and she was ultimately enrolled in hospice.

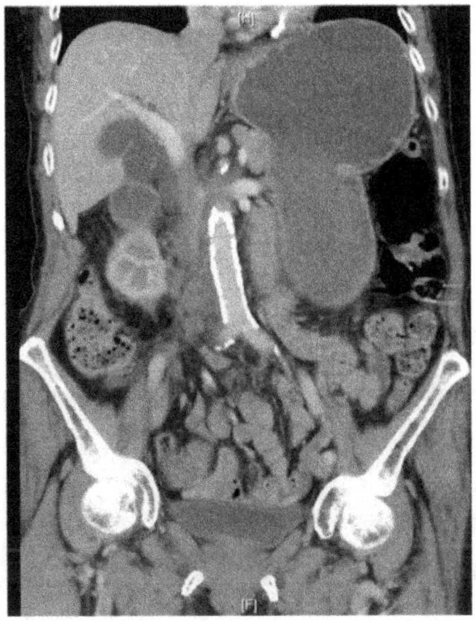

Figure 1: Coronal view of CT scan of the abdomen and pelvis showing wall thickening of the 2nd and 3rd parts of the duodenum and proximal distention of the 1st part of the duodenum and stomach.

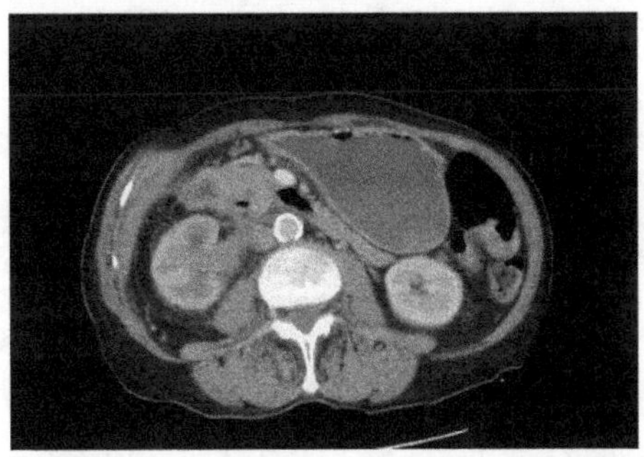

Figure 2: Axial view of the CT scan of the abdomen and pelvis showing a mass in the right renal pelvis.

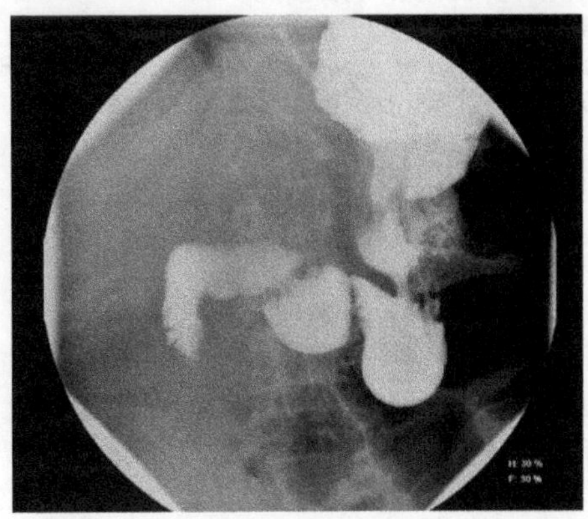

Figure 3: X-ray small bowel follow-through partial obstruction in the 2nd portion of the duodenum as evidenced by narrowing without contrast follow-through.

3. Discussion

Few cases of UTUC as the cause of GOO have been reported [1, 3]. Urothelial carcinoma (UC), also known as transitional cell carcinoma, is the most common cause of bladder cancer [4]. UTUC is a rare form of UC and arises from the renal pelvis and ureter. It makes up approximately 5–10% of all UCs with an incidence of about 3,500 cases per year [5]. UTUC spreads more commonly by direct invasion and extension and through the lymphatic system, unlike UC from the bladder. The thin ureteral walls may allow direct extension of UTUC tumors to occur more commonly than with bladder malignancies [6]. Diagnosis is usually made through a combination of cross-sectional imaging, ureteropyeloscopy with cystoscopy, brush biopsy, and urine cytology. Brush biopsy, as proved to be the case here, has a higher rate of false-negative results in cases of poorly differentiated UTUC compared to well-differentiated UTUC [7].

About 85% of patients with newly diagnosed urothelial carcinomas present with gross or microscopic hematuria occurring in the majority of patients [8]. However, more advanced disease may present in an atypical fashion, as outlined in this case. GOO is a clinical and pathophysiological syndrome as a consequence of a disease process resulting in mechanical obstruction. The most common malignant cause of GOO occurs when a gastrointestinal cancer causes intraluminal obstruction. Pancreatic cancer is the most common cause of obstruction, but other primary gastrointestinal cancers, such as gastric, duodenal, ampullary, and cholangiocarcinoma, have been documented. To our knowledge, this is the third case of UTUC causing GOO, and it demonstrates the challenge diagnosing UTUC can pose. It should also serve as a reminder that a broad differential should be entertained when determining the etiology of GOO.

Acknowledgments

This case report was presented at the 2018 American College of Gastroenterology Annual Scientific Meeting.

References

[1] M. Bandireddy and N. Baffy, "An uncommon cause of gastric outlet obstruction," *Medicine (Baltimore)*, vol. 96, no. 23, Article ID e7059, 2017.

[2] B. Brimhall and D. G. Adler, "Enteral stents for malignant gastric outlet obstruction," *Gastrointestinal Endoscopy Clinics of North America*, vol. 21, no. 3, pp. 389–403, 2011.

[3] L. Stroman, N. Sharma, and M. Sullivan, "Upper ureteric transitional cell carcinoma, extending to the renal pelvis, presenting as duodenal obstruction," *BMJ Case Reports*, vol. 2015, 2015.

[4] N. Malats and F. X. Real, "Epidemiology of bladder cancer," *Hematology/Oncology Clinics of North America*, vol. 29, no. 2, pp. 177–189, 2015.

[5] J. J. Leow, K. T. Chong, S. L. Chang, and J. Bellmunt, "Upper tract urothelial carcinoma: a different disease entity in terms of management," *ESMO Open*, vol. 1, Article ID e000126, 2017.

[6] A. Froemming, T. Potretzke, N. Takahashi, and B. Kim, "Upper tract urothelial cancer," *European Journal of Radiology*, vol. 98, pp. 50–60, 2018.

[7] R. Gupta, G. P. Paner, and M. B. Amin, "Neoplasms of the upper urinary tract: a review with focus on urothelial carcinoma of the pelvicalyceal system and aspects related to its diagnosis and reporting," *Advances in Anatomic Pathology*, vol. 15, no. 3, pp. 127–139, 2008.

[8] D. Kasper, A. Fauci, S. Hauser, L. J. Jameson, and J. Loscalzo, *Harrison's Principles of Internal Medicine*, McGraw-Hill Education, New York, NY, USA, 19th edition, 2015.

Cutaneous Metastasis in the Setting of Both Colon and Breast Primary Malignancies

Mary Junak, Hunter Jecius, and Jennifer Erdrich

Institutional Mailing Address, University of Arizona, Department of Surgery, Tucson, AZ 85724, USA

Correspondence should be addressed to Mary Junak; mjunak@email.arizona.edu

Academic Editor: Shiro Kikuchi

Colorectal cancer (CRC) is the third most diagnosed cancer in the United States, and many patients unfortunately have metastases at the time of their diagnosis. Cutaneous metastases of CRC have been reported in few journals and primarily as case reports due to their rarity. Here, we present the case of an 83-year-old woman with recently resected colon cancer, T4aN1bMx stage IIIB. She presented to our clinic for evaluation of a right midback mass, and a punch biopsy revealed dermal involvement by invasive, poorly differentiated carcinoma with epidermoid features. The mass was excised, and we ordered a PET scan in search of the primary tumor, which at that time was suspected to be of skin cancer origin. Surprisingly, this revealed a second malignancy triple-negative invasive ductal carcinoma of the left breast. The back mass stained positive for CK20, which was compatible with a metastasis from a colonic primary. After initially declining adjuvant therapy, the patient completed one cycle of capecitabine and oxaliplatin, which she tolerated poorly. She continued to further decline, developed widespread cutaneous metastases, and went home on hospice. Cutaneous lesions are an exceedingly rare site of metastasis for colon adenocarcinoma, and their clinical presentation can vary widely. It is important for providers to investigate any new skin lesion in a patient with a recent or remote history of malignancy, even if there were no sites of distant metastasis at initial diagnosis.

1. Introduction

Colorectal cancer (CRC) is the fourth leading cause of cancer-related deaths worldwide and the third most diagnosed cancer in the United States [1]. Overall incidence of CRC has decreased in recent decades secondary to implementation of effective screening guidelines and early detection of primary malignancies. However, most patients diagnosed with CRC die from the malignancy itself, and the National Institutes of Health Surveillance, Epidemiology, and End Results Program (SEER) estimates over 51,000 deaths in 2019 due to CRC alone [2, 3]. Development of metastatic disease largely contributes to this figure, and many patients unfortunately have metastases at the time of their diagnosis [4, 5]. The liver is the most common site of CRC metastases presumably due to venous blood flow, but recent studies suggest that anatomic location and histological subtype significantly affect the pattern of metastases when considering organs beyond the liver. The most common nonhepatic colorectal metastases are to the thorax, nervous system, skeletal system, and peritoneum [6]. Brain, ovary, adrenal, and skin are rare sites of metastases, and the mechanisms of these progressions are not fully understood. Cutaneous metastasis arising from internal malignancy is extremely rare occurring in 0.001% of all skin biopsies performed [7]. Metastatic cutaneous manifestations have been reported to occur in 0.7–9% of patients with visceral neoplasms, with cutaneous metastases of CRC having a prevalence of 5.8% and signaling advanced disease [8–12]. Cutaneous metastases of CRC have been reported in few journals and primarily as case reports due to their rarity. More often, cases of breast cancer followed by lung, colorectal, renal, ovarian, and bladder cancers involve discussions of cutaneous metastases. These present heterogeneously as slow-growing tumors to rapidly growing dermal or subcutaneous nodules with either intact or ulcerated epidermis [13]. We present a unique case of a patient with a past medical history of basal and squamous cell carcinoma who presented with what was ultimately found to be cutaneous metastases from a colon primary without hepatic involvement in the context of a new synchronous diagnosis of an invasive ductal carcinoma of the breast.

2. Case Presentation

An 83-year-old woman with a history of basal cell carcinoma and squamous cell carcinoma presented to our clinic for evaluation of a right midback mass. She initially presented to her dermatologist with what appeared to be an inflamed sebaceous cyst, but after a failed trial of Keflex, a punch biopsy performed at an outside institution revealed dermal involvement by invasive, poorly differentiated carcinoma with epidermoid features. By immunohistochemistry, the tumor cells expressed high-molecular weight keratin, BerEP4, and EMA but were negative for P63, GCDFP15, estrogen receptor, progesterone receptor, TTF-1, CEA, cytokeratin 7, and cytokeratin 20. At this point, the etiology of her mass was unclear; however, it should be noted that the patient was 6 weeks post-op from a laparoscopic-assisted left colectomy at an outside institution for an obstructing, poorly differentiated colon adenocarcinoma with squamous differentiation and 3/25 lymph nodes positive for metastatic carcinoma (pT4aN1b). She declined chemotherapy. Her physical exam on presentation was significant for a 4×4 cm firm, nonpigmented mass with a centrally raised 2×3 cm area of erythema surrounding a punctate opening from the recent biopsy with serous drainage (Figure 1). We ordered a PET scan prior to the excision in order to identify the primary tumor. PET scan was remarkable for a large intensely FDG-avid cutaneous/subcutaneous malignant mass in the right midback with FDG-avid right axillary nodal involvement, focal FDG avidity at the left colon anastomotic site, an intensely FDG-avid left peritoneal node in the left lower quadrant adjacent to the surgical bed suspicious for nodal involvement from the colon primary, and an FDG-avid left lateral breast hyperdense mass. The patient subsequently underwent a wide local excision of the cutaneous mass on her back with 1 cm margins and a right axillary sentinel lymph node biopsy in which 3 lymph nodes were removed. Pathology report showed poorly differentiated carcinoma with squamous differentiation, negative margins, and 1/3 lymph nodes positive. Histologically, infiltrating cords and solid nests of malignant epithelial cells were noted (Figure 2).

The patient underwent additional workup for the PET findings. The patient returned to the clinic and reported that her last mammogram was performed over one year ago but was negative for malignancy. She denied breast skin changes, nipple discharge, and noticeable breast masses. Physical exam revealed a round, mobile palpable mass at 1:00 approximately 5 cm from the left nipple-areola complex. While the breast mass appeared benign, a bilateral diagnostic mammogram and left breast ultrasound were ordered to rule out malignancy in light of her current presentation of carcinoma with unknown origin. Mammography confirmed a suspicious mass in the left breast, and pathology from the ultrasound-guided biopsy revealed invasive ductal carcinoma, grade 3 (ER 0%, PR 0%, HER-2 1+, Ki-67 80%). She underwent a left lumpectomy with pathology confirming triple-negative invasive ductal carcinoma with associated high-grade DCIS and margins negative for both invasive and in situ disease, staining positive for mammaglobin. There was no suspicion that this was a colon metastasis. She elected to omit sentinel lymph node biopsy, radiation, and breast-specific chemotherapy.

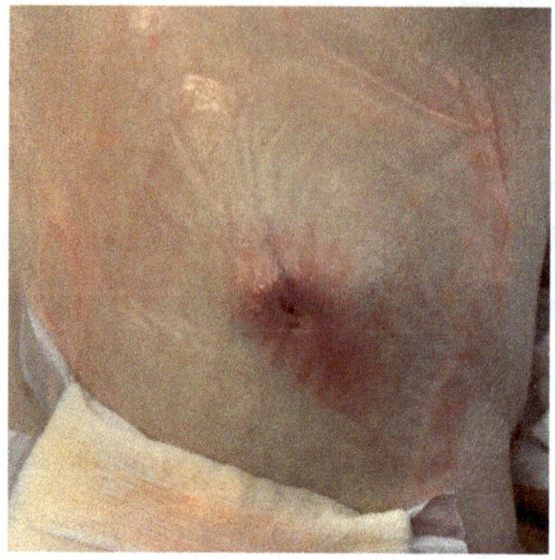

FIGURE 1: Right midback, nonpigmented, raised mass with the central area of erythema and serous drainage.

The final pathology of the back mass continued to be a diagnostic dilemma. To further characterize the origin, the histologic sections from the back and colon specimens were sent for an expert opinion at another institution. A panel of newly performed immunostains showed the neoplastic cells to be positive for CK20 and negative for CDX2, CK7, p63, GATA3, and mammaglobin, which is compatible with a metastasis from colonic primary. The patient was discussed at our multidisciplinary tumor board. We recommended a colon-specific chemotherapy regimen, which the patient declined. She returned to the clinic 4 months after the initial back mass excision and reported pruritus of her right back along the incision line with an associated lump. She also noted a lump in her right axilla, which was painful with arm movement. Exam revealed a well-healed right upper back scar with a 1.5×1.5 cm raised flesh-colored nodule with bluish discoloration proximal to the scar at the midpoint, as well as a well-healed right axillary scar with a firm palpable nodule 5 cm inferior to the scar. The patient was offered a wide resection in the OR, but due to the severe pruritic nature of this lesion, she preferred narrow excision in the office for immediate palliation and diagnosis. Pathology revealed this tissue was morphologically identical to her previous skin lesion, confirming a metastatic poorly differentiated carcinoma of colon primary. Caris testing was performed, and there were no actionable mutations.

The patient represented to medical attention one month later with a large bowel obstruction. Imaging showed recurrence at the colonic anastomosis, and this was managed nonoperatively. At this point, the patient agreed to palliative chemotherapy. She completed one cycle of capecitabine and oxaliplatin but tolerated this regimen poorly and was readmitted to the hospital twice. Subsequently, she declined any further treatment and went home on hospice.

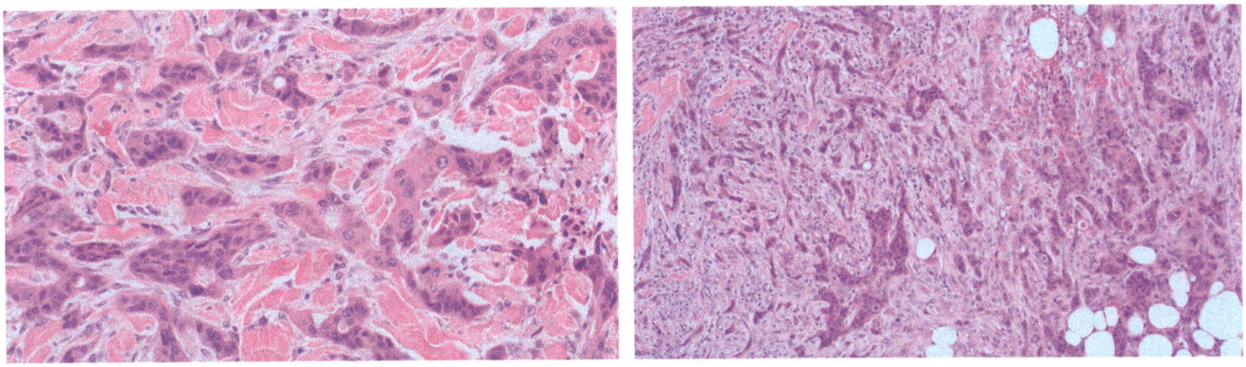

FIGURE 2: Microphotographs of the excisional biopsy of the skin lesion showing infiltrating cords and solid nests of epithelial cells within the deep dermis (H&E, 20x and 40x, respectively).

3. Discussion

At the time of diagnosis, distant metastases are present in approximately 18% of all colorectal cancer cases with 95% of these patients having either liver, lung, bone, or brain lesions [14]. Cutaneous metastases from an internal primary malignancy are uncommon and are a particularly rare manifestation of colon adenocarcinoma. Approximately 4–6% of metastatic colon cancers are associated with cutaneous lesions, which are primarily found on the abdominal skin at the site of postoperative incisional scars likely due to direct seeding [15]. The average time of presentation with skin metastases following a curative operation for CRC is about 2 years, but monitoring for these lesions should begin postoperatively as their presence can be the first detectable sign of disease progression [16].

The morphologic presentation of skin metastases varies widely and seemingly independent of the underlying primary malignancy. Lesions can present as nodules, papules, plaques, masses, or ulcers. Atypical presentations can include alopecia plaques or lesions mimicking morphea, follicular or sebaceous cysts, dermatofibromas, pyogenic granulomas, hemangiomas, herpes zoster eruption, cellulitis, or erysipelas [17]. This variable presentation often leads to a missed or delayed diagnosis. Therefore, providers must practice a high degree of clinical suspicion when investigating any new skin lesion in a patient with a recent or remote history of malignancy, even if there were no sites of distant metastases at initial diagnosis. Nevertheless, given this large variation in the visual appearance of these lesions, a biopsy and pathologic analysis are crucial in making the diagnosis.

Histologically, cutaneous malignant lesions are broadly classified as adenocarcinoma, squamous carcinoma, undifferentiated carcinoma, and other types. However, the morphology of metastatic deposits alone is typically not enough to establish the primary tumor source [18]. This is in part due to the fact that differentiation grade of metastatic tumors can change and obscure typical histologic features [19]. For this reason, the diagnosis of cutaneous metastatic carcinoma depends heavily on immunohistochemical stains to confirm the diagnosis. IHC markers of lower gastrointestinal origin identified in our case included high-molecular weight keratin, BerEP4, and CK20. CK20 is particularly useful in differentiating adenocarcinomas originating from the gastrointestinal tract from nongastrointestinal adenocarcinoma [20].

In general, the median survival after the diagnosis of cutaneous metastases is 6.5 months, with CRC cases of cutaneous lesion survival falling short of that at 4.4 months [21]. This is in comparison to all cases of CRC with distant metastases in which the median survival is between 9 and 19 months depending on whether treatment consists of best supportive care or combination chemotherapy [22]. This clear discrepancy in the length of survival may be due to the fact that cutaneous lesions are rarely the sole site of metastasis in these patients and are typically a sign of advanced disease. In fact, cutaneous metastases usually occur only with concomitant hepatic involvement [8–12]. However, if the skin is the only site of distant metastasis, as in the case of our patient, this may be a more favorable presentation.

While there are no specific guidelines for the management of cutaneous metastases in CRC, it is reasonable to proceed with the standard treatment for any CRC with distant metastases, systemic chemotherapy or targeted therapy, depending on mutational analysis, or a clinical trial. If the cutaneous lesion is the sole site of metastasis, wide local excision should be considered as surgical resection in cases of metastatic CRC is associated with superior outcomes for long-term survival [23].

Cutaneous lesions are an exceedingly rare site of metastasis for colon adenocarcinoma, and their clinical presentation can vary widely. Therefore, it is important for providers to investigate any new skin lesion in a patient with a recent or remote history of malignancy, even if there were no sites of distant metastasis at initial diagnosis. Molecular staining and pathological comparison to the primary tumor, when possible, can aid in the diagnosis of a metastatic skin lesion. Treatment options should include wide local excision if it is a solitary lesion or systemic chemotherapy if there are multiple sites of metastases.

Acknowledgments

The authors would like to thank their patient without whom this work would not be possible. This work was supported by the Department of Surgery at the University of Arizona.

References

[1] D. M. Parkin, F. Bray, J. Ferlay, and P. Pisani, "Global cancer statistics," *CA: A Cancer Journal for Clinicians*, vol. 55, pp. 74–108, 2002.

[2] M. Hamidi, K. Hanna, P. Omesiete et al., "Does it matter where you get your surgery for colorectal cancer?" *International Journal of Colorectal Disease*, vol. 34, no. 12, pp. 2121–2127, 2019.

[3] National Cancer Institute, *SEER Cancer Stat Facts: Colorectal Cancer*, National Cancer Institute, Bethesda, MD, USA, 2020, https://seer.cancer.gov/statfacts/html/colorect.html.

[4] I. J. Fidler, "The pathogenesis of cancer metastasis: the "seed and soil" hypothesis revisited," *Nature Reviews Cancer*, vol. 3, no. 6, pp. 453–458, 2003.

[5] M. Riihimäki, A. Hemminki, M. Fallah et al., "Metastatic sites and survival in lung cancer," *Lung Cancer*, vol. 86, no. 1, pp. 78–84, 2014.

[6] M. Riihimäki, A. Hemminki, J. Sundquist, and K. Hemminki, "Patterns of metastasis in colon and rectal cancer," *Scientific Reports*, vol. 6, no. 1, p. 29765, 2016.

[7] Y. Kemal, E. A. Odabaşı, E. Alis Odabasi, O. Kemal, and M. Bakirtas, "Cutaneous metastasis of colon adenocarcinoma," *Turkish Journal of Surgery*, vol. 34, no. 3, pp. 237–239, 2018.

[8] D. P. Lookingbill, N. Spangler, and F. M. Sexton, "Skin involvement as the presenting sign of internal carcinoma," *Journal of the American Academy of Dermatology*, vol. 22, no. 1, pp. 19–26, 1990.

[9] H. L. Abrams, R. Spiro, and N. Goldstein, "Metastases in carcinoma.Analysis of 1000 autopsied cases," *Cancer*, vol. 3, no. 1, pp. 74–85, 1950.

[10] J. E. McWhorter and A. W. Cloud, "Malignant tumors and their metastases," *Annals of Surgery*, vol. 92, no. 3, pp. 434–443, 1930.

[11] I. M. Reingold, "Cutaneous metastases from internal carcinoma," *Cancer*, vol. 19, no. 2, pp. 162–168, 1966.

[12] J. Marcoval, A. Moreno, and J. Peyrí, "Cutaneous infiltration by cancer," *Journal of the American Academy of Dermatology*, vol. 57, no. 4, pp. 577–580, 2007.

[13] S. Nambiar and A. Karippot, "Multiple cutaneous metastases as initial presentation in advanced colon cancer," *Case Reports in Gastrointestinal Medicine*, vol. 2018, p. 1, Article ID 8032905, 2018.

[14] M. Qiu, J. Hu, D. Yang, D. P. Cosgrove, and R. Xu, "Pattern of distant metastases in colorectal cancer: a SEER based study," *Oncotarget*, vol. 6, no. 36, pp. 38658–38666, 2015.

[15] Y. Hashimi and S Dholakia, "Facial cutaneous metastasis of colorectal adenocarcinoma," *BMJ Case Reports*, vol. 2013, Article ID bcr2013009875, 2013.

[16] B. Aravind, R. Kumar, and P. Basnyat, "Cutaneous metastases secondary to colorectal carcinoma may not be as ominous as previously thought: a case report and review of the literature," *BMJ Case Reports*, vol. 2013, Article ID bcr2013008556, 2013.

[17] I. Alcaraz, L. Cerroni, A. Rütten, H. Kutzner, and L. Requena, "Cutaneous metastases from internal malignancies," *The American Journal of Dermatopathology*, vol. 34, no. 4, pp. 347–393, 2012.

[18] R. A. Krathen, I. F. Orengo, and T. Rosen, "Cutaneous metastasis: a meta-analysis of data," *Southern Medical Journal*, vol. 96, no. 2, pp. 164–167, 2003.

[19] M. R. A. Hussein, "Skin metastasis: a pathologist's perspective," *Journal of Cutaneous Pathology*, vol. 37, no. 9, pp. e1–e20, 2010.

[20] M. Miettinen, "Keratin 20: immunohistochemical marker for gastrointestinal, urothelial, and Merkel cell carcinomas," *Modern Pathology: An Official Journal of the United States and Canadian Academy of Pathology, Inc*, vol. 8, no. 4, pp. 384–388, 1995.

[21] P. Schoenlaub, A. Sarraux, E. Grosshans, E. Heid, and B. Cribier, "Survie après métastases cutanées: étude de 200 cas [Survival after cutaneous metastasis: a study of 200 cases]," *Annals of Dermatology and Venereology*, vol. 128, no. 12, pp. 1310–1315, 2001.

[22] M. A. Rodriguez-Bigas, E. H. Lin, and C. H. Crane, "Stage IV colorectal cancer," in *Holland-frei Cancer Medicine*, D. W. Kufe, R. E. Pollock, R. R. Weichselbaum et al., Eds., BC Decker, Hamilton, ON, USA, 6th edition, 2003.

[23] S. Y. Oh, D. Y. Kim, and K. W. Suh, "Oncologic outcomes following metastasectomy in colorectal cancer patients developing distant metastases after initial treatment," *Annals of Surgical Treatment and Research*, vol. 88, no. 5, pp. 253–259, 2015.

42

Topical Capsaicin for Treating Cannabinoid Hyperemesis Syndrome

Ansar Aziz,[1] **Tayyab Waheed**,[1] **Olubunmi Oladunjoye**,[1] **Adeolu Oladunjoye**,[2] **Midhat Hanif**,[3] **and Fareena Latif**[3]

[1]*Reading Hospital Tower Health, West Reading, PA, USA*
[2]*Boston Children's Hospital, Boston, MA, USA*
[3]*Independent Researcher, West Reading, PA, USA*

Correspondence should be addressed to Ansar Aziz; ansar.aziz@towerhealth.org

Academic Editor: Matteo Neri

Introduction. Cannabinoid hyperemesis syndrome (CHS), associated with chronic cannabis use, presents with cyclic abdominal pain, nausea, and vomiting. With increasing use of marijuana, the incidence of CHS is expected to increase. Most patients with CHS make frequent visits to the emergency room and are usually refractory to conventional treatment. We, therefore, present a case of CHS successfully treated with topical capsaicin application. *Case Presentation.* A 41-year-old female with a recent excess use of cannabis presented to the emergency department for evaluation of recurrent excruciating epigastric pain accompanied by severe nausea and vomiting. She had similar, milder symptoms a year ago and underwent endoscopic evaluation which was negative except for mild reflux esophagitis for which she was started on a proton pump inhibitor. On this presentation, basic laboratory workup, EKG, and CT scan of abdomen and pelvis were unremarkable. A detailed abdominal exam was only positive for mild epigastric tenderness. She was instructed to continue pantoprazole and pain medication and outpatient repeat esophagogastroduodenoscopy. The patient returned the next day with extreme retching, nausea, and vomiting and was admitted for further evaluation. Intravenous fluids, antiemetics, and morphine were started for pain control with no symptomatic improvement. A diagnosis of cannabis hyperemesis syndrome was made based on history of chronic marijuana use and otherwise negative workup. A trial of topical capsaicin, over the epigastric region, was tried that provided dramatic relief within 24 hours. Repeat endoscopic evaluation had no evidence of ulcers, celiac disease, or esophagitis. She was discharged on topical capsaicin and counselled on marijuana abstinence, with no return of symptoms. *Conclusion.* Based on the dramatic resolution of symptoms with topical capsaicin, our case supports this promising intervention and provides an alternate approach to antiemetics and narcotics routinely used in patients with cannabis hyperemesis syndrome.

1. Introduction

Cannabinoid hyperemesis syndrome (CHS) is a known condition associated with chronic cannabis use. It usually presents with cyclic abdominal pain, nausea, and vomiting and often followed by a temporary relief with a hot shower bath. As increased use of marijuana is observed since its legalization, the incidence of CHS is expected to be on the rise [1–4]. Unfortunately, most patients with CHS make frequent visits to the emergency room and get several medical tests and imaging studies done which eventually turn out to be negative or lead to delay in diagnosing CHS [5–8]. In addition, some of these patients end up receiving multiple medications including antiemetics with potential side effects and are still refractory to treatment [6, 9].

The pathophysiology of CHS is not well understood. However, there are receptors implicated called transient receptor potential vanilloid 1 (TRPV-1) receptors which respond to high temperature and substance P regulation (a nausea and vomiting mediator). This might explain the reason why hot shower bath provides temporary symptomatic relief in CHS patients [5, 10, 11]. TRPV-1 is also found in the peripheral nervous system and is thought to be involved in dysregulation of the endocannabinoid system in the hypothalamus. Capsaicin is known to exert its effects on this system and can potentially provide symptomatic relief [12, 13].

Here, we present a case of CHS successfully treated with topical capsaicin application.

2. Case Report

A 41-year-old female with significant past medical history of cannabis use, tobacco use, bipolar disorder, chronic obstructive pulmonary disease, hypertension, and reflux esophagitis, but no alcohol use, presented to the emergency department for evaluation of recurrent excruciating epigastric pain accompanied by severe nausea and vomiting. Previously, she has had a similar but milder symptom for which she was evaluated. Previous esophagogastroduodenoscopy revealed no evidence of Barrett's esophagus or sprue; however, reflux esophagitis was detected for which she was started on a proton pump inhibitor.

The patient had been relatively symptom-free over the course of the two years until recently when she started experiencing severe epigastric pain with retching and nausea. She was then given pantoprazole and was discharged to follow up as an outpatient. The patient returned to the emergency department a few days later with similar epigastric pain with nausea and vomiting. Electrocardiogram (EKG) was without any significant ST or T wave changes ruling out acute coronary artery syndrome. CT scan abdomen and pelvis was performed and was negative for any acute pathology. The patient was treated with pantoprazole and pain medications and was later discharged after stabilization. The next day, the patient returned to the emergency department complaining of severe crampy abdominal pain with severe nausea and intermittent vomiting. The patient described her pain as being more severe with a rating of 10/10, twisting in nature, and some sensations of "butterflies" going up in the chest. Her pain was worse with eating, and she had been unable to tolerate any solid or liquid diet. She reported no relief with pantoprazole. Her review of systems was negative for heart burn or reflux-type symptoms, diarrhea, melena, or hematochezia. She also denied headache or history of migraine.

A detailed abdominal examination was also done which was negative for guarding or rebound tenderness. The patient, however, had moderate tenderness to palpation in her epigastrium. Other workups including EKG, complete blood count (CBC), electrolytes, urinalysis, and kidney and liver functions were all within normal limits. The urinary pregnancy test was also negative.

The patient was then admitted to the hospital with initial differential diagnosis of gastritis, severe gastroesophageal reflux, cyclic vomiting syndrome, and peptic ulcer disease. She was given intravenous fluids, antiemetics, and initial one dose of morphine to decrease the pain and anxiety. The next morning, the patient's symptoms were unchanged. A urine drug screen was ordered which came back positive for marijuana. The patient admitted to its chronic use with increasing use over the past 2 weeks.

Concerns for cannabis hyperemesis syndrome were raised given the repeated bouts of abdominal pain, nausea, and vomiting with benign abdominal exam in the setting of recent increased use of marijuana. The patient was continued on pantoprazole with addition of metoclopramide for nausea control but there was no improvement in her symptoms. Esophagogastroduodenoscopy was repeated that was evident only for mild gastropathy that could not fully explain her symptoms. After discussion with the patient and her spouse, a trial of capsaicin 0.1% topical cream, one application 3 times daily, was ordered with which the patient had dramatic relief with near complete resolution of her symptoms.

3. Discussion

CHS is subdivided into three phases: prodromal, vomiting, and recovery phases. The prodromal phase is characterized by nausea and abdominal discomfort. The vomiting phase is characterized by severe nausea, vomiting, and retching that can occur several times in an hour [14]. During the vomiting phase, the patient shows compulsive desire to bath in hot water which often times gives them temporary relief. However, most patients will present in the emergency room when they no longer can control their symptoms [15]. The recovery phase is when the patient stops taking cannabis and begins to see cessation of symptoms within a week [14, 16, 17].

The pathophysiology of CHS is not well understood. However, in the available literature, it has been proposed that CHS maybe caused by dysregulation of endocannabinoid systems called endogenous cannabinoid receptors CB-1 and CB-2 found in the brain, peripheral nervous system, and gastrointestinal system [16]. These receptors such as CB-1 receptors are found close to TRPV-1 which might explain their effective relationship [18]. The accumulation of tetrahydrocannabinol (THC), the active component of marijuana, is thought to bind to the receptors in the gastrointestinal tract leading to gastrointestinal motility, nausea, and vomiting, hence the presentation in CHS [5, 12, 19–21].

TRPV-1 is also found in the peripheral nervous system and is thought to be involved in the dysregulation of the endocannabinoid system in the hypothalamus, and capsaicin is known to exert its effects on this system [12, 13]. Capsaicin binds TRPV-1 with high specificity and responds to high temperature and substance P regulation [22]. Capsaicin is thought to inhibit substance P action at the postrema area by overactivation of TPRV-1 and leading to antiemesis [4].

Recent trials have emerged with the use of capsaicin or 8 methyl-*N*-vanillyl-6- nonenamide, an active ingredient of chili pepper as a viable option to treat CHS [4]. It is an alkaloid extract from capsicum a flowering plant [10]. It is available in different concentrations such as 0.025 0.075, and 0.1% topical cream, and it is being reported that higher concentration formulations are more effective than lower concentration formulations [22, 23]. Capsaicin is used as a topical cream that produces heat sensation on the skin, thereby relieving significant symptoms of nausea and vomiting in CHS patients. An advantage of capsaicin is that it is noninvasive and cost-effective and has a low risk of adverse effects. However, capsaicin is not without side effects. Such side effects include burning sensation, skin irritation, and blisters at application site. Others less common side effects are diarrhea, nausea, back pain, dizziness, headache, and hypertension [24].

In a case series in 2016 by Burillo-Putze and colleagues [25, 26], which supports our study findings, they reported successful resolution of symptoms after other antiemetics such as metoclopramide and granisetron failed. Another study in 2017 by Dezieck et al. [4] reported similar findings that after the use of several antiemetics failed, their patients experienced resolution of symptoms with the use of topical capsaicin. In the case of our patient, she received antiemetics earlier with no relief which warranted the physicians to change to topical capsaicin that resulted in near resolution of symptoms. Some case reports and case series have also suggested the use of haloperidol to be effective [27–30].

A documented limitation of capsaicin use is the patient's insight and compliance to capsaicin application. It is reported that some patients could not relate their relief of symptoms to the use of topical capsaicin [4]. This may be attributed to their impaired judgement because of their chronic cannabis use. Another potential limitation is that topical capsaicin may also have affected pain sensitivity by acting on TRPV-1 receptors. However, the main stay of treatment remains cessation of cannabis use. Future studies and trials are needed to further explore the role of capsaicin use in cannabinoid hyperemesis syndrome.

4. Conclusion

Use of topical capsaicin for treatment of CHS seems promising as previously reported in several case reports and studies. However, further studies are warranted to support this finding to be used as a first-line treatment option for CHS management.

References

[1] A. Azofeifa, M. E Mattson, G. Schauer, T. McAfee, A. Grant, and R. Lyerla, "National estimates of marijuana use and related indicators-national survey on drug use and health, United States, 2002–2014," *MMWR Surveillance Summaries*, vol. 65, no. 11, pp. 1–28, 2016.

[2] S. T. Wilkinson, S. Yarnell, R. Radhakrishnan, S. A. Ball, and D. C. D'Souza, "Marijuana legalization: impact on physicians and public health," *Annual Review of Medicine*, vol. 67, no. 1, pp. 453–466, 2016.

[3] H. S. Kim, J. D. Anderson, O. Saghafi, K. J. Heard, and A. A. Monte, "Cyclic vomiting presentations following marijuana liberalization in Colorado," *Academic Emergency Medicine*, vol. 22, no. 6, pp. 694–699, 2015.

[4] L. Dezieck, Z. Hafez, A. Conicella et al., "Resolution of cannabis hyperemesis syndrome with topical capsaicin in the emergency department: a case series," *Clinical Toxicology*, vol. 55, no. 8, pp. 908–913, 2017.

[5] C. J. Sorensen, K. DeSanto, L. Borgelt, K. T. Phillips, and A. A. Monte, "Cannabinoid hyperemesis syndrome: diagnosis, pathophysiology, and treatment-a systematic review," *Journal of Medical Toxicology*, vol. 13, no. 1, pp. 71–87, 2017.

[6] J. R. Richards, "Cannabinoid hyperemesis syndrome: pathophysiology and treatment in the emergency department," *The Journal of Emergency Medicine*, vol. 54, no. 3, pp. 354–363, 2018.

[7] H. S. Kim and A. A. Monte, "Colorado cannabis legalization and its effect on emergency care," *Annals of Emergency Medicine*, vol. 68, no. 1, pp. 71–75, 2016.

[8] J. C. Maxwell and B. Mendelson, "What do we know now about the impact of the laws related to marijuana?" *Journal of Addiction Medicine*, vol. 10, no. 1, pp. 3–12, 2016.

[9] J. Graham, M. Barberio, and G. S. Wang, "Capsaicin cream for treatment of cannabinoid hyperemesis syndrome in adolescents: a case series," *Pediatrics*, vol. 140, no. 6, Article ID e20163795, 2017.

[10] J. R. Richards, J. M. Lapoint, and G. Burillo-Putze, "Cannabinoid hyperemesis syndrome: potential mechanisms for the benefit of capsaicin and hot water hydrotherapy in treatment," *Clinical Toxicology*, vol. 56, no. 1, pp. 15–24, 2018.

[11] A. A. Izzo and K. A. Sharkey, "Cannabinoids and the gut: new developments and emerging concepts," *Pharmacology & Therapeutics*, vol. 126, no. 1, pp. 21–38, 2010.

[12] R. Waterson Duncan and M. Maguire, "Capsaicin topical in emergency department treatment of cannabinoid hyperemesis syndrome," *The American Journal of Emergency Medicine*, vol. 35, no. 12, pp. 1977-1978, 2017.

[13] R. Biary, A. Oh, J. Lapoint, L. Nelson, R. Hoffman, and M. Howland, "Topical capsaicin cream used as a therapy for cannabinoid hyperemesis syndrome," *Clinical Toxicology*, vol. 52, no. 7, p. 787, 2014.

[14] S. L. Price, C. Fisher, R. Kumar, and A. Hilgerson, "Cannabinoid hyperemesis syndrome as the underlying cause of intractable nausea and vomiting," *The Journal of the American Osteopathic Association*, vol. 111, no. 3, pp. 166–169, 2011.

[15] S. Pingle, J. Matta, and G. Ahern, "Capsaicin receptor: TRPV1 a promiscuous TRP channel. transient receptor potential (TRP) channels," *Handbook of Experimental Pharmacology*, vol. 179, pp. 155–171, 2007.

[16] N. A. Darmani, "Cannabinoid-induced hyperemesis: a conundrum-from clinical recognition to basic science mechanisms," *Pharmaceuticals*, vol. 3, no. 7, pp. 2163–2177, 2010.

[17] J. A. Galli, R. Sawaya, and F. Friedenberg, "Cannabinoid hyperemesis syndrome," *Current Drug Abuse Reviews*, vol. 4, no. 4, pp. 241–249, 2011.

[18] F. Yang and J. Zheng, "Understand spiciness: mechanism of TRPV1 channel activation by capsaicin," *Protein & Cell*, vol. 8, no. 3, pp. 169–177, 2017.

[19] K. A. Sharkey, N. A. Darmani, and L. A. Parker, "Regulation of nausea and vomiting by cannabinoids and the endocannabinoid system," *European Journal of Pharmacology*, vol. 722, pp. 134–146, 2014.

[20] Y. Lee, J. Jo, H. Y. Chung, C. Pothoulakis, and E. Im, "Endocannabinoids in the gastrointestinal tract," *American Journal of Physiology-Gastrointestinal and Liver Physiology*, vol. 311, no. 4, pp. G655–G666, 2016.

[21] C. Hasenoehrl, U. Taschler, M. Storr, and R. Schicho, "The gastrointestinal tract-a central organ of cannabinoid signaling in health and disease," *Neurogastroenterology & Motility*, vol. 28, no. 12, pp. 1765–1780, 2016.

[22] F. Yang, X. Xiao, W. Cheng et al., "Structural mechanism underlying capsaicin binding and activation of the TRPV1 ion channel," *Nature Chemical Biology*, vol. 11, no. 7, pp. 518–524, 2015.

[23] S. Derry, A. S. Rice, P. Cole, T. Tan, and R. A. Moore, "Topical capsaicin (high concentration) for chronic neuropathic pain in adults," *Cochrane Database of Systematic Reviews*, vol. 1, no. 1, Article ID CD007393, 2017.

[24] N. Ellison, C. L. Loprinzi, J. Kugler et al., "Phase III placebo-controlled trial of capsaicin cream in the management of surgical neuropathic pain in cancer patients," *Journal of Clinical Oncology*, vol. 15, no. 8, pp. 2974–2980, 1997.

[25] F. Román, P. Llorens, and G. Burillo-Putze, "Capsaicina tópica en el tratamiento del síndrome de hiperemesis por cannabinoides," *Medicina Clínica*, vol. 147, no. 11, pp. 517-518, 2016.

[26] G. Burillo-Putze and P. Llorens, "Perspectivas en el tratamiento del síndrome de hiperemesis por cannabis," *Adicciones*, vol. 29, no. 2, pp. 134-135, 2017.

[27] J. L. Hickey, J. C. Witsil, and M. B. Mycyk, "Haloperidol for treatment of cannabinoid hyperemesis syndrome," *The American Journal of Emergency Medicine*, vol. 31, no. 6, pp. 1003.e5–1003.e6, 2013.

[28] J. C. Witsil and M. B. Mycyk, "Haloperidol, a novel treatment for cannabinoid hyperemesis syndrome," *American Journal of Therapeutics*, vol. 24, no. 1, pp. e64–e67, 2017.

[29] J. L. Jones and K. E. Abernathy, "Successful treatment of suspected cannabinoid hyperemesis syndrome using haloperidol in the outpatient setting," *Case Reports in Psychiatry*, vol. 2016, no. 2, 3 pages, Article ID 3614053, 2016.

[30] F. Inayat, H. U. H. Virk, W. Ullah, and Q. Hussain, "Is haloperidol the wonder drug for cannabinoid hyperemesis syndrome?" *BMJ Case Reports*, vol. 2017, Article ID bcr2016218239, 2017.

43

Gastric Mucormycosis: An Infection of Fungal Invasion into the Gastric Mucosa in Immunocompromised Patients

Haider A. Naqvi,[1,2,3,4] Muhammad Nadeem Yousaf,[1,2,3,4] Fizah S. Chaudhary,[1,2,3,4] and Lawrence Mills[5]

[1]*Department of Medicine, Medstar Union Memorial Hospital, Baltimore, MD 21218, USA*
[2]*Department of Medicine, MedStar Good Samaritan Hospital, Baltimore, MD 21239, USA*
[3]*Department of Medicine, MedStar Franklin Square Medical Center, Baltimore, MD 21237, USA*
[4]*Department of Medicine, MedStar Harbor Hospital, Baltimore, MD 21225, USA*
[5]*Department of Gastroenterology, MedStar Good Samaritan Hospital, Baltimore, MD 21239, USA*

Correspondence should be addressed to Haider A. Naqvi; haider.a.naqvi@medstar.net

Academic Editor: Hirotada Akiho

Primary gastric mucormycosis is a rare but potentially lethal fungal infection due to the invasion of Mucorales into the gastric mucosa. It may result in high mortality due to increased risk of complications in immunocompromised patients. Common predisposing risk factors to develop gastric mucormycosis are prolonged uncontrolled diabetes mellitus with or without diabetic ketoacidosis (DKA), solid organ or stem cell transplantation, underlying hematologic malignancy, and major trauma. Abdominal pain, hematemesis, and melena are common presenting symptoms. The diagnosis of gastric mucormycosis can be overlooked due to the rarity of the disease. A high index of suspicion is required for early diagnosis and management of the disease, particularly in immunocompromised patients. Radiological imaging findings are nonspecific to establish the diagnosis, and gastric biopsy is essential for histological confirmation of mucormycosis. Prompt treatment with antifungal therapy is the mainstay of treatment with surgical resection reserved in cases of extensive disease burden or clinical deterioration. We presented a case of acute gastric mucormycosis involving the body of stomach in a patient with poorly controlled diabetes and chronic renal disease, admitted with acute onset of abdominal pain. Complete resolution of lesion was noted with 16 weeks of medical treatment with intravenous amphotericin B and posaconazole.

1. Introduction

Gastric mucormycosis is a rare but lethal fungal infection due to invasion of Mucorales (a filamentous fungus) into the gastric mucosa that may result in high mortality (up to 54%) in immunocompromised patients [1]. An estimated 75% of mucormycosis (formally known as zygomycosis) infection is caused by the fungi class of zygomycetes and particularly Mucor, Rhizopus, or Rhizomucor species [1–3]. Common sites of mucormycosis are upper respiratory tract, nasal or paranasal sinuses, skin, orbit, and brain; however, the gastrointestinal tract is rarely infected [4]. Serologic biomarkers are nonspecific; however, a biopsy from the affected site is the gold standard to establish histologic diagnosis of mucormycosis. A positive culture or polymerase chain reaction (PCR) on biopsy specimen is occasionally required for diagnosis confirmation. Medical management with antifungal therapy such as lipid formulation of amphotericin B, posaconazole, and newer agents isavuconazole or triazole is the mainstay option for treating gastric mucormycosis [5, 6]. For patients with severe disease such as tissue necrosis and those with late presentation, a combination of both medical management with early surgical resection may improve the outcome of disease. We present a case of an immunocompetent individual who developed gastric mucormycosis.

2. Case Presentation

A 55-year-old female with past medical history of insulin-dependent uncontrolled diabetes mellitus and stage IIIb chronic kidney disease presented to the emergency room with acute abdominal pain for two weeks. The abdominal pain was epigastric, 7/10 in severity, and nonradiating, without precipitating or relieving factors. It was associated with nausea and multiple episodes of nonbiliary, nonbloody emesis. On physical examination, vitals were unremarkable. Epigastric tenderness was noted on abdominal examination. Laboratory workup was remarkable for leukocytosis (11.2 k/ul), elevated lipase (589 u/L), and elevated creatinine (1.62 mg/dL). Computed tomography (CT) of the abdomen and pelvis (Figure 1) demonstrated transmural thickening at gastric body and fundus, with associated perigastric inflammation and reactive adenopathy. Esophagogastroduodenoscopy (EGD) revealed multiple ulcerated sessile masses in the gastric fundus with a large exudate covering mass (Figure 2). Biopsy of mass revealed polymorphonuclear neutrophils indicating inflammation of gastric mucosa and fragments of invasive fungal hyphae (zygomycetes) with polymerase chain reaction (PCR) and culture of the biopsy specimens detecting *Rhizopus microsporus* DNA (Figures 3(a) and 3(b)). The patient was not amenable to the surgical resection because of multiple comorbidities and high risk for surgical complications. She was medically treated with intravenous amphotericin B 5 mg/kg daily that was later switched to posaconazole 300 mg daily due to worsening renal function and poor tolerance. Surveillance of the gastric lesions was performed with serial EGDs. Complete resolution of gastric mucormycosis with the absence of hyphae was noted on endoscopic gastric biopsies after 16 weeks of antifungal therapy (Figure 4).

3. Discussion

An estimated prevalence of mucormycosis is 0.16 (0.12 to 0.20) per 10,000 patients [7]. The prevalence rate of mucormycosis amongst patients with uncontrolled diabetes is 36% [8]. We presented a case of acute gastric mucormycosis in a patient with poorly controlled diabetes and chronic renal disease, admitted with acute onset of abdominal pain. An uncontrolled diabetes and CKD stage IIIb were major risk factors predisposing to the development of gastric mucormycosis. The patient's symptoms were not amenable to proton pump inhibitors which prompted further investigation including abdominal radiological imaging and upper endoscopy. Radiological imaging findings were nonspecific; however, EGD revealed multiple ulcerated sessile masses located at greater curvature and gastric fundus. These mucosal lesions were covered with a large grayish exudate, highly suspicious for gastric mucormycosis. The diagnosis of gastric mucormycosis was confirmed with histological examination, culture, and PCR of biopsy specimen.

Gastrointestinal mucosal involvement could be the sole manifestations of mucormycosis that accounts for approximately 7% of all reported cases [1]. Among gastrointestinal mucormycosis, the stomach is the most commonly affected organ (67%), followed by the colon (21%), small intestine (4%), and esophagus (2%) [1, 4, 8, 9]. The invasion of Mucorales into the body occurs through inhalation, ingestion, or inoculation of the spores [8]. The ingestion of the spores possibly from being present in fermented milk, dried bread products, fermented porridges, and alcoholic beverages derived from infected corn is the primary mode of Mucorales entry into the gastrointestinal tract. And even possibly from infected tongue depressors at physician clinics [2]. An iatrogenic gastric mucormycosis has been reported in a study from using a wooden tongue depressor and wooden applicators for crushing and mixing medication for a critically ill patient on tube feeding [10]. While immunocompetent hosts can fight off the invasion of Mucorales after ingestion of the spores into the alimentary tract, immunocompromised individuals are not able to resist mucosal invasion due to poor defence mechanism and are prone to develop severe infection. The pathogenesis of infection in diabetic patients with or without diabetic ketoacidosis (DKA) remains to be elusive at this time. The proposed mechanism of gastric mucormycosis infection is the phagocytic dysfunction, impaired chemotaxis, and defective intracellular destruction of Mucorales in the presence of acidic environment of the stomach [11]. Uncontrolled diabetes and CKD may produce slightly acidic environment in the body similar to a diabetic ketoacidosis and predispose patients to mucormycosis.

In the current literature, multiple case reports on gastric mucormycosis have shown abdominal pain as the most common presenting symptom followed by hematemesis, melena, hematochezia, nausea, vomiting, dysphagia, and odynophagia (Table 1) [4, 9, 12–44]. The predisposing risk factors to develop gastric mucormycosis are prolonged uncontrolled diabetes mellitus with or without diabetic ketoacidosis (DKA), solid organ or stem cell transplantation, underlying hematologic malignancy, major trauma, utility of steroids, disseminated chronic infections, iron overload states, and severe neutropenia (Table 1) [4, 9, 12–44]. The gastric body is the most commonly affected location of gastric mucormycosis. The invasion of blood vessels under the mucosal surface may result in life-threatening gastrointestinal hemorrhage and is a poor prognostic factor of disease [4].

The radiological modalities such as CT scan or MRI of the abdomen usually reveal nonspecific findings such as mucosal wall thickening, mass, and reactive lymphadenopathy and prompts additional investigation with endoscopic or surgical biopsy of the lesions. EGD finding of ulcerated patchy mucosal lesions with overlying greenish or greyish exudate is a characteristic feature of gastric mucormycosis; however, biopsy of lesions is essential to differentiate it from gastric malignancy [4, 8, 21]. EGD alone does not help to make a definitive diagnosis, and additional testing with biopsy specimens is required. Histopathological and culture testing is the most definite in establishing the diagnosis. Direct microscopy, using optical brighteners, and

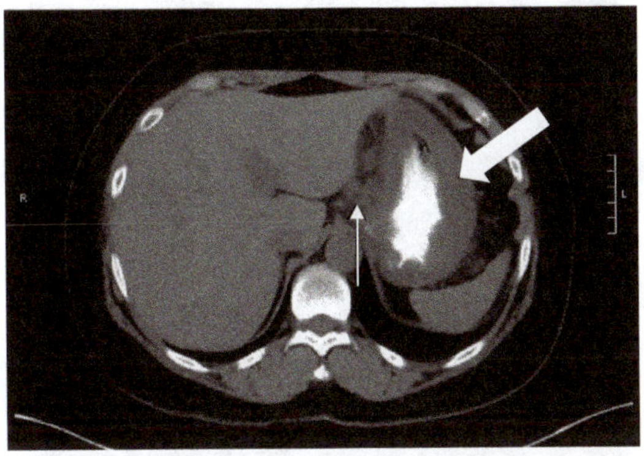

FIGURE 1: CT scan of the abdomen displaying the transmural thickening of the stomach (white blocked arrow) and the perigastric inflammation with reactive adenopathy (white arrow).

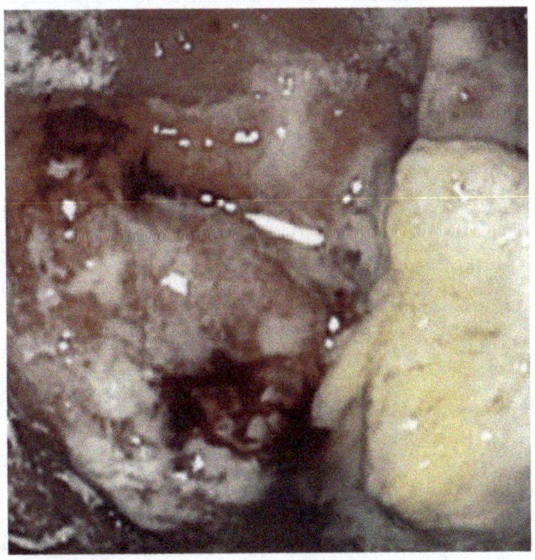

FIGURE 2: Upper endoscopy showing ulcerated lesion in the gastric fundus with the overlaying bleeding and exudative material.

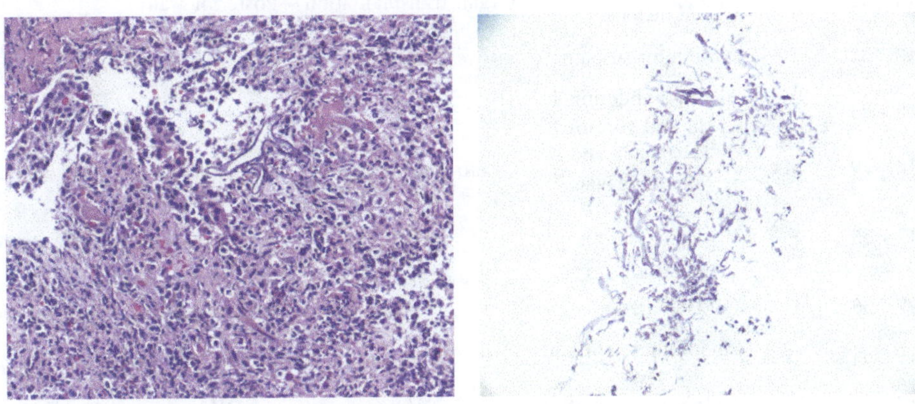

(a) (b)

FIGURE 3: Histological examination of lesion showing polymorphonuclear neutrophils indicating inflammation of gastric mucosa (a) and fragments of invading fungal hyphae (b).

hematoxylin and eosin stains have shown rapid visualization of the morphological structure of fungi for diagnosis of mucormycosis [45]. In addition, neutrophilic infiltration can also be seen on histological examination. PCR and fungal cultures of the specimen are occasionally needed for absolute confirmation of diagnosis. The cultures are performed on the

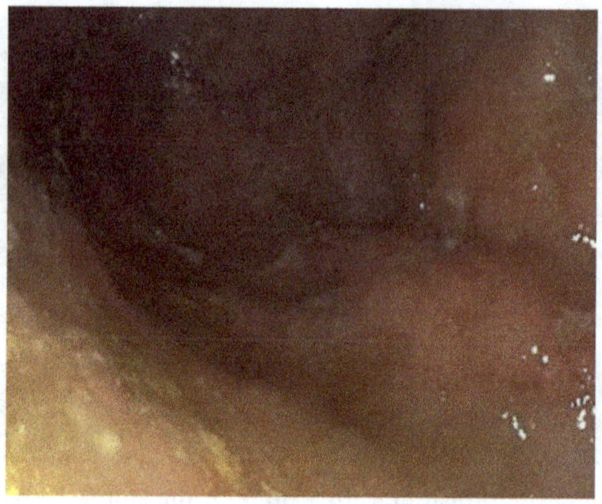

Figure 4: Repeat EGD showing cleared infection and ulceration in the fundus of the stomach.

Table 1: Clinical presentation and management of gastric mucormycosis.

Study	Year	Age	Gender	Presenting symptoms	Predisposing factor	Location	Treatment	Outcome
Sharma [12]	2020	66	F	Abdominal pain	N/A	Body	Total gastrectomy and amphotericin B	Alive
Madireddy [13]	2020	28	M	Melena	Diabetes mellitus	Fundus	Gastrectomy, amphotericin B, and posacanozole	Alive
Buckholz and Kaplan [14]	2020	63	M	Epigastric pain	Hematological malignancy	Body and fundus	Total gastrectomy and amphotericin B	Died
Platt et al. [15]	2019	33	F	Epigastric pain, nausea, and vomiting	Immunosuppressive medication	Cardia	Amphotericin B and surgical debridement	Died
Yusuf et al. [16]	2019	51	M	Hematemesis	Hematological malignancy	Cardia	Amphotericin B	N/A
Adhikari et al. [17]	2019	57	F	Hematemesis	N/A	N/A	Amphotericin B and posacanozole	Alive
Uchida et al. [4]	2019	82	F	Epigastric pain and melena	Immunosuppressive medication	Upper body and fundus	Amphotericin B	Died
Guddati et al. [18]	2019	42	M	Hematemesis	N/A	Multiple sites	Total gastrectomy	Alive
Sehmbey et al. [19]	2019	48	M	Coffee ground emesis	Trauma	Body and fundus	Amphotericin B	Died
Alfano et al. [20]	2018	42	F	Abdominal pain and melena	Organ transplantation	Posterior wall	Amphotericin B and posacanozole	Alive
Termos et al. [9]	2018	52	F	Abdominal pain	Diabetes	N/A	Amphotericin B and total gastrectomy	Died
Abreu et al. [50]	2018	23	F	Diffuse abdominal pain and vomiting	N/A	N/A	Total gastrectomy and amphotericin B	Alive
Gani et al. [21]	2018	79	M	Dysphagia and odynophagia	Organ transplantation	N/A	Isavuconazole	Alive
Sánchez-Velázquez et al. [22]	2017	53	F	Hematemesis	N/A	Cardia	Total gastrectomy	Died
Kgomo et al. [23]	2017	38	F	Hematemesis	HIV	Entire stomach	Amphotericin B	Died
Chow et al. [24]	2017	34	M	Abdominal pain and fever	Trauma	Fundus and cardia	Subtotal gastrectomy	Died
Nasa et al. [25]	2017	31	M	Abdominal distention	N/A	N/A	Amphotericin B	Died
Lee and Lee [26]	2016	41	F	Melena	Trauma	N/A	Amphotericin B	Died
Kim et al. [27]	2016	45	M	Weakness	Diabetic ketoacidosis	Entire stomach	Amphotericin B and gastrectomy	Alive
El Hachem et al. [28]	2016	67	M	Dysphagia and epigastric pain	N/A	Greater curvature	Amphotericin B and posacanozole	Alive
Sethi et al. [29]	2016	58	M	Hematemesis	Organ transplantation	Antrum and distal body	Amphotericin B	Alive

Table 1: Continued.

Study	Year	Age	Gender	Presenting symptoms	Predisposing factor	Location	Treatment	Outcome
Putrus et al. [30]	2015	65	M	Abdominal pain	Diabetes mellitus	Cardia and body	Amphotericin B and total gastrectomy	Died
Alvarado-Lezama et al. [31]	2015	32	M	Abdominal pain	Diabetic ketoacidosis	N/A	Total gastrectomy	Died
Raviraj et al. [32]	2015	19	F	Fever, vomiting, and diarrhea	N/A	N/A	Amphotericin B and posacanozole	Alive
Kulkarni and Thakur [33]	2014	50	M	Abdominal pain and distention	Diabetes	Gastric body	Surgical intervention	Died
Lee et al. [34]	2014	55	M	Severe abdominal pain	N/A	N/A	Subtotal gastrectomy and amphotericin B	Alive
Katta et al. [35]	2013	60	M	Unconsciousness	N/A	Cardia and fundus	Amphotericin B and posacanozole	Alive
Dutta et al. [36]	2012	64	F	Abdominal distention and odynophagia	N/A	Fundus and body	Amphotericin B	Alive
Chhaya et al. [37]	2011	53	F	Melena	N/A	Body	Amphotericin B	Alive
Berne et al. [38]	2009	55	M	Postoperative fever	N/A	Greater curvature	Total gastrectomy and amphotericin B	Died
Prasad and Nataraj [39]	2008	28	M	Abdominal pain, bloody diarrhea, and fever	N/A	Lesser curvature	Amphotericin B	Died
Ho et al. [40]	2007	58	W	Hematemesis	N/A	Posterior wall	Amphotericin B	Alive
Paulo De Oliveria and Milech [41]	2002	17	F	Epigastric pain	Diabetic ketoacidosis	Greater curvature and posterior wall	Amphotericin B	Died
Sheu et al. [42]	1998	70	M	Fever, epigastric pain, and melena	Organ transplantation	Greater curvature	Amphotericin B	Died
Winkler et al. [43]	1996	37	F	Melena	Organ transplantation	N/A	Amphotericin B	Alive
Sasaki et al. [44]	1993	80	F	Pancytopenia	Hematological malignancy	N/A	N/A	Died

Sabouraud agar, and rapid growth of fungi can be seen within three to seven days. Molecular-based assays, such as PCR, have shown sensitivity and specificity closer to 100% in comparison to microscopic and histopathological assays and have been noted to yield faster test results [45].

Early initiation of antifungal therapy within 6 days was found to have better patient outcomes and lower mortality rates [9, 46]. Multiple studies have shown the medical management with antifungal therapy is the mainstay treatment; however, a combination of antifungal with surgical management with either debridement or gastrectomy of mucormycosis lesions may be required in a significant number of cases specifically in those with severe disease and multiple comorbidities (Table 1) [4, 9, 12–44]. In vitro studies have shown the resistance of Mucorales to many antifungal medications such as fluconazole, ketoconazole, voriconazole, itraconazole, flucytosine, and echinocandins [47]. Commonly used antifungal medications are lipid formulation of amphotericin B (45% to 52%) and posaconazole (45%) in hospitalized patients with mucormycosis [7]. The dosage of amphotericin B remained under debate for a long time, and decision to use low versus high dose should be based upon individual patient factors including drug tolerability, side effects, and disease response to medical therapy. Currently, a dose of 5 mg/kg body is recommended by majority of physicians with a gradual escalation of dose up to 10 mg/kg for effective control of disease [45, 48, 49]. Among patients with poor tolerability of amphotericin B and those with the risk of potential side effects such as nephrotoxicity, an alternative antifungal, posaconazole, is recommended. Posaconazole is an oral agent which can also be used as maintenance agent and for long-term prophylaxis in the management of gastric mucormycosis. Although it is better tolerated than amphotericin B, in patients with hematological malignancy and gastric mucormycosis, erratic absorption of drug is concerning which may result in breakthrough infection due to suboptimal concentration of serum posaconazole. In our case, the patient was initially started on first-line antifungal agent liposomal amphotericin B. It was stopped in two weeks due to development of worsening renal function and poor tolerability. It was switched with posaconazole 300 mg daily that was also used as maintenance and salvage therapy. Posaconazole was continued for roughly four months thereafter when repeat EGD showed complete resolution of gastric mucormycosis. The duration of antifungal therapy at this time appears to be controversial given insufficient data. Serial EGD surveillance of gastric lesions is required to determine the effect of the therapy. Newer antifungal agents isavuconazole and triazole are also being utilized; however, their efficacy in resolution of the disease is still under investigation.

At times, management is not only sufficient with antifungal therapy alone and certain patients require surgical intervention. A combination of antifungal and surgical resection of lesions is indicated in case of extensive disease, angioinvasion, mucosal necrosis, and those with failed medical therapy [26, 45]. Aggressive surgical resection of necrotic lesions and negative tissue margins of fungal invasion may prevent dissemination of disease and its complications such as bowel perforation, peritonitis, and massive hemorrhage [2].

4. Conclusion

Mucormycosis is a fatal opportunistic fungal infection which may result in high mortality in untreated patients. A high index of suspicion and awareness of physicians is required for early diagnosis and management of disease particularly in immunocompromised patients. A typical presentation such as worsening abdominal pain should be investigated with CT scan or MRI and EGD in those with inconclusive finding on radiological imaging. Biopsy of the suspected mucosal lesions is the diagnostic of gastric mucormycosis. Immediate medical management with antifungal agents such as liposomal amphotericin B or posaconazole is required given the invasive nature of disease and high mortality. Serial EGD may be essential to monitor healing of gastric mucormycosis and determine duration of medical management. A combination of medical and surgical resection of mucosal lesions is warranted in the case of poor response to antifungal therapy and those with extensive disease burden.

Authors' Contributions

Haider A. Naqvi and Muhammad Nadeem Yousaf were responsible for manuscript writing, figures, and review of data. Fizah S. Chaudhary contributed to data review and proofreading. Lawrence Mills was responsible for the overall supervision of the manuscript.

References

[1] M. M. Roden, T. E. Zaoutis, W. L. Buchanan et al., "Epidemiology and outcome of zygomycosis: a review of 929 reported cases," *Clinical Infectious Diseases*, vol. 41, no. 5, pp. 634–653, 2005.

[2] G. Petrikkos, A. Skiada, O. Lortholary, E. Roilides, T. J. Walsh, and D. P. Kontoyiannis, "Epidemiology and clinical manifestations of mucormycosis," *Clinical Infectious Diseases* vol. 54, no. 1, pp. S23–S34, 2012.

[3] D. Neofytos, D. Horn, E. Anaissie et al., "Epidemiology and outcome of invasive fungal infection in adult hematopoietic stem cell transplant recipients: analysis of multicenter prospective antifungal therapy (PATH) alliance registry," *Clinical Infectious Diseases*, vol. 48, no. 3, pp. 265–273, 2009.

[4] T. Uchida, M. Okamoto, and K. Fujikawa, "Gastric mucormycosis complicated by a gastropleural fistula: a case report and review of the literature," *Medicine (Baltimore)*, vol. 98, Article ID e18142, 2019.

[5] F. M. Marty, L. Ostrosky-Zeichner, O. A. Cornely et al., "Isavuconazole treatment for mucormycosis: a single-arm open-label trial and case-control analysis," *The Lancet Infectious Diseases*, vol. 16, no. 7, pp. 828–837, 2016.

[6] D. P. Kontoyiannis and R. E. Lewis, "How I treat mucormycosis," *Blood*, vol. 118, no. 5, pp. 1216–1224, 2011.

[7] D. P. Kontoyiannis, H. Yang, and J. Song, "Prevalence, clinical and economic burden of mucormycosis-related hospitalizations in the United States: a retrospective study," *BMC Infectious Diseases*, vol. 16, p. 730, 2016.

[8] A. Vera, S. G. Hubscher, P. McMaster, and J. A. C. Buckels, "Invasive gastrointestinal zygomycosis in a liver transplant recipient," *Transplantation*, vol. 73, no. 1, pp. 145–147, 2002.

[9] S. Termos, F. Othman, M. Alali et al., "Total gastric necrosis due to mucormycosis: a rare case of gastric perforation," *American Journal of Case Reports*, vol. 19, pp. 527–533, 2018.

[10] E. Maraví-Poma, J. L. Rodríguez-Tudela, J. G. de Jalón et al., "Outbreak of gastric mucormycosis associated with the use of wooden tongue depressors in critically ill patients," *Intensive Care Medicine*, vol. 30, no. 4, pp. 724–728, 2004.

[11] A. S. Ibrahim and D. P. Kontoyiannis, "Update on mucormycosis pathogenesis," *Current Opinion in Infectious Diseases*, vol. 26, no. 6, pp. 508–515, 2013.

[12] D. Sharma, "Successful management of emphysematous gastritis with invasive gastric mucormycosis," *BMJ Case Report*, vol. 13, 2020.

[13] N. P. R. Madireddy, S. G. Uppin, and M. S. Uppin, "A rare case of gastric zygomycosis mimicking malignancy: case report with review of literature," *Journal of Bacteriology and Mycology*, vol. 7, p. 1126, 2020.

[14] A. Buckholz and A. Kaplan, "Gastrointestinal mucormycosis presenting as emphysematous gastritis after stem cell transplant for myeloma," *Mayo Clinic Proceedings*, vol. 95, no. 1, pp. 33-34, 2020.

[15] J. M. Platt, J. N. Chu, and J. C. Yarze, "Gastric mucormycosis and pneumatosis in a patient with APECED: 2717," *The American Journal of Gastroenterology*, vol. 114, 2019.

[16] A. Yusuf, L. Castellani, X. Xiong, M. Muller, and G. May, "A165 invasive gastric mucormycosis-case report of a rare cause of upper gastrointestinal bleeding," *Journal of the Canadian Association of Gastroenterology*, vol. 2, no. 2, pp. 326-327, 2019.

[17] S. Adhikari, A. R. Gautam, B. Paudyal, K. R. Sigdel, and B. Basnyat, "Case report: gastric Mucormycosis-a rare but important differential diagnosis of upper gastrointestinal bleeding in an area of Helicobacter pylori endemicity," *Wellcome Open Research*, vol. 4, p. 5, 2019.

[18] H. Guddati, C. Andrade, P. Muscarella, and H. Hertan, "An unusual cause of massive upper gastrointestinal bleeding-gastric mucormycosis," *Oxford Medical Case Reports*, vol. 2019, no. 2, p. 135, 2019.

[19] G. Sehmbey, R. Malik, and D. Kosa, "Gastric ulcer and perforation due to mucormycosis in an immunocompetent patient," *ACG Case Reports Journal*, vol. 6, Article ID e00154, 2019.

[20] G. Alfano, F. Fontana, D. Francesca et al., "Gastric mucormycosis in a liver and kidney transplant recipient: case report and concise review of literature," *Transplantation Proceedings*, vol. 50, no. 3, pp. 905–909, 2018.

[21] I. Gani, A. Doroodchi, and K. Falkenstrom, "Gastric mucormycosis in a renal transplant patient treated with

isavuconazole monotherapy," *Case Reports in Transplantation*, vol. 2019, Article ID 9839780, , 2019.

[22] P. Sánchez Velázquez, M. Pera, and J. Gimeno, "Mucormycosis: an unusual cause of gastric perforation and severe bleeding in immunocompetent patients," *Revista Española de Enfermedades Digestivas*, vol. 109, pp. 223–225, 2017.

[23] M. K. Kgomo, A. A. Elnagar, K. Mashoshoe, P. Thomas, and W. G. V. Hougenhouck-Tulleken, "Gastric mucormycosis: a case report," *World Journal of Clinical Infectious Diseases*, vol. 8, no. 1, pp. 1–3, 2018.

[24] K. L. Chow, D. P. McElmeel, H. G. Brown, M. S. Tabriz, and E. C. Omi, "Invasive gastric mucormycosis: a case report of a deadly complication in an immunocompromised patient after penetrating trauma," *International Journal of Surgery Case Reports*, vol. 40, pp. 90–93, 2017.

[25] M. Nasa, Z. Sharma, L. Lipi, and R. Sud, "Gastric angioinvasive mucormycosis in immunocompetent adult, a rare occurrence," *The Journal of the Association of Physicians of India*, vol. 65, no. 12, pp. 103-104, 2017.

[26] S. W. Lee and H. S. Lee, "Gastric mucormycosis followed by traumatic cardiac rupture in an immunocompetent patient," *The Korean Journal of Gastroenterology*, vol. 68, no. 2, pp. 99–103, 2016.

[27] J. H. Kim, H. J. Lee, J. H. Ha et al., "A case of gastric mucormycosis induced necrotic gastric ulcer in patients with diabetic ketoacidosis," *The Korean Journal of Helicobacter and Upper Gastrointestinal Research*, vol. 16, no. 4, pp. 230–234, 2016.

[28] G. El Hachem, N. Chamseddine, and G. Saidy, "Bone marrow necrosis: an unusual initial presentation of sickle cell anemia," *Clinical Lymphoma Myeloma and Leukemia*, vol. 16, no. 1, pp. S195–S198, 2016.

[29] S. S. N. Sethi, J. S. Sandhu, S. Kaur, V. Makkar, and P. M. Sohal, "Gastric mucormycosis: an unusual transplant infection," *International Journal of Medical Science and Public Health*, vol. 6, pp. 819–821, 2017.

[30] A. A.-G. A. Putrus, M. A. AlSamman, M. Castro-Borobio, M. B. Khan, and S. C. Ng, "Gastric mucormycosis: a devastating fungal infection in an immunocompromised patient," *Gastroenterology*, vol. 148, p. S321, 2015.

[31] J. Alvarado-Lezama, O. Espinosa-González, E. García-Cano, and G. Sánchez-Córdova, "Gastritis enfisematosa secundaria a mucormicosis gástrica," *Cirugía Y Cirujanos*, vol. 83, no. 1, pp. 56–60, 2015.

[32] K. S. Raviraj, P. Miglani, A. Garg, and P. K Agarwal, "Gastric mucormycosis with hemolytic uremic syndrome," *The Journal of the Association of Physicians of India*, vol. 63, no. 10, pp. 75-76, 2015.

[33] R. V. Kulkarni and S. S. Thakur, "Invasive gastric mucormycosis-a case report," *Indian Journal of Surgery*, vol. 77, no. S1, pp. 87–89, 2015.

[34] S. H. Lee, Y. G. Son, S. S. Sohn, and S. W. Ryu, "Successful treatment of invasive gastric mucormycosis in a patient with alcoholic liver cirrhosis: a case report," *Experimental and Therapeutic Medicine*, vol. 8, no. 2, pp. 401–404, 2014.

[35] J. Katta, S. G. Gompf, T. Narach et al., "Gastric mucormycosis managed with combination antifungal therapy and no surgical debridement," *Infectious Diseases in Clinical Practice*, vol. 21, no. 4, pp. 265–268, 2013.

[36] A. Dutta, M. Roy, and T. D. Singh, "Gastric mucormycosis in an immunocompetent patient," *Journal of Medical Society*, vol. 26, pp. 192–194, 2012.

[37] V. Chhaya, S. Gupta, and A. Arnaout, "Mucormycosis causing giant gastric ulcers," *Endoscopy*, vol. 43, no. S 02, pp. E289–E290, 2011.

[38] J. D. Berne, D. H. Villarreal, T. M. McGovern, S. A. Rowe, F. O. Moore, and S. H. Norwood, "A fatal case of posttraumatic gastric mucormycosis," *The Journal of Trauma: Injury, Infection, and Critical Care*, vol. 66, no. 3, pp. 933–935, 2009.

[39] B. S. S. A. Prasad and K. S. Nataraj, "Primary gastrointestinal mucormycosis in an immunocompetent person," *Journal of Postgraduate Medicine*, vol. 54, pp. 211–213, 2008.

[40] Y.-H. Ho, B.-G. Wu, Y.-Z. Chen, and L.-S. Wang, "Gastric mucormycosis in an alcoholic with review of the literature," *Tzu Chi Medical Journal*, vol. 19, no. 3, pp. 169–172, 2007.

[41] J. E. Paulo De Oliveira and A. Milech, "A fatal case of gastric mucormycosis and diabetic ketoacidosis," *Endocrine Practice*, vol. 8, pp. 44–46, 2002.

[42] B. S. Sheu, P. C. Lee, and H. B. Yang, "A giant gastric ulcer caused by mucormycosis infection in a patient with renal transplantation," *Endoscopy*, vol. 30, pp. S60–S61, 1998.

[43] S. Winkler, S. Susani, B. Willinger et al., "Gastric mucormycosis due to Rhizopus oryzae in a renal transplant recipient," *Journal of Clinical Microbiology*, vol. 34, no. 10, pp. 2585–2587, 1996.

[44] A. Sasaki, M. Tsukaguchi, and K. Takayasu, "Myelodysplastic syndrome developing acute myelocytic leukemia with gastric mucormycosis," *Rinsho Byori*, vol. 41, pp. 1054–1058, 1993.

[45] A. Skiada, C. Lass-Floerl, and N. Klimko, "Challenges in the diagnosis and treatment of mucormycosis," *Medical Mycology*, vol. 56, pp. 93–101, 2018.

[46] G. Chamilos, R. E. Lewis, and D. P. Kontoyiannis, "Delaying amphotericin B-based frontline therapy significantly increases mortality among patients with hematologic malignancy who have zygomycosis," *Clinical Infectious Diseases*, vol. 47, no. 4, pp. 503–509, 2008.

[47] N. G. Almyroudis, D. A. Sutton, A. W. Fothergill, M. G. Rinaldi, and S. Kusne, "In vitro susceptibilities of 217 clinical isolates of zygomycetes to conventional and new antifungal agents," *Antimicrobial Agents and Chemotherapy*, vol. 51, no. 7, pp. 2587–2590, 2007.

[48] F. Tissot, S. Agrawal, L. Pagano et al., "ECIL-6 guidelines for the treatment of invasive candidiasis, aspergillosis and mucormycosis in leukemia and hematopoietic stem cell transplant patients," *Haematologica*, vol. 102, no. 3, pp. 433–444, 2017.

[49] O. A. Cornely, M. Cuenca-Estrella, J. F. Meis, and A. J. Ullmann, "European society of clinical microbiology and infectious diseases (ESCMID) fungal infection study group (EFISG) and European confederation of medical mycology (ECMM) 2013 joint guidelines on diagnosis and management of rare and emerging fungal diseases," *Clinical Microbiology and Infection*, vol. 20, no. 3, pp. 1–4, 2014.

[50] B. F. B. B. D. Abreu, M. L. Duarte, L. R. D. Santos, A. Sementilli, and F. N. Figueiras, "A rare case of gastric mucormycosis in an immunocompetent patient," *Revista da Sociedade Brasileira de Medicina Tropical*, vol. 51, no. 3, pp. 401-402, 2018.

44

Improvising in Endoscopy: Endoscopic Removal of Sharp Foreign Bodies in the Upper GI Tract, using a Handmade Protective Device

Konstantinos Miltiadou,[1] Zisimangelos Solomos,[2] Dimitrios Lygkos,[1] Alexandros Chatzidakis,[1] Evripidis Rizos,[1] Ioannis S. Papanikolaou,[1] and Konstantinos Triantafyllou[1]

[1]*Hepatogastroenterology Unit, 2nd Department of Internal Medicine-Propaedeutic, Research Institute and Diabetes Center, Medical School, National and Kapodistrian University, Attikon University General Hospital, Athens 124 62, Greece*
[2]*Doctors of the World, Greek Delegation, Athens 105 53, Greece*

Correspondence should be addressed to Zisimangelos Solomos; zisimosmed@gmail.com

Academic Editor: Yoshiro Kawahara

Introduction. Foreign body ingestion is a common problem in large-volume endoscopic departments. Several techniques and devices have been described for the safe endoscopic removal of these objects. However, these devices may not be suitable in every clinical setting or—as in our case—they may not even be available. *Case Presentation.* We report the case of a 34-year-old patient, presenting with sharp foreign body ingestion. The foreign bodies were safely removed using a handmade protective hood due to lack of a commercial device. In our case, improvisation proved to be of great benefit for the patient as well as for the endoscopist. *Discussion.* Improvised interventions can be of special interest in the setting of insufficiently funded or equipped endoscopic departments.

1. Introduction

Ingestion of foreign bodies is a common problem in large-volume endoscopic departments. In adults, it is usually related to elderly, psychosocial-developmental problems, intoxication, and incarceration. Although up to 80% of them will pass spontaneously, the ingestion of sharp foreign bodies can be technically challenging for the endoscopist and dangerous for the patient, because the risk of complications (esophagogastric/pharyngeal damage and aspiration) is as high as 35%, especially if not removed in time [1–4]. Therefore, several techniques have been proposed [5–12] and the use of protective devices is recommended, to avoid these complications during extraction of sharp foreign bodies [4].

A variety of protective devices are available to safely aid endoscopic removal of such objects [13]. However, these devices may not be suitable in every clinical setting [5] and sometimes, they may not even be available. In such occasions, a case-by-case approach or even improvisation can be beneficial for the patient (and perhaps the endoscopist). Examples of such handmade devices (caps, condoms, gloves, and tubes) have been reported in the literature [14–18].

Herein, we present a case of sharp foreign bodies removed from the stomach of a patient, using a handmade rubber hood, fashioned from a plastic transfusion pressure infusor.

2. Case Presentation

A 34-year-old male patient with no prior medical history presented at the Emergency Department reporting ingestion of several metallic objects one hour before. The clinical examination was unremarkable, and the patient was in overall excellent condition. X-ray studies revealed at least 4 metallic objects in various parts of the GI tract (Figure 1).

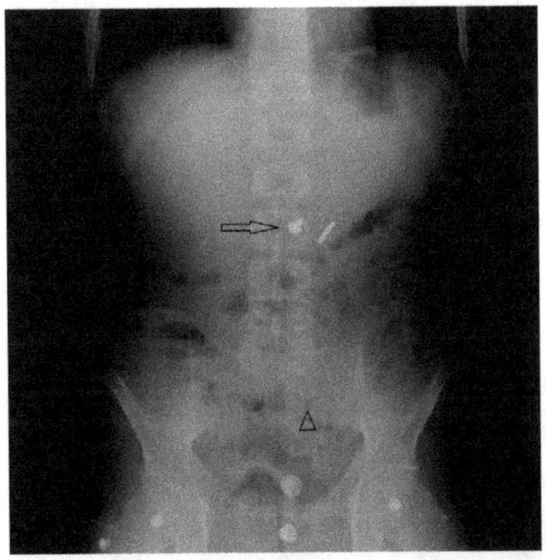

FIGURE 1: Abdominal X-ray: arrow showing 3 metallic objects (screw, coin, and plastic head pin) in the stomach, and arrow head showing another plastic head pin well into the small intestine. Note that the small metal scrap that was later seen on endoscopy is not evident here.

Considering the timing of ingestion and the type of the ingested materials, endoscopic extraction was decided. Esophagogastroduodenoscopy (EGD) was performed approximately 2 hours after the ingestion. Four objects were visualized at the time of endoscopy (one screw in the first part of the duodenum, one elongated pin impacted in the antrum wall, one coin, and one small metal scrap in the stomach). The coin was easily removed from the stomach using a Roth Net. An overtube was then introduced in order to safely retrieve the remaining 2 larger sharp objects. None of the remaining objects could fit in the overtube, and the patient's tolerance to the procedure was poor despite maximal sedation. No other protective devices such as rubber hoods were available at the time of endoscopy. Therefore, any further efforts to extract the objects were abandoned, and the patient was returned to the surgical ward for monitoring. Recognizing that complication rates could be high in this patient and that referral to another better equipped facility would require time, such that it would expose the patient to the risks of delayed intervention, we improvised a handmade rubber hood, constructed from a plastic transfusion pressure infusor (Figure 2). This material was chosen because it was flexible enough to invert back on itself in the cardia upon withdrawal of the scope, yet thick enough to withstand puncturing. The hood was fastened with silk tape to the distal end of a 9.8 mm gastroscope (GIF-Q165 Olympus Corporation, Tokyo, Japan), in a coned fashion (to facilitate the entrance of the foreign body into the bell of the hood), and then inverted (Figures 3(a) and 3(b)). A test was carried out before scope insertion to make sure that the foreign body fits in the hood (Figure 4).

The patient was called for the second EGD three hours after the first one. The two larger foreign bodies were still in the stomach, whilst the small metal scrap had migrated distally. With the help of mild sedation (3 mg of midazolam), the pin and the screw were captured using rat-tooth forceps, pulled into the hood, and extracted (Figure 5). The hood inverted back on itself as expected, with no tissue injury upon second endoscopic look. The procedure lasted only 15 minutes with excellent tolerance from the patient.

The patient was returned to the ward for monitoring because two sharp objects were still in his small bowel. Repeat X-ray studies the following days confirmed successful discharge of the foreign bodies per rectum without any complications.

3. Discussion

We have presented a case of successful endoscopic sharp foreign body extraction, using a handmade protective hood. To our knowledge, this is the first time that the specific device has been used, although examples of similar handmade devices (caps, condoms, gloves, and tubes) have been successfully used and reported in the literature [14–18]. In our case, it was very helpful in a moment of need, when a commercial protective hood was unavailable. It proved beneficial for both the patient and the frustrated endoscopist.

This scenario could also be relevant in the setting of small, remote, inadequately equipped or funded endoscopic departments, especially if an anesthesiologist is not readily available to intubate or heavily sedate the young patient who cannot tolerate large overtubes.

The device seems to offer some advantages: it practically comes at no cost; it can be constructed in a matter of minutes; it offers good visualization of the lumen; and it seems to be safe. On the other hand, it is a handmade, nonvalidated device which cannot be duplicated in the exact same form, and therefore, its performance is unpredictable. There are concerns that the device may not invert in the cardia, or even dislodge from the endoscope, adding one more foreign body in the stomach. However, if one is found in a situation of limited options such as ours, it seems relatively safe to give it a try and abandon the extraction if the device does not fold properly, or easily extract the device with a Roth Net if dislodged in the stomach.

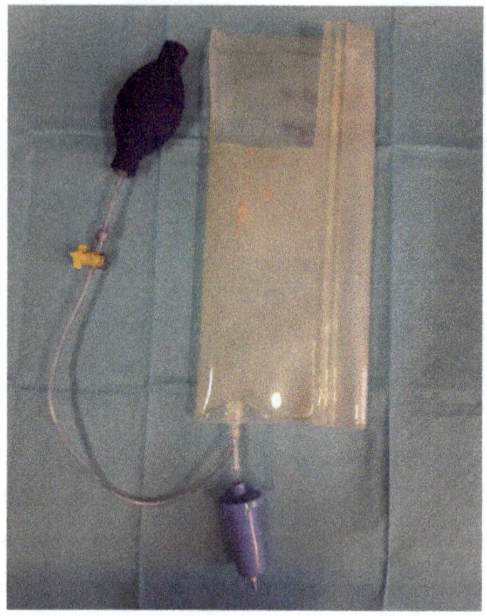

Figure 2: A plastic transfusion pressure infusor. Note the missing rubber part used to construct the hood.

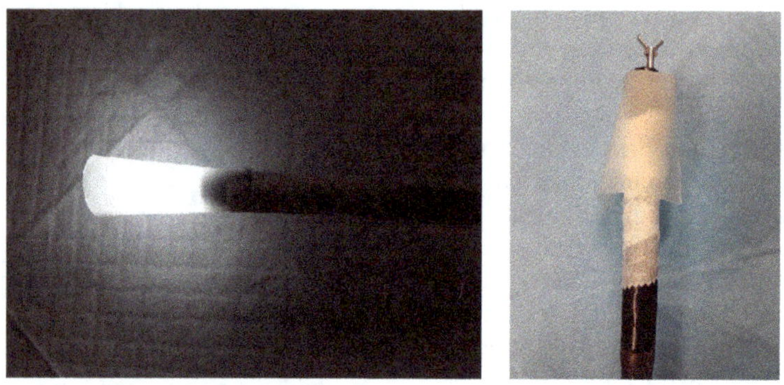

(a) (b)

Figure 3: (a) Rubber folded in coned fashion forming a bell-shaped hood and secured with silk tape. (b) Hood-inverted back on itself before scope insertion.

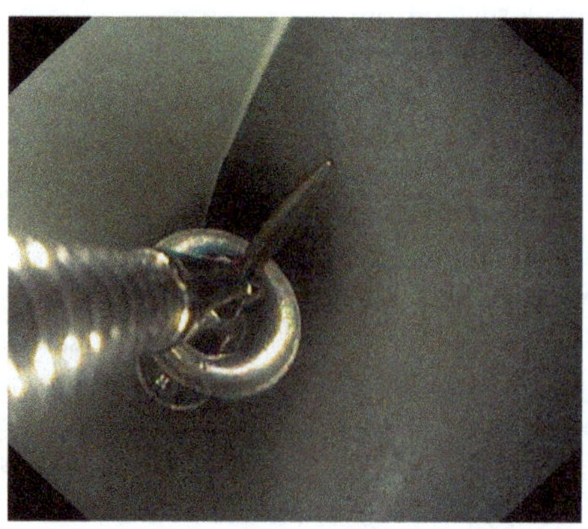

Figure 4: Testing if the foreign body fits in the hood before inserting the scope.

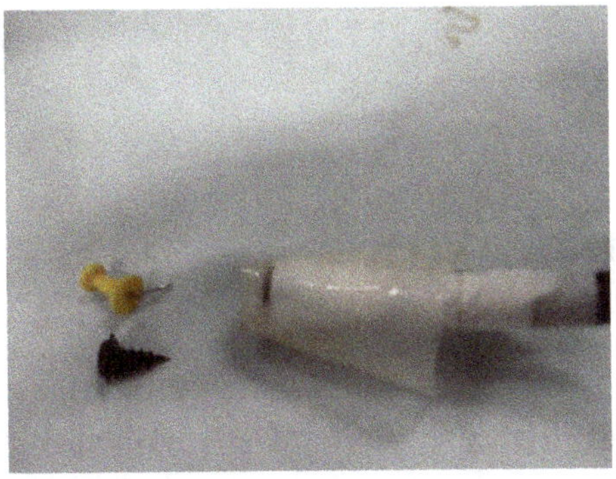

FIGURE 5: Elongated pin and thick screw safely extracted. Note the bended tip of the pin which was impacted in the antrum wall.

4. Conclusion

In our case, improvisation proved to be of great benefit for the patient as well as for the endoscopist. Such interventions can be of special interest in the setting of insufficiently funded or equipped endoscopic departments.

Authors' Contributions

Miltiadou K and Triantafyllou K conducted the endoscopy of the upper GI tract of the patient and drafted the manuscript. Lygkos D, Chatzidakis A, Rizos E, and Papanikolaou IS reviewed the literature and contributed to manuscript drafting. Solomos Z revised, corrected, and submitted the manuscript. All authors issued final approval for the version to be submitted.

References

[1] S. O. Ikenberry, T. L. Jue, M. A. Anderson et al., "Management of ingested foreign bodies and food impactions," *Gastrointestinal Endoscopy*, vol. 73, no. 6, pp. 1085–1091, 2011.

[2] L. Carp, "Foreign bodies in the intestine," *Annals of Surgery*, vol. 85, no. 4, pp. 575–591, 1927.

[3] W. Rösch and M. Classen, "Fiberendoscopic foreign body removal from the upper gastrointestinal tract," *Endoscopy*, vol. 4, no. 4, pp. 193–197, 1972.

[4] M. Birk, P. Bauerfeind, P. Deprez et al., "Removal of foreign bodies in the upper gastrointestinal tract in adults: European Society of Gastrointestinal Endoscopy (ESGE) Clinical Guideline," *Endoscopy*, vol. 48, no. 5, pp. 489–496, 2016.

[5] G. Bertoni, R. Sassatelli, R. Conigliaro, and G. Bedogni, "A simple latex protector hood for safe endoscopic removal of sharp-pointed gastroesophageal foreign bodies," *Gastrointestinal Endoscopy*, vol. 44, no. 4, pp. 458–461, 1996.

[6] B. H. Rogers, C. Kot, S. Meiri, and M. Epstein, "An overtube for the flexible fiberoptic esophagogastroduodenoscope," *Gastrointestinal Endoscopy*, vol. 28, no. 4, pp. 256-257, 1982.

[7] J.-S. Shin, B.-S. Sheu, X.-Z. Lin, C.-Y. Chen, and T.-C. Leow, "Longitudinal linear-incised overtube for endoscopic removal of larger ingested foreign bodies," *Gastrointestinal Endoscopy*, vol. 41, no. 6, p. 618, 1995.

[8] H. H. Tuen, E. C. S. Lai and S. T. Fan, Endoscopic retrieval of ingested broken glass in the esophagus and stomach by end-hood and suction technique," *Gastrointestinal Endoscopy*, vol. 35, no. 4, pp. 357-358, 1989.

[9] L. Witzel, U. Scheurer, A. Mühlemann, and F. Halter, "Removal of razor blades from stomach with fibreoptic endoscope," *Bmj*, vol. 2, no. 5918, p. 539, 1974.

[10] R. W. Werth, C. Edwards, and W. C. Jennings, "A safe and quick method for endoscopic retrieval of multiple gastric foreign bodies using a protective sheath," *Surgery, Gynecology & Obstetrics*, vol. 171, no. 5, pp. 419-420, 1990.

[11] W. C. Martin, S. A. Jones, N. Nagai, and E. C. Texter, "Fiberendoscopic removal of long foreign bodies from the stomach using a colon stiffening tube as a protective sheath," *The American Journal of Gastroenterology*, vol. 71, no. 5, pp. 505–507, 1979.

[12] J. Garrido and J. S. Barkin, "Endoscopic modification for safe foreign body removal," *The American Journal of Gastroenterology*, vol. 80, no. 12, pp. 957-958, 1985.

[13] D. O. Faigel, B. R. StotlandM. L. Kochman et al., Device choice and experience level in endoscopic foreign object retrieval: an in vivo study," *Gastrointestinal Endoscopy*, vol. 45, no. 6, pp. 490–492, 1997.

[14] K.-W. Chiu, L.-S. Lu, T.-C. Wu, and S.-S. Chiou, "Novel low-cost endoscopic cap for esophageal foreign objects: a case report," *Medicine (Baltimore)*, vol. 94, no. 17, 2015.

[15] Y. Tateno and R. Suzuki, "Cut endotracheal tube for endoscopic removal of an ingested push-through pack," *World Journal of Gastrointestinal Endoscopy*, vol. 8, no. 13, pp. 472–476, 2016.

[16] L. S. Kao, T. Nguyen, J. Dominitz, H. L. Teicher, and D. J. Kearney, "Modification of a latex glove for the safe endoscopic removal of a sharp gastric foreign body," *Gastrointestinal Endoscopy*, vol. 52, no. 1, pp. 127–129, 2000.

[17] L. F. Lin, "Condoms used to assist difficult endoscopic removal of impacted upper esophageal foreign bodies," *Advances in Digestive Medicine*, vol. 3, no. 1, pp. 24–27, 2016.

[18] S. Zhang, J. Wang, J. Wang, B. Zhong, M. Chen, and Y. Cui, "Transparent cap-assisted endoscopic management of foreign bodies in the upper esophagus: a randomized, controlled trial," *Journal of Gastroenterology and Hepatology*, vol. 28, no. 8, pp. 1339–1342, 2013.

45

A Rare Case of Colonic Sarcoidosis Presenting as a Mass

Haozhe Sun,[1] **Jasbir Makker**,[1,2] **Harish Patel**,[1,2] **Nikhitha Mantri**,[1] **Ali N. Hussain**,[2] **and Naeem Abbas**[3]

[1]*Department of Internal Medicine, Bronx Care Health Systems–Affiliate of Mount Sinai Hospital Systems, 1650 Grand Concourse, Bronx, NY 10457, USA*
[2]*Division of Gastroenterology, Bronx Care Health Systems–Affiliate of Mount Sinai Hospital Systems, 1650 Grand Concourse, Bronx, NY 10457, USA*
[3]*Department of Gastroenterology, Advantage Care Physician, 260 W Sunrise Highway Stream Valley, Rosedale, NY 11581, USA*

Correspondence should be addressed to Haozhe Sun; hsun@bronxcare.org

Academic Editor: Tetsuo Hirata

Introduction. Sarcoidosis is a common multisystem chronic inflammatory disease of an unidentified inciting etiology. The most common initial manifestations of this disease involve the pulmonary system, and involvement of the gastrointestinal tract is rare. Sarcoidosis of the gastrointestinal tract occurs in an oral-anal gradient, with the esophagus and stomach being the most commonly involved sites, while colonic involvement remains extremely rare. *Case Presentation*. We present a case of a 24-year-old African American man who was evaluated for persistent abdominal pain, chronic diarrhea, and weight loss. Workup for infectious etiologies and celiac disease was unrevealing. An inflammatory mass in the hepatic flexure was found during colonoscopy, and a computed tomography (CT) scan of the abdomen was significant for circumferential thickening of the cecum and ascending colon, along with nodular thickening of the peritoneum without enhancement. Malignancy and inflammatory bowel disease were the initial differentials. A peritoneal biopsy was also performed. Pathology of the colon and peritoneal biopsy was significant for the presence of noncaseating granulomas and confluent granulomatous inflammation. The patient was diagnosed with colonic sarcoidosis, and treatment with corticosteroids was initiated. Symptoms resolved with treatment, and a follow-up colonoscopy five months later showed interval healing. *Conclusion*. Although rare, colonic sarcoidosis should be considered as one of the differential diagnoses when evaluating a patient with chronic diarrhea and a mass on colonoscopy. Histopathology is the key to diagnosis as it distinguishes malignancy from sarcoidosis. Corticosteroids remain as an option for treating colonic sarcoidosis.

1. Introduction

Chronic diarrhea is defined as loose stool with increased frequency or urgency of more than four-week duration [1]. It is estimated that 5% of the population in the United States suffer from chronic diarrhea [2]. The predominant etiologies of chronic diarrhea include inflammatory bowel disease, irritable bowel syndrome, malabsorption syndrome, chronic pancreatitis, and intestinal infections. Most cases of chronic diarrhea require an extensive workup in order to reach a diagnosis. The unusual etiologies of chronic diarrhea continue to pose a diagnostic challenge [3–5]. Malignancy of the colon, while rare, can also manifest as chronic diarrhea [6].

Sarcoidosis is a chronic inflammatory granulomatous disease of young, middle-aged individuals with multisystem involvement that predominantly affects females [7]. The lung is the most common affected organ. Symptomatic gastrointestinal tract involvement is rare and occurs in less than 1% of patients with sarcoidosis [8]. If the gastrointestinal tract is involved, an oral-anal gradient is observed, and approximately 80% of such cases would involve the upper gastrointestinal tract. Therefore, involvement of the colon is rare in gastrointestinal sarcoidosis [9]. Abdominal pain is the most common presenting symptom for colonic sarcoidosis followed by diarrhea and weight loss [10].

We report a case of a 24-year-old African American male, who presented with persistent abdominal pain, diarrhea, and weight loss. Colonoscopy revealed a colonic mass concerning for malignancy. Initial imaging was significant for colonic wall thickening with possible peritoneal involvement. However, pathology results from the colonic and peritoneal biopsy were consistent with the diagnosis of colonic sarcoidosis. This patient did not have any pulmonary symptoms on presentation, and sarcoidosis was not in the array of the differentials until pathology results were obtained. The patient responded clinically to medical therapy, and resolution of colonic lesions was observed on repeat biopsy by colonoscopy.

2. Case Presentation

Our patient is a 24-year-old black male, who presented to us for the evaluation of persistent abdominal pain, diarrhea, and weight loss. He describes a six-month history of episodic, diffuse, and crampy abdominal pain. Each episode would last about five to ten minutes and was mild to moderate in intensity. The pain would resolve spontaneously, and there were no associated symptoms, aggravating, or alleviating factors. Three months prior to his presentation, he started experiencing loose, watery diarrhea which would occur every two to three days. He described having three to four loose bowel movements per day, with no presence of mucus or blood. He also complained of anorexia and a 10 lb weight loss over the previous three months.

A comprehensive review of systems was otherwise negative. He denied any fever, chills, or any relation of his diarrhea to food intake, and there was no history of nocturnal diarrhea. There was no recent antibiotic use and no history of recent travel or sick contacts. He denies any joint pain, skin rash, or mouth ulcers. There was no history of shortness of breath, cough, wheezing, chest pain, or urinary symptoms.

His past medical history was significant for Lyme disease in childhood and attention-deficit hyperactive disorder. There was no history of surgery in the past. He denied any history of smoking, alcohol use, or recreational drug use. There was no family history of inflammatory bowel disease (IBD), colon cancer, or any other GI malignancies.

On physical examination, the patient appeared malnourished, evident by temporal wasting. His vital signs were generally unremarkable. He weighed 134 lb (60.8 kg) which puts him at a BMI of 17.80 kg/m^2. Examination of the gastrointestinal system was unremarkable, with a soft, nontender abdomen, with no visceromegaly. There was no scleral icterus or conjunctival pallor. The remainder of the physical exam was normal.

Results of routine hematology and biochemistry investigations including liver enzymes were all within normal limits. Celiac serology was negative, and stool workup including fecal leukocytes, stool culture, ova and parasites, giardia, and cryptosporidium were all negative. His carcinoembryonic antigen (CEA) was within normal limits.

Colonoscopy showed a circumferentially encasing, partially obstructing, stenotic mass, with overlying granular and inflammatory mucosa in the hepatic flexure (Figures 1(a)–1(c)). The colonoscope could not be negotiated through the mass to evaluate the cecum. The colonic biopsy revealed soft consistency of the mass, and there was excess of bleeding from the biopsy site (Figure 1(c)). The colonic mucosa of the remaining part of the colon appeared normal, and random colon biopsy was obtained. The histopathology of the hepatic flexure mass was significant for focal active chronic colitis with ulceration, polypoid granulation tissue formation, reactive epithelial changes, and noncaseating granulomata formation that was consistent with granulomatous inflammation (Figure 2(a)). Special stains for tuberculosis, fungi, and other microorganisms were all negative. The crypt architecture was preserved (Figure 2(c)), and the histopathological findings were devoid of the basal cell plasmacytosis to conclude to inflammatory bowel disease. Esophagogastroduodenoscopy was performed and was unremarkable; biopsies of gastric and duodenal tissues and subsequent testing for *Helicobacter pylori* infection, celiac disease, and Whipple disease were all negative.

An abdominal CT scan of the abdomen performed with contrast was remarkable for circumferential thickening of the cecum and ascending colon without any evidence of obstruction. There were perihepatic and pelvic ascites in the cul-de-sac and nodular thickening of the peritoneum in the right lateral abdominal wall and minimally at the omentum. The patient subsequently underwent a laparoscopic peritoneal biopsy. The biopsy specimen showed noncaseating granulomas and confluent granulomatous inflammation. Special stains for tuberculosis and fungi were negative.

A CT scan of the chest was performed and revealed a slightly irregular 1 cm pulmonary nodule in the superior segment of the right lower lobe. The area of nodular sarcoid cannot be excluded. There was also minimal fissural nodularity which could represent underlying sarcoid.

A diagnosis of colonic sarcoidosis was made, and the patient was treated medically with oral prednisone, starting at 40 mg daily for one week with a gradual taper to a target maintenance dose of 5 mg daily over the course of eight weeks. Upon starting prednisone, the patient improved clinically with the resolution of his abdominal pain and diarrhea, along with a 20 lb weight gain, and remained in sustained symptomatic remission after three months of treatment. A colonoscopy performed five months after treatment revealed interval improvement of colonic stenosis resolution of the inflammatory mass, and the scope could be traversed through the stricture (Figure 3(a)). Some mucosal inflammation and granularity could be noted; however, there was significant improvement as compared to the index colonoscopy (Figure 3(b)). The biopsy specimens from the previously involved areas showed chronic mucosal injury with no evidence of dysplasia, malignancy, or noncaseating granulomas (Figure 4).

3. Discussion

Sarcoidosis presenting initially with solely gastrointestinal symptoms is extremely rare, with the current literature based on a few case reports [9]. Sarcoidosis is more prevalent in blacks with an incidence of 35.5 per 100,000 as compared to

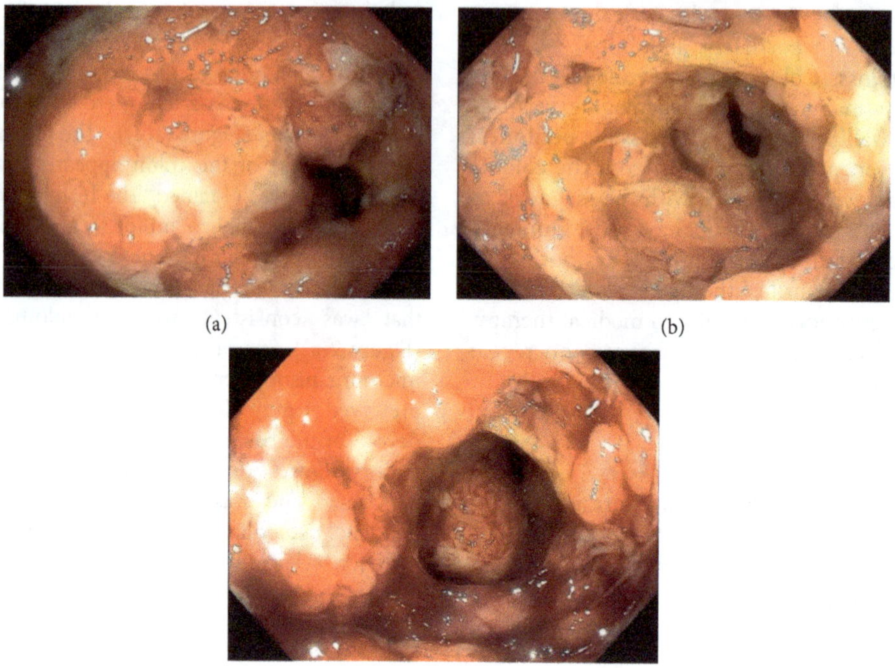

(a) (b) (c)

Figure 1: Colonoscopic findings of the hepatic flexure, demonstrating circumferential inflammatory and stenotic mass.

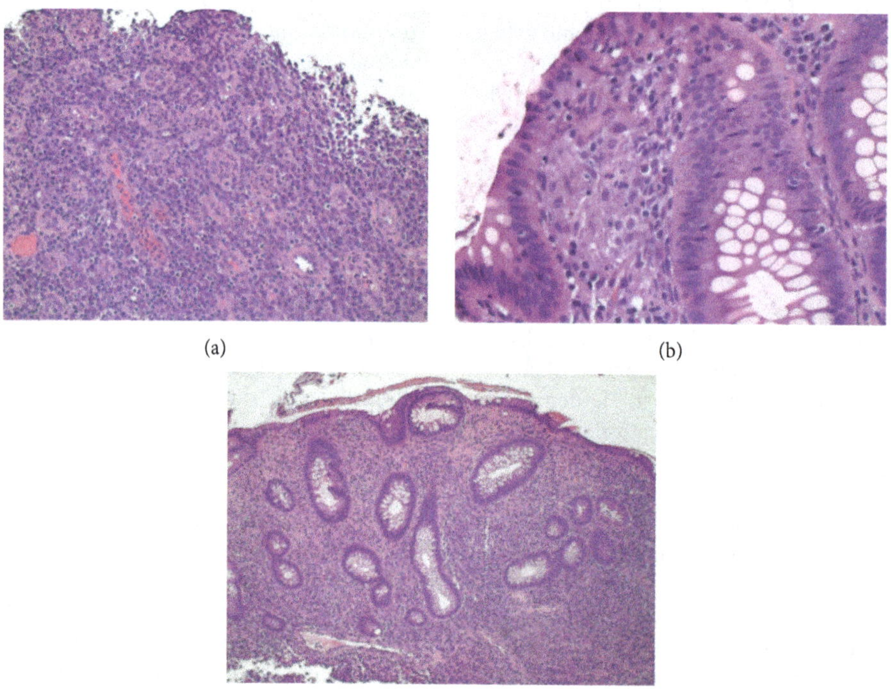

(a) (b) (c)

Figure 2: Hematoxylin and eosin (H&E) staining of the hepatic flexure mass, revealing focal active chronic colitis with ulceration, polypoid granulation tissue formation, reactive epithelial, and noncaseation granulomatous changes. Basal cell plasmacytosis could not be demonstrated. Hematoxylin and eosin (H&E) staining of the normal-appearing colon revealing the chronic colitis and preserved crypt architecture.

the trailing incidence of 10.9 per 100,000 in whites [11]. Women are more affected than men. However, based on the review of 31 cases of colon sarcoidosis, it is difficult to gauge ethnic or gender predominance [9].

Patients with colonic sarcoidosis often present with nonspecific signs and symptoms, such as abdominal pain, diarrhea, weight loss, and in some cases, iron deficiency anemia, hematochezia, or colonic obstruction. Combined

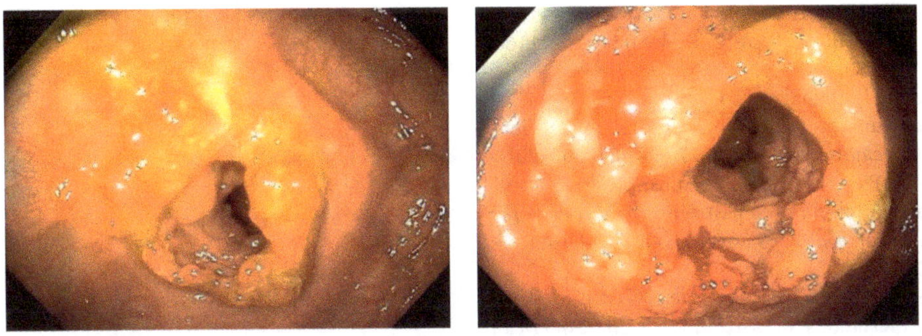

(a) (b)

FIGURE 3: Posttreatment colonoscopy reveals interval improvement of colonic stenosis resolution of the inflammatory mass.

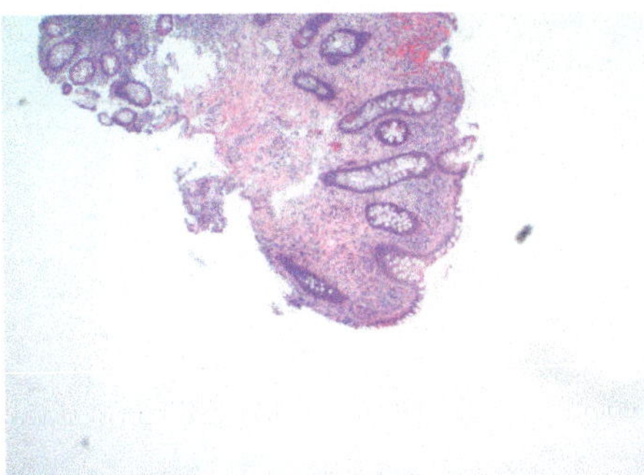

FIGURE 4: H&E staining of the colonic mucosa (poststeroid treatment) showing focal active chronic colitis without any evidence of dysplasia, metaplasia, or noncaseating granulomas.

with abdominal imaging findings of a mass, or signs of luminal obstruction, an extensive workup for a neoplastic process is often warranted.

Apart from colorectal malignancy, another important differential to consider would include the granulomatous inflammatory bowel diseases such as ulcerative colitis and particularly Crohn's disease. Both sarcoidosis and inflammatory bowel disease can share similarities in terms of extraintestinal manifestations such as erythema nodosum, arthropathy, and uveitis. Other differentials would also include colonic granulomatous disorders, hypersensitivity to foreign antigens, or infectious etiologies such as tuberculosis, syphilis, and fungal infections. It is also important to consider that these diseases could be primarily responsible for the clinical manifestations, and the coexistence of sarcoidosis is just an incidental finding.

The diagnosis of colonic sarcoidosis remains challenging, and the demonstration of noncaseating granulomas on biopsy is necessary. The resolution of granulomatous inflammation and significant clinical improvement with corticosteroid therapy point to a diagnosis of sarcoidosis in our reported case. However, in equivocal cases, clinicians should be prudent in excluding other alternative diagnoses. In such cases, diligent follow-up and re-evaluation of the patient could prove to be a sensible strategy.

The therapeutic approach to colonic sarcoidosis would usually involve surgery due to the lack of a definitive diagnosis by endoscopic biopsy or a concern for a neoplastic process. There are a few reports of responsiveness to corticosteroid therapy in gastrointestinal sarcoidosis and one with methotrexate [12]. There is no consensus with regard to the appropriate follow-up period of colonic sarcoidosis; however, the resolution of colonic masses with steroids in our case is reassuring and rules out the possibility of an alternative diagnosis.

4. Conclusion

Colonic involvement is an extremely rare initial presentation of sarcoidosis. Colonic sarcoidosis may present with colonic masses with peritoneal lesions and require a tissue diagnosis to rule out the alternative diagnosis of malignancy. Corticosteroids are a viable therapeutic option, and based on our current case report, surveillance is suggested to interval resolution.

References

[1] L. R. Schiller, D. S. Pardi, and J. H. Sellin, "Chronic diarrhea: diagnosis and management," *Clinical Gastroenterology and Hepatology*, vol. 15, no. 2, pp. 182–193, 2017.

[2] L. R. Schiller, "Diarrhea," *Medical Clinics of North America*, vol. 84, no. 5, pp. 1259–1274, 2000.

[3] J. Qu, X. Lü, Q. Gao, and Y. Zhang, "Good syndrome, a rare cause of refractory chronic diarrhea and recurrent pneumonia in a Chinese patient after thymectomy," *Clinical and Vaccine Immunology*, vol. 20, no. 7, pp. 1097-1098, 2013.

[4] S. Proksell, J. Chennat, and J. G. Hashash, "A rare cause of chronic diarrhea and weight loss," *Clinical Gastroenterology and Hepatology*, vol. 12, no. 8, pp. A21–A22, 2014.

[5] R. Gil Borrás, O. Juan Vidal, M. I. Talavera Encinas, and M. Bixquert Jiménez, "Diarrea crónica de causa infrecuente," *Gastroenterología Y Hepatología*, vol. 28, no. 3, pp. 110–113, 2005.

[6] B.-A. Adelstein, P. Macaskill, S. F. Chan, P. H. Katelaris, and L. Irwig, "Most bowel cancer symptoms do not indicate colorectal cancer and polyps: a systematic review," *BMC Gastroenterology*, vol. 11, no. 1, p. 65, 2011.

[7] Statement on Sarcoidosis, "Joint statement of the American thoracic society (ATS), the European respiratory society (ERS) and the world association of sarcoidosis and other granulomatous disorders (WASOG) adopted by the ATS board of

directors and by the ERS executive committee," *American Journal of Respiratory and Critical Care Medicine*, vol. 160, no. 2, pp. 736–755, 1999.

[8] K. L. MacArthur, F. Forouhar, and G. Y.-H. Wu, "Intra-abdominal complications of sarcoidosis," *Journal of the Formosan Medical Association*, vol. 109, no. 7, pp. 484–492, 2010.

[9] P. Brito-Zerón, K. Bari, R. P. Baughman, and M. Ramos-Casals, "Sarcoidosis involving the gastrointestinal tract," *The American Journal of Gastroenterology*, vol. 114, no. 8, pp. 1238–1247, 2019.

[10] E. C. Ebert, M. Kierson, and K. D. Hagspiel, "Gastrointestinal and hepatic manifestations of sarcoidosis," *The American Journal of Gastroenterology*, vol. 103, no. 12, pp. 3184–3192, 2008.

[11] K. W. Thomas and G. W. Hunninghake, "Sarcoidosis," *Jama*, vol. 289, no. 24, pp. 3300–3303, 2003.

[12] S. S. S. Hidenobu, P. Om, and A. Kamyar, "Colon sarcoidosis responds to methotrexate: a case report with review of literature," *Journal of Pulmonary & Respiratory Medicine*, vol. 3, 2013.

Nonfatal Hyperammonemic Encephalopathy as a Late Complication of Roux-en-Y Gastric Bypass

Juan D. Salcedo,[1] Jordan S. Goldstein,[1] Jose M. Quinonez,[2] and Maria Antonietta Mosetti[3]

[1] *Department of Internal Medicine, University of Miami Miller School of Medicine, Miami, FL, USA*
[2] *University of Miami Miller School of Medicine, Miami, FL, USA*
[3] *Division of Hospital Medicine, University of Miami Medical Towers, University of Miami Miller School of Medicine, Miami, FL, USA*

Correspondence should be addressed to Juan D. Salcedo; juan.salcedobetanco@jhsmiami.org

Academic Editor: Yoshihiro Moriwaki

Roux-en-Y gastric bypass (RYGB) is the most common weight loss procedure performed in the US. Gastric bypass–related hyperammonemia (GaBHA) is a potentially fatal entity, characterized by encephalopathy associated with hyperammonemia and various nutritional deficiencies, which can present at variable time intervals after RYGB. Twenty-five cases of hyperammonemic encephalopathy after bariatric surgery have been previously reported in the literature. We describe the case of a 48-year-old Hispanic woman with no prior history of liver disease, presenting with nonfatal hyperammonemic encephalopathy as a late postoperative complication 20 years after undergoing a RYGB. Hyperammonemic encephalopathy in the absence of known hepatic dysfunction presents a diagnostic dilemma. An early diagnosis and intervention are crucial to decrease morbidity and mortality.

1. Introduction

Roux-en-Y gastric bypass (RYGB) is the most common weight loss procedure performed in the US [1, 2]. It achieves successful and sustained weight loss in morbidly obese patients, through restrictive and malabsorptive mechanisms [3].

Although RYGB has lower morbidity and mortality rates compared to other bariatric procedures, there are numerous postoperative complications which may occur [4]. Early postoperative complications include gastrointestinal leaks, venous thromboembolic disease, pulmonary and cardiovascular complications, and tracheal reintubation [5]. The average 30-day mortality rate reported for RYGB is 0.2% [6]. Late postoperative complications include anastomotic stricture, bowel obstruction, fistula formation, intussusception, marginal ulcers, gallstone formation, dumping syndrome, hypoglycemia, malnutrition, fat malabsorption, and vitamin deficiencies [7].

Neurologic complications after bariatric surgery have a reported prevalence of 5% [8], including optic neuropathy, polyradiculoneuropathy, myelopathy, and encephalopathy. Of these, encephalopathy is a rare complication, usually occurring early, and generally attributed to thiamine deficiency [9]. Gastric bypass–related hyperammonemia (GaBHA) has been recently recognized as a life-threatening distinct entity, characterized by encephalopathy associated with hyperammonemia, elevated plasma glutamine, hypoalbuminemia, reactive hypoglycemia, low zinc, and other nutritional deficiencies. This condition has a high fatality rate reported around 50% and has a predilection for middle-aged women without prior liver disease who have achieved successful weight loss after RYGB [10]. It can occur at variable time intervals after RYGB, ranging from 1 month to 28 years after the surgery [11]. Hyperammonemic encephalopathy in the absence of known hepatic dysfunction presents a diagnostic dilemma. Therefore, an early diagnosis and intervention are crucial to prevent a rapid decline that may occur when the diagnosis is unrecognized.

2. Methods

We conducted a MEDLINE database query by combining the search terms "Hyperammonemia", "Encephalopathy", and "Bariatric surgery". The resultant seven articles

[10–16] were pulled from the literature. English language article titles and abstracts were screened and the appropriate articles reviewed. As far as we could determine in our search, twenty-five cases of hyperammonemic encephalopathy after bariatric surgery have been previously reported in the literature.

3. Case Presentation

A 48-year-old Hispanic female with a past medical history of multiple bariatric surgical procedures, presented with increasing lower extremity edema secondary to worsening chronic lymphedema.

During her hospitalization she developed altered mental status in the setting of elevated serum ammonia levels, despite having no history of liver disease.

Vertical banded gastroplasty was initially performed at age 28, but it failed to produce adequate weight loss. Consequently, three years later, she underwent open surgical revision which was converted to an open RYGB with concomitant cholecystectomy. She had lost over 100 kg since the first bariatric procedure (166 kg preoperatively to 63 kg on presentation). However, she developed multiple complications, including chronic lower extremity lymphedema, small bowel obstruction requiring multiple surgical interventions, malabsorption secondary to short bowel syndrome, multiple vitamin deficiencies, wet beriberi requiring chronic thiamine replacement, osteoporosis causing a left hip fracture, and chronic low back pain.

In July 2018, she initially presented to the emergency department with increasing lower extremity edema secondary to chronic lymphedema. On arrival, her vital signs were within normal limits. Her physical exam was remarkable for bilateral lower extremity pitting edema extending to the hips and an otherwise unremarkable exam. A chest x-ray disclosed no cardiomegaly, pulmonary congestion or pleural effusion. Her last echocardiogram showed an ejection fraction of 60% with no wall motion abnormalities.

During the admission, the patient received intravenous bumetanide with significant improvement. However, she developed waxing and waning episodes of confusion, and on day 3 of her hospitalization became overtly encephalopathic. She was disoriented to person, time, and space, with bizarre affect as well as incoherent speech, unable to recognize her close relatives. On physical exam patient was lethargic and had asterixis. According to her family members, the patient had previous episodes where she would become lethargic, but never to this degree.

Laboratory results were significant for an elevated plasma ammonia level of 173 μmol/L (normal range 11 - 50 μmol/L), despite downtrending transaminases (aspartate transaminase of 32 U/L and alanine transaminase of 55 U/L). Results were also significant for macrocytic anemia (hemoglobin 10.3 g/dL and mean corpuscular volume 107/5), a low serum albumin of 2.3 g/dL, low serum protein of 4.1 g/dL, alkaline phosphatase of 122 U/L, total bilirubin of 0.5 mg/dL, and an elevated international normalized ratio (INR) of 1.65. Serum glucose and zinc levels were borderline low at 62 and 54 (normal range 56 – 134 μg/dL), respectively. The laboratory findings are further outlined in Table 1. Additionally, her plasma salicylate level, acetaminophen level, and urine toxicology were all negative. Despite a history of vitamin deficiencies, she was receiving chronic thiamine and vitamin B12 replacement at home, with normal values on admission. Noncontrast computed tomography (CT) imaging of the head disclosed no evidence of acute infarction, intracranial hemorrhage, or mass effect. The patient had no history of prior liver conditions or cirrhosis, and even though she presented elevation of transaminases and the INR, these abnormalities resolved once her condition improved. The patient had no other laboratory findings for compatible signs of cirrhosis (no thrombocytopenia or hyperbilirubinemia), neither physical stigmata suggestive of acute or chronic liver disease. Abdominal ultrasound was performed to further elucidate liver panel abnormalities and demonstrated only mild hepatic steatosis with no evidence of cirrhosis or ascites.

She was treated with supportive care and lactulose. The following day she had numerous bowel movements, and her serum ammonia level came down to 24 μmol/L. Given the fast clinical improvement and resolution of laboratory abnormalities after supportive treatment, a liver biopsy was not indicated. Once her clinical condition improved and her mental status returned to normal, the patient was discharged from the hospital.

4. Discussion

Ammonia is extremely toxic to the central nervous system [17]. It is a bi-product of protein catabolism from amino acid deamination (whether from a high-protein diet, prolonged starvation, or naturally produced by gut flora) [18]. The urea cycle catabolizes toxic ammonia into urea, a process that occurs predominantly in the liver. Urea is nontoxic and is ultimately excreted by the kidneys [18].

In the urea cycle (Figure 1), ammonia is the source of the first amino group, required in the synthesis of carbamoyl phosphate, which happens in the hepatocyte mitochondria. The second amino group comes from glutamate in the formation of aspartate, which happens in the hepatocyte cytoplasm. This reaction produces α-ketoglutarate, which then becomes available for the Krebs cycle [18]. In the muscle and peripheral tissues (including the brain astrocytes), glutamate accepts free ammonia produced by amino acid catabolism. Glutamine transports ammonia from the peripheral tissues to the liver, where glutamine is broken back to glutamate and ammonia via glutaminase [19, 20]. An increase in free blood ammonia has shown to accumulate glutamine within the astrocytes, which has osmotic effects and causes astrocyte swelling and cerebral edema [21]. The normal rate of urea cycle far exceeds the ammonia production rate by protein catabolism. Therefore, slight elevations in the serum free ammonia concentration (>60 μmol/L) reflect an impairment in the urea cycle, independent of the etiology [19]. This impairment may cause a wide range of neurologic manifestations including asterixis, changes in behavior, slurred speech,

TABLE 1: Laboratory findings during admission.

Laboratory	Day of Admission	Day 3	Day 4 (discharge)	Normal range
Ammonia (μmol/L)	NA	173	24	11 - 50 μmol/L
Hemoglobin (g/dL)	10.3	10.5	10.5	11.1 - 14.6 g/dL
Mean Corpuscular Volume	107.5	106.5	107.9	79.9 - 95.0 fL
Platelets (103/uL)	152	179	341	140 – 400 103/uL
White Blood Cells (103/uL)	7.0	7.5	5.3	4.0 - 10.5 103/uL
Glucose (mg/dl)	81	62	85	65 - 99 mg/dL
Zinc (μg/dL)	54	NA	NA	56-134 μg/dL
Vitamin B1 (nmol/L)	191.9	ND	ND	66.5-200.5 (nmol/L)
Vitamin B12 (pg/mL)	>2,000	ND	ND	232 - 1,245 (pg/mL)
Sodium (mmol/L9	142	145	147	135 - 146 mmol/L
Potassium (mmol/L)	4.1	3.9	3.9	3.5 - 5.5 mmol/L
Chloride (mmol/L)	108	106	108	98 - 110 mmol/L
CO2 (mmol/L)	21	28	25	19 - 34 mmol/L
Anion Gap	13	11	14	6 to 22
Blood Urea Nitrogen (mg/dL)	20	25	30	6 - 20 mg/dL
Osmolality mOsm/Kg	285	291	298	275 - 295 mOsm/kg
Creatinine (mg/dL)	1.09	0.77	0.58	0.40 - 1.10 mg/dL
Calcium, Serum (mg/dL)	7.8	7.8	7.8	8.6 - 10.3 mg/dL
Protein, Total (g/dL)	4.3	4.1	3.9	6.1 - 8.1 g/dL
Albumin (g/dL)	2.6	2.3	1.7	3.5 - 5.2 g/dL
Bilirubin, Total (mg/dL)	0.3	0.5	0.5	0.0 - 1.2 mg/dL
AST (SGOT) (U/L)	66	32	31	10 - 40 U/L
ALT (SGPT) (U/L)	70	55	50	0 - 33 U/L
Alkaline Phosphatase (U/L)	115	122	102	35 - 105 U/L
Magnesium (mg/dL)	1.7	1.6	1.8	1.6 - 2.6 mg/dL
Prothrombin time (sec)	20	NA	NA	12.0 - 14.5 sec
International Normalized Ratio	1.65	NA	1.1	NA
activated partial thromboplastin time (sec)	26.1	NA	NA	23.7 - 35.3 sec

ALT, alanine aminotransferase; AST, aspartate aminotransferase; NA, not available.

sleep disorders, lethargy, stupor, coma, cerebral edema, and even death [18].

Several mechanisms have been proposed in the developing of GaBHA, which seems to be multifactorial [10]. This syndrome occurs almost exclusively in women, and previous reports have found functional ornithine transcarbamylase (OTC) deficiency given a low enzymatic activity [11, 15], even in the presence of normal OTC sequencing genetic testing [11, 15]. Others have reported cases of GaBHA with late-onset carbamoyl phosphate synthase 1 (CPS1) deficiency [15]. Nutritional deficits may lead to functional inhibition of urea cycle enzymes, producing accumulation of ammonia [13]. Low arginine levels inhibit the urea cycle [22] as well as low zinc concentrations, possibly by interfering with the OTC function [23]. Therefore, in adult patients who develop GaBHA, OTC deficiency and other urea cycle abnormalities should be strongly considered. RYGB has been associated with hyperinsulinemia and reactive hypoglycemia, which may contribute to the catabolic state and ammonia excess [24]. Also, the gastric-small bowel pouch in RYGB may cause overgrowth of intestinal flora favoring the production of ammonia by urease-producing bacteria [11].

In general, conservative management of hyperammonemic encephalopathy has been traditionally supportive with prevention of seizures and cerebral edema and lactulose and rifaximin [13], achieving reductions in plasma ammonia levels. Other proposed therapies for GaBHA patients have been the repletion of deficient amino acids, zinc, micro nutrients, and intravenous glucose infusion, attempting to improve the catabolic state [10].

5. Conclusion

We present the case of a middle-aged woman without prior liver disease, who developed nonfatal hyperammonemic encephalopathy as a late postoperative complication 20 years after RYGB procedure. GaBHA is an underrecognized potentially fatal syndrome, for which early active treatment may be life-saving. It is thought to be associated with hypoalbuminemia, hypoglycemia, and low zinc plasma levels,

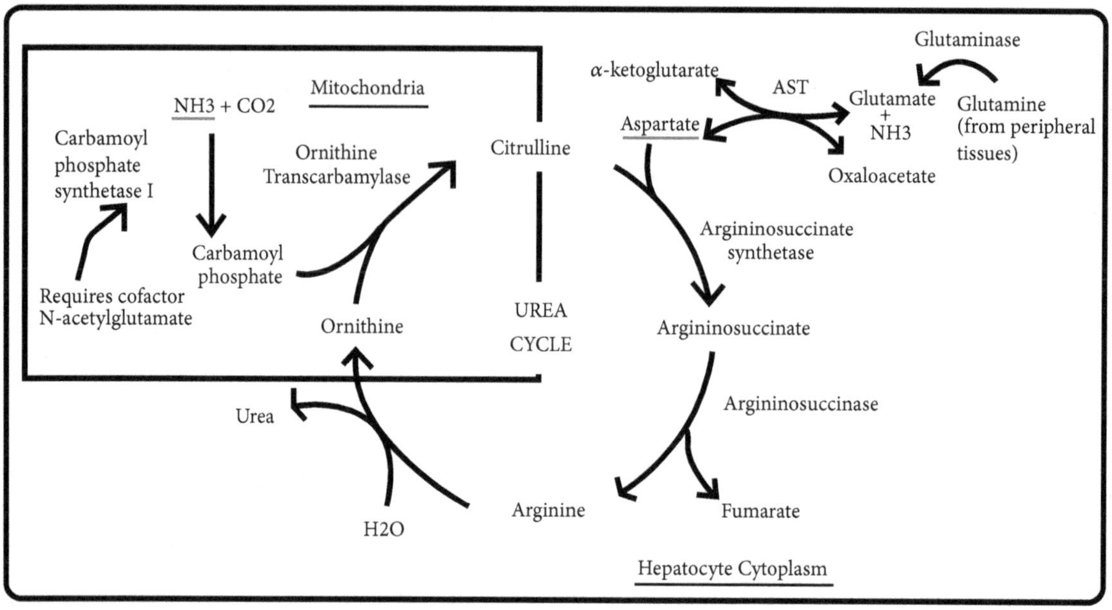

FIGURE 1: Urea cycle. Ammonia is the source of the first amino group in the urea cycle, required in the synthesis of carbamoyl phosphate (CPS), which happens in the hepatocyte mitochondria. The second amino group comes from glutamate in the formation of aspartate, which happens in the hepatocyte cytoplasm. This reaction produces α-ketoglutarate, which then becomes available for the Krebs cycle. The synthesis of argininosuccinate links the Krebs cycle and urea cycle. In the peripheral tissues, glutamate accepts free ammonia from amino acid catabolism. Glutamine transports ammonia from the peripheral tissues to the liver, where glutamine is broken back to glutamate and ammonia via glutaminase. AST, aspartate transaminase.

indicating severe nutritional deficiency. In high-risk patients, a rigorous screening for plasma ammonia, zinc, and serum albumin may facilitate an early diagnosis and treatment of this entity.

Authors' Contributions

Author contributions: J.Salcedo and J. Goldstein wrote and edited the manuscript. J. Salcedo and J. Quinonez collected the patient's clinical data. M. Mosetti is the article guarantor.

References

[1] I. Samuel, E. E. Mason, K. E. Renquist, Y. Huang, M. B. Zimmerman, and M. Jamal, "Bariatric surgery trends: an 18-year report from the International Bariatric Surgery Registry," *The American Journal of Surgery*, vol. 192, no. 5, pp. 657–662, 2006.

[2] N. T. Nguyen, J. Root, K. Zainabadi et al., "Accelerated growth of bariatric surgery with the introduction of minimally invasive surgery," *Archives of Surgery*, vol. 140, no. 12, pp. 1198–1202, 2005.

[3] H. Buchwald, Y. Avidor, E. Braunwald et al., "Bariatric surgery: a systematic review and meta-analysis," *The Journal of the American Medical Association*, vol. 292, no. 14, pp. 1724–1737, 2004.

[4] H. Buchwald and J. N. Buchwald, "Evolution of operative procedures for the management of morbid obesity 1950–2000," *Obesity Surgery*, vol. 12, no. 5, pp. 705–717, 2002.

[5] D. R. Flum, S. H. Belle, and W. C. King, "Perioperative safety in the longitudinal assessment of bariatric surgery," *The New England Journal of Medicine*, vol. 361, no. 5, pp. 445–454, 2009.

[6] M. A. Maggard, L. R. Shugarman, M. Suttorp et al., "Meta-analysis: surgical treatment of obesity," *Annals of Internal Medicine*, vol. 142, no. 7, pp. 547–559, 2005.

[7] K. Seeras and P. P. Lopez, "Roux-en-Y Gastric Bypass, Chronic Complications," in *Treasure Island (FL)*, StatPearls Publishing, 2018, https://www.ncbi.nlm.nih.gov/books/NBK519489/.

[8] B. M. Koffman, L. J. Greenfield, I. I. Ali, and N. A. Pirzada, "Neurologic complications after surgery for obesity," *Muscle & Nerve*, vol. 33, no. 2, pp. 166–176, 2006.

[9] K. Juhasz-Pocsine, S. A. Rudnicki, R. L. Archer, and S. I. Harik, "Neurologic complications of gastric bypass surgery for morbid obesity," *Neurology*, vol. 68, no. 21, pp. 1843–1850, 2007.

[10] A. Nagarur and A. Z. Fenves, "Late presentation of fatal hyperammonemic encephalopathy after roux-En-Y gastric bypass," *Baylor University Medical Center Proceedings*, vol. 30, no. 1, pp. 41–43, 2017.

[11] A. Z. Fenves, O. A. Shchelochkov, and A. Mehta, "Hyperammonemic syndrome after Roux-en-Y gastric bypass," *Obesity*, vol. 23, no. 4, pp. 746–749, 2015.

[12] A. Fenves, C. R. Boland, R. Lepe, P. Rivera-Torres, and S. J. Spechler, "Fatal hyperammonemic encephalopathy after gastric bypass surgery," *American Journal of Medicine*, vol. 121, no. 1, pp. el–e2, 2008.

[13] J. Estrella, G. Yee, B. Wilcken, M. Tchan, and M. Talbot, "Hyperammonemic encephalopathy complicating bariatric surgery: a case study and review of the literature," *Surgery for Obesity and Related Diseases*, vol. 10, no. 3, pp. e35–e38, 2014.

[14] M. L. Kromas, O. Y. Mousa, and S. John, "Hyperammonemia-induced encephalopathy: A rare devastating complication of bariatric surgery," *World Journal of Hepatology*, vol. 7, no. 7, p. 1007, 2015.

[15] W. T. Hu, O. H. Kantarci, J. L. Merritt II et al., "Ornithine transcarbamylase deficiency presenting as encephalopathy during

adulthood following bariatric surgery," *JAMA Neurology*, vol. 64, no. 1, pp. 126–128, 2007.

[16] K. L. Borreggine, D. K. Hosker, T. A. Rummans, and D. M. Manning, "Psychiatric manifestations of hyperammonemic encephalopathy following roux-en-y gastric bypass," *Psychosomatics*, vol. 59, no. 1, pp. 90–94, 2018.

[17] W. L. Stone and G. B. Jaishankar, "Urea cycle disorders," in *StatPearls*, StatPearls Publishing, 2018, https://www.ncbi.nlm.nih.gov/books/NBK482363/.

[18] W. Barmore and W. L. Stone, "Physiology, urea cycle," in *StatPearls*, Treasure Island (FL): StatPearls Publishing, 2018, https://www.ncbi.nlm.nih.gov/books/NBK513323/.

[19] R. M. Cohn and K. S. Roth, "Hyperammonemia, bane of the brain," *Clinical Pediatrics*, vol. 43, no. 8, pp. 683–689, 2004.

[20] D. Xiao, L. Zeng, K. Yao, X. Kong, G. Wu, and Y. Yin, "The glutamine-alpha-ketoglutarate (AKG) metabolism and its nutritional implications," *Amino Acids*, vol. 48, no. 9, pp. 2067–2080, 2016.

[21] S. W. Brusilow, "Hyperammonemic encephalopathy," *Medicine*, vol. 81, no. 3, pp. 240–249, 2002.

[22] C. Bachmann, "Mechanisms of hyperammonemia," *Clinical Chemistry and Laboratory Medicine*, vol. 40, no. 7, 2002.

[23] E. Aquilio, R. Spagnoli, D. Riggio, and S. Seri, "Effects of zinc on hepatic ornithine transcarbamylase (OTC) activity," *Journal of Trace Elements and Electrolytes in Health and Disease*, vol. 7, no. 4, pp. 240-241, 1993.

[24] Z. Li, M. L. Yarmush, and C. Chan, "Insulin concentration during preconditioning mediates the regulation of urea synthesis during exposure to amino acid-supplemented plasma," *Tissue Engineering Part A*, vol. 10, no. 11-12, pp. 1737–1746, 2004.

47

Octreotide Use in a Patient with MEN-1 Syndrome and Multifocal Pancreatic Neuroendocrine Tumors: A Case Report and Review of the Literature

Matthew H. Kemm, Cory D. Manly, Thanh D. Hoang, Vinh Q. Mai, and Mohamed K. M. Shakir

Division of Endocrinology, Department of Medicine, Walter Reed National Military Medical Center, Bethesda, USA

Correspondence should be addressed to Thanh D. Hoang; tdhdthanh@gmail.com

Academic Editor: Yoshifumi Nakayama

We report a patient with multiple endocrine neoplasia type 1 with pancreatic polypeptide (PP) secreting subcentimeter pancreatic neuroendocrine tumors (pNETs) treated with octreotide and review the current literature that pertains to the management of these patients. Clinical data, laboratory results, and imaging were reviewed. A literature search was performed in PUBMED using combinations of the terms "multiple endocrine neoplasia type 1," "somatostatin," octreotide," "pancreatic polypeptide," and "pancreatic tumor." Relevant references were selected and reviewed. A 43-year-old male with a history of MEN1 and multiple subcentimeter neuroendocrine tumors with elevation of PP was treated with octreotide therapy leading to a reduction and normalization of PP levels. The patient tolerated octreotide therapy but self-discontinued octreotide after 24 months with a rise in PP levels off therapy. Tumors remained stable in size through 40 months of imaging follow-up. In patients with MEN1 and subcentimeter pNETs, octreotide therapy is well tolerated and can lead to a significant drop in PP levels with no change in lesion size. There is insufficient data to suggest long-term benefit with octreotide therapy but it may be considered versus standard conservative management.

1. Introduction

Multiple endocrine neoplasia type 1 (MEN1) is a rare, autosomal dominant syndrome causing a predisposition to tumors of the parathyroid glands, anterior pituitary, and enteropancreatic endocrine cells with an estimated prevalence of 2 to 20 per 100,000 individuals [1]. The malignant potential of pancreatic neuroendocrine tumors (pNETs) is now the primary life-threatening manifestation of MEN1 [2]. Functioning enteropancreatic endocrine tumors such as gastrinomas, insulinomas, or the rarely seen VIPomas or glucagonomas may be readily diagnosed based on clinical symptomatology alone [1]. However, nonfunctional tumors may constitute the bulk of these enteropancreatic tumors with studies suggesting a prevalence of 30-80% and with current screening protocols being likely discovered very early in the disease process [3, 4]. These asymptomatic, enteropancreatic tumors may be malignant and capable of causing liver metastases with evidence to suggest a worsened prognosis compared to functional tumors.

Current recommendations for screening for enteropancreatic neuroendocrine tumors include both biochemical evaluation and radiological screening [1]. Cost effective imaging may include magnetic resonance imaging (MRI), computed tomography (CT), or endoscopic ultrasound. It is recommended that annual biochemical evaluation includes measurement of serum gastrin, glucagon, vasoactive intestinal polypeptide, pancreatic polypeptide, chromogranin A, and insulin levels in addition to a fasting blood glucose. There are few studies evaluating the utility of these peptides in the setting of MEN1 patients. Pancreatic polypeptide (PP), a 36-amino-acid peptide produced and secreted by PP cells of the pancreas, has been shown to have a low sensitivity and specificity for pNETs in patients with MEN1, with one study reporting 36% sensitivity and 74% specificity [5–7]. However, a separate study found that, in MEN1 patients with elevated

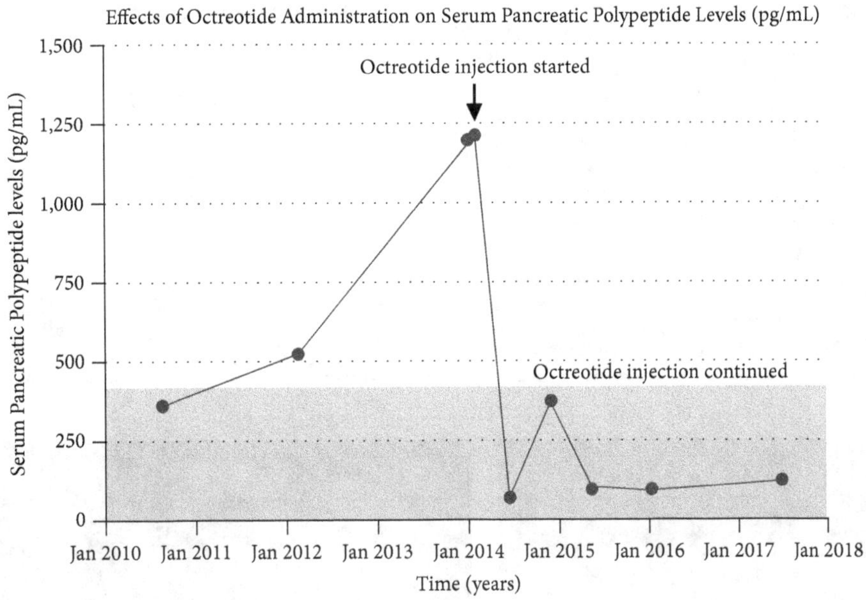

FIGURE 1: Showing serum pancreatic polypeptide (PP) levels (pg/mL) over time. Octreotide treatment was initiated in February 2014. Since initiation of octreotide treatment, the PP levels remain stable. Reference range PP (0.0-418.0 pg/mL).

PP, a level 3.0 times the normal age-specific value was 95% sensitive and 88% specific for an imageable islet cell tumor [7].

The management of pNETs is variable due to the heterogeneity of the disease. The role of surgery for nonfunctional pancreatic tumors (NFPETs) in MEN1 is controversial with the endocrine society clinical practice guideline suggesting surgery for tumors greater than 1 cm and/or demonstrating significant growth over 6-12 months [1]. For nonresectable tumors, treatment includes somatostatin analogs (SSA), targeted radionucleotide therapy, locoregional treatments, and chemotherapy. Treatment of small pancreatic tumors in asymptomatic individuals has yet to be fully delineated in the guidelines due to lack of long-term data comparing treatment options. Observational data suggest a low potential for metastasis and no increased mortality in NFPETs under 2 cm [8]. Additionally, pNETs under 2 cm appear to grow slowly and those under 1 cm may grow even slower whereas surgical resection at any tumor size can carry substantial risks [9, 10].

Here we describe a middle-aged patient with a history of MEN1 who presented with a markedly elevated serum PP level, leading to the discovery of multiple subcentimeter pancreatic lesions found on screening CT, and with prolonged stability on SSA medical therapy.

2. Case Presentation

A 43-year-old male reported to endocrine clinic for evaluation of pancreatic lesions. His past history was relevant for total parathyroidectomy for parathyroid hyperplasia, with forearm autograph implantation at the age of 16 years. The patient has a strong family history of pancreatic and parathyroid disorders in his paternal grandfather, two paternal aunts, a paternal uncle, his father, and sister. Additionally, menin gene mutation was confirmed in his father and paternal uncle. The patient underwent a genetic testing at the age of 40 years and this confirmed menin gene mutation. Patient had no symptoms to suggest hypoglycemia, peptic ulcer disease, diarrhea, or other symptoms of endocrine disorders. Review of systems was unremarkable. On physical examination, the vital signs were normal and examination of the heart, lungs, and abdomen was also normal. He has no clinical features of hypogonadism or Cushing syndrome. The patient is married without children and does not smoke or drink alcohol. Additional blood test showed normal serum calcium, testosterone levels, FSH, LH, prolactin, and IGF-I. Additionally evaluation for Cushing syndrome was also negative. Serum gastrin, chromogranin A, vasoactive intestinal polypeptide levels, and 24-hour urine 5-HIAA levels were also normal, and a 48-hour fast did not confirm hypoglycemia. However, fasting serum pancreatic polypeptide level was elevated (520 pg/mL, reference 0-418). A CT scan of the abdomen showed multiple subcentimeter lesions. The patient refused any treatment initially; 11 months later the serum pancreatic polypeptide levels rose to 1198 pg/mL (range 912-1588), and 5 weeks later the value was 1215 pg/mL (Figure 1). At this time a repeat CT scan showed 3 hyperenhancing lesions in the head and tail of the pancreas measuring 10, 9, and 4 mm (Figure 2). These lesions correlated with 111–Indium Octreotide scan (Figure 3). Since the patient refused any surgical treatment, he was offered octreotide treatment. Initially the patient was treated with the short-acting octreotide 100 μg 3 times daily, and this was later transitioned to a long-acting octreotide 20 mg monthly. Following the octreotide treatment, the serum pancreatic polypeptide levels normalized to 62 pg/mL in approximately 6 weeks (Figure 1). A follow-up CT scan at 9 and 33 months later confirmed stability of the pancreatic lesions without evidence of metastasis. Additionally, the

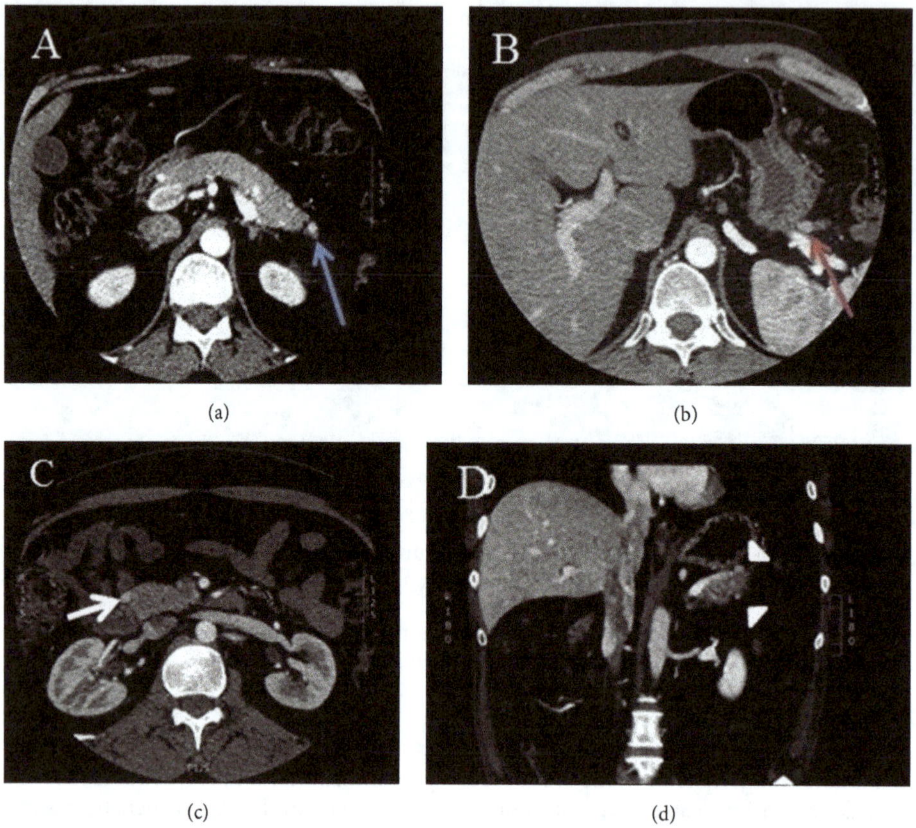

FIGURE 2: CT of the pancreas showing three hyperenhancing lesions. (a) 4 mm lesion in the inferior aspect of the pancreatic tail (blue arrow). (b) 9 mm lesion in the superior aspect of the pancreatic tail (red arrow). (c) 10 mm lesion in the pancreatic head (white arrow). (d) Coronal view revealing both pancreatic tail lesions (arrow heads).

serum pancreatic polypeptide levels remained within normal limits (91.6 pg/mL) (Figure 1). The patient continued to feel well and has tolerated octreotide without any adverse effects over the entire period of treatment. A most recent gallium-68 DOTATATE PET/CT scan (Figure 4) performed 3 years later, while the patient was on octreotide therapy, further confirmed the stability of the pancreatic lesions. Additionally, serum pancreatic polypeptide remained normal along with normal levels of somatostatin, glucagon, gastrin, vasoactive intestinal polypeptide, and chromogranin A during the entire course of octreotide treatment.

3. Discussion

Use of somatostatin analogs in the treatment of pNETs is based on investigations showing that the natural 14-amino-acid peptide binds to G-protein-coupled somatostatin receptors (SSTRs) that are expressed on most NETs with SSTR-2 expressed in approximately 80% of pNETs [11, 12]. Octreotide and lanreotide bind with a high affinity to SSTR-2 [13, 14]. Binding to these receptors can lead to antisecretory and antiproliferative effects. It has been shown that significant improvement in patients with gastrinoma, VIPoma, and glucagonoma can occur following somatostatin analog treatment [15]. In the phase III CLARINET trial of 204 patients, lanreotide 120 mg, in patients with advanced, well or moderately differentiated nonfunctional GI and pancreatic NETs with SSTR avid disease, leading to significantly prolonged median progression-free survival (>24 mo.) vs. placebo (18 mo.) [16]. Given the relative good safety profile of somatostatin analog therapy, the results of the CLARINET trial significantly question the utility of observation in patients with locally, advanced, unresectable, or metastatic NETs and support the inclusion of SSA treatment in early stage NET management. National Comprehensive Cancer Network (NCCN) guidelines now state that treatment can be considered for these patients with sporadic NFPETs [17]. Whether this would be the case in an NFPET in MEN1 is unknown. Results from the Dutch MEN1 and the French Endocrine Tumor study groups have recently shown that surgical treatment of NFPET nodules <2cm versus observation resulted in no significant increase in survival over time but did cause a significant number of postoperative complications [8, 18]. If surgery is no longer a reasonable treatment option for this group of patients and observation is not a reasonable option for a patient, SSA therapy may be an appropriate alternative. The currently available data suggest that there may be a benefit in these small, <2 cm, nonfunctional nodules. In a single study in twenty MEN1 patients on SSA therapy over 12-75 months of follow-up with tumors <2 cm, stable disease was found in 80% of patients, tumor shrinkage in 10%, and hormonal suppression

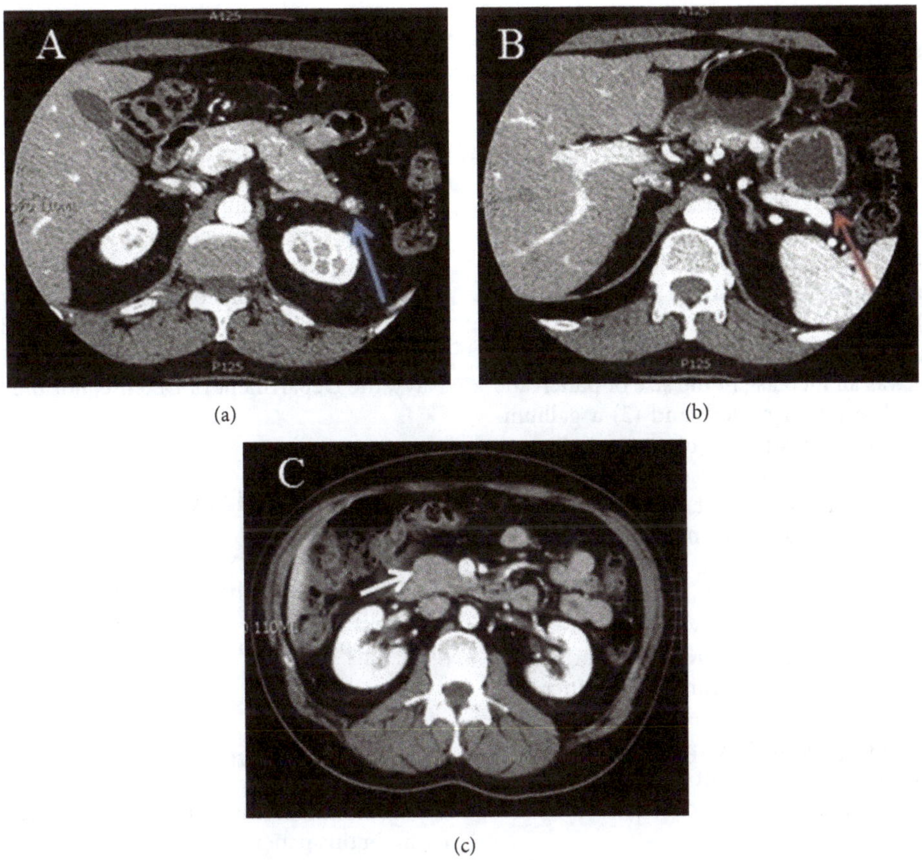

FIGURE 3: CT of the pancreas showing three hyperenhancing lesions which have remained stable 38 months after initiating octreotide. (a) Stable 4 mm tumor in the inferior aspect of the pancreatic tail (blue arrow). (b) Stable lesion in the superior aspect of the pancreatic tail (red arrow). (c) Stable lesion in the pancreatic head.

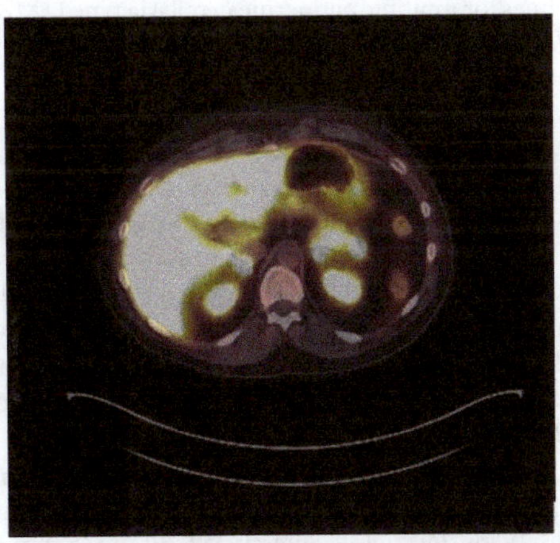

FIGURE 4: Gallium-68 DOTATATE PET/CT scan showing stability of the pancreatic tumors over time.

in all 6 patients with elevated CgA or gastrin levels [19]. Cioppi et al. (LARO-MEN1 study) investigated whether early treatment with long-acting somatostatin analog could act as a preventive approach in relatively small MEN1-related gastroenteropancreatic neuroendocrine tumors. In 8 patients with small (<2 cm) neuroendocrine tumors and abnormal laboratory values of at least one of the gastroenteropancreatic hormones, administration of octreotide acetate slow-release formulation (LAR) (10 mg intramuscularly every 28 days) was effective in decreasing gastroenteropancreatic hormone levels and stabilizing tumor size. Furthermore the treatment was safe in the majority of patients up to six years of treatment [20]. Additional data in this select population is likely many years away but a phase 3 trial in Europe comparing SSA therapy vs. no treatment in MEN1 patients with NFPET will be opening soon for enrollment [21].

Additionally, there is insufficient evidence to clarify whether a decline in PP level correlates with a reduction in tumor burden. We would argue that the significant decline in PP level, a nonspecific tumor marker, in addition to the lack of tumor growth and stable follow-up PP level is indicative of a treatment effect as has been seen with other hormonally active NETs treated with SSA therapy. We speculate that if the level of PP continues to rise off therapy, the patient would experience further nodular growth, which could have adverse health consequences. Typical management of sub-centimeter NFPETs has typically involved serial imaging and biochemical testing. SSA therapy in addition to serial testing represents a reasonable treatment option that is well tolerated in this patient population although its high-cost may hinder its utilization.

Furthermore, basal and meal-stimulated pancreatic polypeptide has been shown to be useful for early detection of pancreatic involvement in 75% of patients with MEN-1. Our patient's basal fasting pancreatic polypeptide levels were not only elevated but actually doubled at one-year follow-up. The stability of the pancreatic tumors along with the normalization of serum PP level confirms the effectiveness of SSA therapy in this patient. It may be stated that the pancreatic lesions would have remained stable without octreotide treatment; however, octreotide was effective in our patient for several reasons: (1) the serum PP level doubled over the 11-month observation period when he did not receive octreotide treatment; (2) there was an increase in the size of pancreatic tumors during this observation period; and (3) a gallium-68 DOTATATE scan showed stability of tumor size over the course of treatment. Therefore, these findings support the effectiveness of octreotide treatment. As the benefits of pancreatic surgery for small lesions (<2cm) are not clear, the morbidity, mortality, and long-term complications of surgery must be considered. Our patient was thus offered medical therapy with long-acting octreotide, which was recently shown to provide 90% objective tumor response and stability in MEN-1 patients with early nonfunctional pancreatic NET [19]. Discontinuation of octreotide and reassessment of serum pancreatic polypeptide level and tumor growth would have confirmed the effectiveness of octreotide therapy; however, we felt it may be unethical to discontinue octreotide therapy.

4. Conclusion

The malignant potential of pNETs is the primary life-threatening manifestation of MEN1 but treatment for NFPET <1 cm has not been clearly defined by the guidelines. We describe the case of a middle-aged patient with a history of MEN1 who presented with elevated serum PP levels and multiple subcentimeter pancreatic lesions found on imaging who was treated with SSA therapy for 24 months leading to a marked reduction in PP level during treatment with stability in lesion size after 40 months of follow-up. SSA therapy represents a reasonable and potential alternative to watchful waiting in this patient population but further research is necessary to better define long-term outcomes.

Abbreviations

CgA:	Chromogranin A
CT:	Computed tomography
MEN1:	Multiple endocrine neoplasia type 1
NFPET:	Nonfunctional pancreatic tumor
pNET:	Pancreatic neuroendocrine tumor
PP:	Pancreatic polypeptide
VIP:	Vasoactive intestinal peptide
PET:	Positron emission tomography.

Disclosure

We certify that the document represents valid work; that if we used information derived from another source, we obtained all necessary approvals to use it and made appropriate acknowledgments in the document; and that each author takes public responsibility for it. The authors are employees of the United States Government. This work was prepared as part of their official duties. Title 17 U.S.C. §105 provides that 'Copyright protection under this title is not available for any work of the United States Government.' Title 17 U.S.C. §101 defines a U.S. Government work as a work prepared by a military service member or employee of the U.S. Government as part of that person's official duties. The views expressed in this article are those of the authors and do not necessarily reflect the official policy or position of the Department of the Navy, the Department of Defense, nor the U.S. Government.

Authors' Contributions

All individuals who qualify as authors have been listed; each has participated in the conception and design of this work, the analysis of data, the writing of the document, and the approval of the submission of this version.

Acknowledgments

We would like to thank Mr. Jay McDaniel for preparing the figure in this paper.

References

[1] R. V. Thakker, P. J. Newey, G. V. Walls et al., "Clinical practice guidelines for multiple endocrine neoplasia type 1 (MEN1)," *The Journal of Clinical Endocrinology & Metabolism*, vol. 97, no. 9, pp. 2990–3011, 2012.

[2] T. Ito, H. Igarashi, H. Uehara, M. J. Berna, and R. T. Jensen, "Causes of death and prognostic factors in multiple endocrine neoplasia type 1: A prospective study:Comparison of 106 MEN1/zollinger-ellison syndrome patients with 1613 literature men1 patients with or without pancreatic endocrine tumors," *Medicine (United States)*, vol. 92, no. 3, pp. 135–181, 2013.

[3] F. Triponez, D. Dosseh, P. Goudet et al., "Epidemiology data on 108 MEN 1 patients from the GTE with isolated nonfunctioning tumors of the pancreas," *Annals of Surgery*, vol. 243, no. 2, pp. 265–272, 2006.

[4] M. A. Kouvaraki, S. E. Shapiro, G. J. Cote et al., "Management of pancreatic endocrine tumors in multiple endocrine neoplasia type 1," *World Journal of Surgery*, vol. 30, no. 5, pp. 643–653, 2006.

[5] W. Qiu, I. Christakis, A. Silva et al., "Utility of chromogranin A, pancreatic polypeptide, glucagon and gastrin in the diagnosis and follow-up of pancreatic neuroendocrine tumours in multiple endocrine neoplasia type 1 patients," *Clinical Endocrinology*, vol. 85, no. 3, pp. 400–407, 2016.

[6] J. M. de Laat, C. R. Pieterman, M. Weijmans et al., "Low accuracy of tumor markers for diagnosing pancreatic neuroendocrine tumors in multiple endocrine neoplasia type 1 patients," *The Journal of Clinical Endocrinology & Metabolism*, vol. 98, no. 10, pp. 4143–4151, 2013.

[7] M. G. Mutch, M. M. Frisella, M. K. DeBenedetti et al., "Pancreatic polypeptide is a useful plasma marker for radiographically evident pancreatic islet cell tumors in patients with multiple endocrine neoplasia type 1," *Surgery*, vol. 122, no. 6, pp. 1012–1020, 1997.

[8] F. Triponez, S. M. Sadowski, F. Pattou et al., "Long-term Follow-up of MEN1 patients who do not have initial surgery for small ≤2 cm nonfunctioning pancreatic neuroendocrine tumors, an AFCE and GTE study: Association Francophone de Chirurgie Endocrinienne & Groupe d'Etude des Tumeurs Endocrines," *Annals of Surgery*, vol. 268, pp. 158–164, 2018.

[9] W. F. W. Kappelle, G. D. Valk, M. Leenders et al., "Growth rate of small pancreatic neuroendocrine tumors in multiple endocrine neoplasia type 1: Results from an endoscopic ultrasound based cohort study," *Endoscopy*, vol. 49, no. 1, pp. 27–34, 2017.

[10] Y. N. You, G. B. Thompson, W. F. Young Jr. et al., "Pancreatoduodenal surgery in patients with multiple endocrine neoplasia type 1: Operative outcomes, long-term function, and quality of life," *Surgery*, vol. 142, no. 6, pp. 829–836, 2007.

[11] M. Papotti, M. Bongiovanni, M. Volante et al., "Expression of somatostatin receptor types 1-5 in 81 cases of gastrointestinal and pancreatic endocrine tumors. A correlative immunohistochemical and reverse transcriptase polymerase chain reaction analysis," *Virchows Archiv*, vol. 440, no. 5, pp. 461–475, 2002.

[12] J. C. Reubi, B. Waser, J.-C. Schaer, and J. A. Laissue, "Somatostatin receptor sst1–sst5 expression in normal and neoplastic human tissues using receptor autoradiography with subtype-selective ligands," *European Journal of Nuclear Medicine and Molecular Imaging*, vol. 28, no. 7, pp. 836–846, 2001.

[13] W. Bauer, U. Briner, W. Doepfner et al., "SMS 201-995: a very potent and selective octapeptide analog of somatostatin with prolonged action," *Life Sciences*, vol. 31, no. 11, pp. 1133–1140, 1982.

[14] H. Shojamanesh, F. Gibril, A. Louie et al., "Prospective study of the antitumor efficacy of long-term octreotide treatment in patients with progressive metastatic gastrinoma," *Cancer*, vol. 94, no. 2, pp. 331–343, 2002.

[15] R. Eldor, B. Glaser, M. Fraenkel, V. Doviner, A. Salmon, and D. J. Gross, "Glucagonoma and the glucagonoma syndrome - Cumulative experience with an elusive endocrine tumour," *Clinical Endocrinology*, vol. 74, no. 5, pp. 593–598, 2011.

[16] M. E. Caplin, M. Pavel, J. B. Ćwikła et al., "Lanreotide in metastatic enteropancreatic neuroendocrine tumors," *The New England Journal of Medicine*, vol. 371, no. 3, pp. 224–233, 2014.

[17] M. H. Kulke, M. H. Shah, A. B. Benson 3rd et al., "Neuroendocrine tumors," *Journal of the National Comprehensive Cancer Network*, vol. 13, pp. 78–108, 2015.

[18] S. Nell, H. M. Verkooijen, C. R. C. Pieterman et al., "Management of MEN1 related nonfunctioning pancreatic NETs: A shifting paradigm: results from the DutchMEN1 study group," *Annals of Surgery*, vol. 267, no. 6, pp. 1155–1160, 2018.

[19] V. Ramundo, M. Del Prete, V. Marotta et al., "Impact of long-acting octreotide in patients with early-stage MEN1-related duodeno-pancreatic neuroendocrine tumors," *Clinical Endocrinology*, vol. 80, no. 6, pp. 850–855, 2014.

[20] F. Cioppi, L. Cianferotti, L. Masi et al., "The LARO-MEN1 study: a longitudinal clinical experience with octreotide Long-Acting Release in patients with Multiple Endocrine Neoplasia type 1 Syndrome," *Clinical Cases in Mineral and Bone Metabolism*, vol. 14, no. 2, pp. 123–130, 2017.

[21] A. Selberherr, *Non-functioning pancreatic neuroendocrine tumors in MEN1: somatostatin analogs versus no treatment (SANO)*, 2018, https://clinicaltrials.gov/ct2/show/NCT02705651?cond=Non-functioning+Pancreatic+Neuroendocrine+Tumors+in+MEN1&rank=1.

48

Zollinger Ellison Syndrome in a Patient with Multiple Endocrine Neoplasia Type 1: A Classic Presentation

Ishani Shah,[1] **Neil Vyas**,[2] **and Kambiz S. Kadkhodayan**[2]

[1]*Department of Internal Medicine, Creighton University St. Joseph's Hospital and Medical Center, Phoenix, AZ, USA*
[2]*Department of Gastroenterology, Creighton University St. Joseph's Hospital and Medical Center, Phoenix, AZ, USA*

Correspondence should be addressed to Ishani Shah; ishani1991@gmail.com

Academic Editor: Tetsuo Hirata

Zollinger Ellison Syndrome (ZES) is characterized by a wide spectrum of conditions including severe gastroesophageal reflux disease, peptic ulcer disease, watery diarrhea, and weight loss. We present a case of a 60-year-old woman being evaluated for severe dyspepsia, vomiting, and chronic diarrhea, who was diagnosed to have ZES associated with a pancreatic neuroendocrine tumor, in the setting of multiple endocrine neoplasia (MEN) type 1. Although cases of ZES have been reported previously, we believe that our case is a classic presentation of ZES diagnosed on the basis of typical radiologic, endoscopic, and endosonographic features.

1. Introduction

Zollinger Ellison Syndrome (ZES) is caused by ectopic hypersecretion of gastrin from pancreatic or duodenal neuroendocrine tumors (NETs), commonly referred to as gastrinomas. Such high gastrin levels cause gastric acid overproduction, leading to a typical presentation, usually consisting of peptic ulcer disease and severe diarrhea. We present a classic case of ZES in a patient with multiple endocrine neoplasia (MEN) type 1.

2. Case Presentation

A 60-year-old woman presented to our hospital with severe nausea, vomiting, watery diarrhea, and burning epigastric pain for a duration of one week. Her epigastric pain was associated with severe acid reflux, which had been intermittently present for a duration of two years and was resistant to over-the-counter low-dose proton pump inhibitor (PPI) therapy. Her past medical history was negative for any evidence of gastrointestinal (GI) bleed. Interestingly, the patient had a daughter who had been diagnosed with multiple endocrine neoplasia (MEN) type 1 a year prior to presentation. On physical exam, she was afebrile with stable hemodynamics. Abdominal palpation revealed mild epigastric tenderness without any guarding or rigidity. Cardiopulmonary exam was within normal limits.

Significant laboratory findings included WBC count of 15,000/microL, potassium of 3 mmol/L, magnesium of 0.7 mg/dL, and calcium of 11.8 mg/dL. Lipase level was within normal limits. Other pertinent laboratory values included fasting serum gastrin level of 1603 pg/mL (0-180 pg/mL), chromogranin A level of 14600 ng/mL (0-100 ng/mL), prolactin hormone level of 21 ng/mL (2-29 ng/mL), and parathyroid hormone (PTH) level of 473 pg/mL (10-65 pg/mL). She did not have any history of prior gastric surgeries, gastroparesis, or renal disease, to possibly explain her elevated gastrin level. An infectious workup for her diarrhea, including *Clostridium difficile* toxin and a stool PCR panel for common enteric pathogens, was negative. Subsequently, an extensive workup for evaluation of MEN was done, which revealed a unilateral parathyroid adenoma on neck imaging and diffuse stomach wall thickening along with pancreatic cystic lesions in body (1.2 cm) and tail (0.7 cm) on abdominal MRI (Figure 1). Testing for pituitary disease was negative.

An esophagogastroduodenoscopy (EGD) was performed for further evaluation of her symptoms, which revealed severe reflux esophagitis, diffusely hypertrophic gastric rugae and multiple postbulbar ulcers in the duodenum (Figures 2(a),

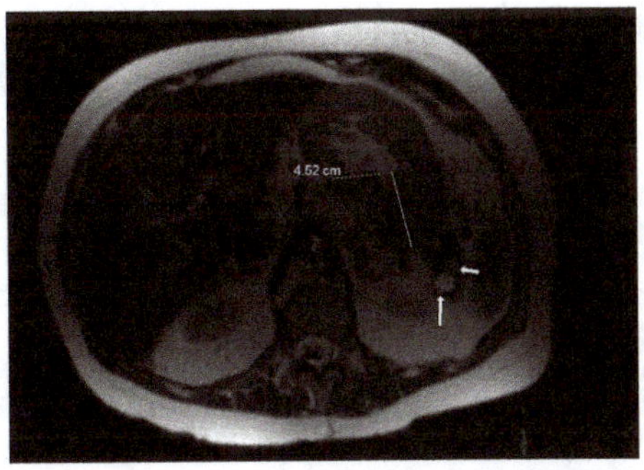

FIGURE 1: MRI abdomen showing diffuse gastric wall thickening (4.52 cm) with a small pancreatic cystic lesion (arrows).

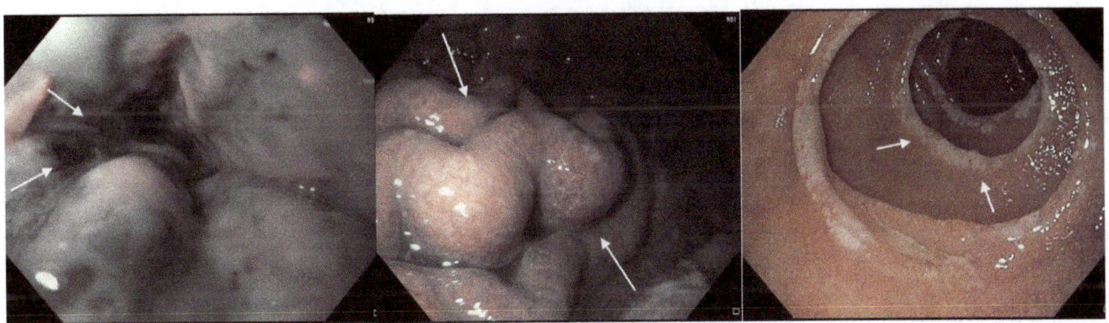

FIGURE 2: EGD showing LA grade D esophagitis in the distal esophagus (a), hypertrophic rugae in the gastric body (b), and multiple postbulbar ulcers in third part of the duodenum (c), as indicated by arrows.

2(b), and 2(c)). Endoscopic ultrasound (EUS) subsequently revealed diffuse thickening of the gastric rugae, predominantly of echo-layers I-III (Figure 3(a)). In addition, the patient was found to have a cystic lesion in the pancreatic neck with thick hypoechoic walls (Figure 3(b)). Random biopsies of the gastric antrum and body revealed patchy chronic gastritis with intestinal metaplasia (Figure 4(a)) while FNA from pancreatic cyst revealed well differentiated NET (Figure 4(b)).

The patient eventually underwent a distal pancreatectomy and parathyroidectomy with clinical improvement. The remainder of her hospital course was uncomplicated and she was discharged home on high-dose PPI and octreotide.

3. Discussion

Patients presenting with gastroesophageal reflux disease (GERD) unresponsive to standard PPI therapy and chronic diarrhea should be evaluated for ZES from gastrin producing NETs, also known as gastrinomas. Gastrinomas leading to ZES are predominantly duodenal; about 25% are pancreatic in origin [1]. The annual incidence of gastrinomas is about 4 to 5 per million population [2]. Most ZES patients present with symptoms of acid reflux (52%-56%) and peptic ulcer disease (73%-98%), while other common symptoms include chronic diarrhea (60%-75%) and weight loss (7%-53%) [3, 4]. Fasting serum gastrin (FSG) levels of more than 10 times the upper limit of normal along with a gastric pH of less than 2 are highly predictive of ZES. However, there is data to suggest that FSG levels can be elevated in various other conditions such as antral gastric cell hyperplasia, *H. Pylori* infection, acute renal failure, gastric outlet obstruction, and short bowel syndrome [5]. Additionally, secretin stimulation testing is commonly used for distinguishing ZES from other causes of hypergastrinemia such as antral G-cell hyperplasia and gastric outlet obstruction. An increase in gastrin level of less than ten times upper limit of normal or gastric pH of <2 essentially indicates an alternate diagnosis. It works on the principle that secretin stimulates gastrin secretion from gastrinoma cells but inhibits normal gastric G cells.

While clinical and laboratory findings can usually be diagnostic of ZES, radiologic and endoscopic investigations are required for localizing gastrinomas and evaluating for metastases. CT, MRI, and somatostatin receptor scintigraphy are often useful; however definitive diagnosis is frequently established via endoscopic evaluation as seen in our case. Similar to our case, upper endoscopy in most cases of ZES shows reflux esophagitis, hypertrophic gastric folds, and multiple ulcers scattered over first (75%) and third (14%) parts of the duodenum and sometimes over the jejunum (11%) [6]. Additionally, EUS is an extremely sensitive (93%) and specific (95%) test for diagnosing pancreatic NETs and has been shown to be superior to CT, MRI, and other invasive diagnostic measures such as angiography and secretin stimulation testing [7–10]. It can detect pancreatic lesions as small as 2 or 3 mm in diameter and provides the opportunity to perform FNA of suspicious lesions.

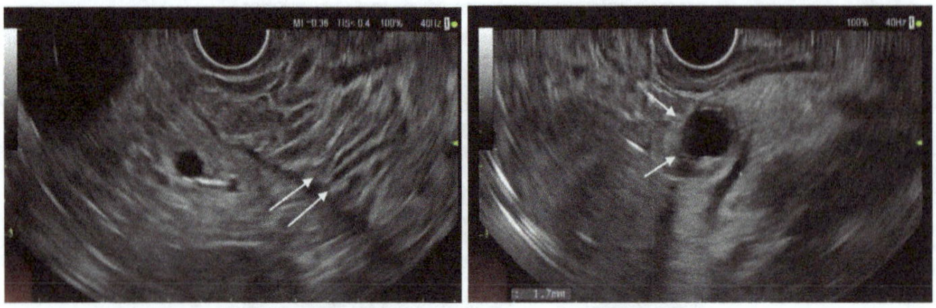

(a) (b)

FIGURE 3: EUS showing hypertrophic gastric rugae (a) and neuroendocrine tumor in the pancreatic neck (b), respectively, as indicated by arrows.

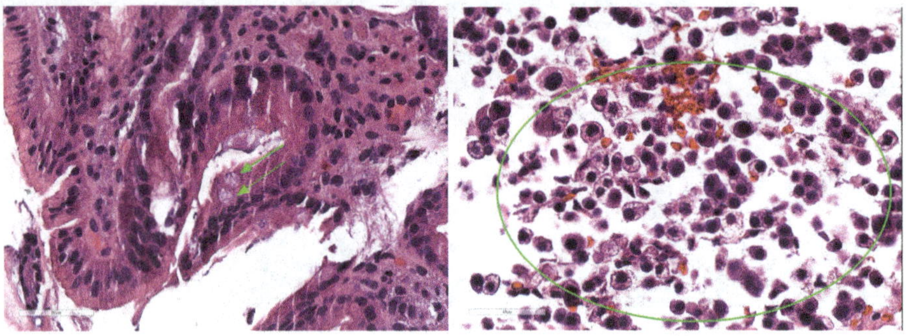

(a) (b)

FIGURE 4: Gastric biopsy (a) showing patchy hypertrophic gastritis and intestinal metaplasia (green arrows) while pancreatic aspirate (b) showing neuroendocrine cells (area enclosed within circle).

Around 80% of gastrinomas are sporadic; however 20% are associated with MEN type 1, an autosomal dominant condition associated with predisposition to tumors in the hyperparathyroidism glands, pancreas, and pituitary [11]. About 40% of patients with MEN type 1 initially present with symptoms of ZES [12]. Therefore, an extensive workup for MEN should be carried out in all patients with ZES. In many studies, EUS has consistently been proven to be superior to other imaging modalities for diagnosing pancreatic NETs in patients with a suspected or established diagnosis of MEN type 1 [8, 13, 14].

In conclusion, our case is a classic blend of clinical, radiologic, endoscopic, and endosonographic features of ZES in a patient with MEN type 1. It highlights the importance of early recognition of these findings for prompt diagnosis and appropriate treatment.

Authors' Contributions

Ishani Shah, MD, is responsible for writing and editing the case report. Neil Vyas, MD, and Kambiz S. Kadkhodayan, MD, are responsible for editing the case report.

References

[1] J. I. Isenberg, J. H. Walsh, and M. I. Grossman, "Progress in gastroenterology, zollinger-ellison syndrome," *Gastroenterology*, vol. 65, p. 140, 1973.

[2] K. Öberg, "Pancreatic endocrine tumors," *Seminars in Oncology*, vol. 37, no. 6, pp. 594–618, 2010.

[3] P. K. Roy, D. J. Venzon, H. Shojamanesh et al., "Zollinger-ellison syndrome. Clinical presentation in 261 patients," *Medicine*, vol. 79, no. 6, pp. 379–411, 2000.

[4] J. A. Norton, D. S. Foster, T. Ito, and R. T. Jensen, "Gastrinomas: medical or surgical treatment," *Endocrinology and Metabolism Clinics*, vol. 47, no. 3, pp. 577–601, 2018.

[5] M. J. Berna, K. M. Hoffmann, J. Serrano, F. Gibril, and R. T. Jensen, "Serum gastrin in Zollinger-Ellison syndrome: I. Prospective study of fasting serum gastrin in 309 patients from the national institutes of health and comparison with 2229 cases from the literature," *Medicine*, vol. 85, no. 6, pp. 295–330, 2006.

[6] H. Tariq, M. U. Kamal, V. Vootla et al., "A rare cause of abdominal pain and mass in an 18-year-old patient: a diagnostic dilemma," *Gastroenterology Research*, vol. 11, no. 1, p. 75, 2018.

[7] T. Rosch, C. J. Lightdale, J. F. Botet et al., "Localization of pancreatic endocrine tumors by endoscopic ultrasonography," *The New England Journal of Medicine*, vol. 326, no. 26, pp. 1721–1726, 1992.

[8] M. A. Anderson, S. Carpenter, N. W. Thompson, T. T. Nostrant, G. H. Elta, and J. M. Scheiman, "Endoscopic ultrasound is highly accurate and directs management in patients with neuroendocrine tumors of the pancreas," *American Journal of Gastroenterology*, vol. 95, no. 9, pp. 2271–2277, 2000.

[9] M. A. Khashab, E. Yong, A. M. Lennon et al., "EUS is still superior to multidetector computerized tomography for detection of pancreatic neuroendocrine tumors," *Gastrointestinal Endoscopy*, vol. 73, no. 4, pp. 691–696, 2011.

[10] P. D. James, A. V. Tsolakis, M. Zhang et al., "Incremental benefit of preoperative EUS for the detection of pancreatic neuroendocrine tumors: A meta-analysis," *Gastrointestinal Endoscopy*, vol. 81, no. 4, pp. 848–856, 2015.

[11] J. A. Norton, "Neuroendocrine tumors of the pancreas and duodenum," *Current Problems in Surgery*, vol. 31, no. 2, pp. 89–156, 1994.

[12] F. Gibril, M. Schumann, A. Pace, and R. T. Jensen, "Multiple endocrine neoplasia type 1 and Zollinger-Ellison syndrome: a prospective study of 107 cases and comparison with 1009 cases from the literature," *Medicine*, vol. 83, no. 1, pp. 43–83, 2004.

[13] S. J. Van Asselt, A. H. Brouwers, H. M. Van Dullemen et al., "EUS is superior for detection of pancreatic lesions compared with standard imaging in patients with multiple endocrine neoplasia type 1," *Gastrointestinal Endoscopy*, vol. 81, no. 1, pp. 159–167, 2015.

[14] P. H. Kann, E. Balakina, D. Ivan et al., "Natural course of small, asymptomatic neuroendocrine pancreatic tumours in multiple endocrine neoplasia type 1: An endoscopic ultrasound imaging study," *Endocrine-Related Cancer*, vol. 13, no. 4, pp. 1195–1202, 2006.

Case Report of Gastrointestinal Bleeding in an Adult with Chronic Visceral Acid Sphingomyelinase Deficiency

David Cassiman,[1] **Louis Libbrecht**,[2,3] **Wouter Meersseman**,[4] **and Alexander Wilmer**[5]

[1] *Department of Gastroenterology-Hepatology and Metabolic Center, University of Leuven, Belgium*
[2] *Laboratory of Hepatology, University of Leuven, Belgium*
[3] *Department of Pathology, University Hospital Saint-Luc, Brussels, Belgium*
[4] *General Internal Medicine-Metabolic Diseases, University Hospital Gasthuisberg, Leuven, Belgium*
[5] *Medical Intensive Care, University Hospital Gasthuisberg, Leuven, Belgium*

Correspondence should be addressed to David Cassiman; david.cassiman@kuleuven.be

Academic Editor: Olga I. Giouleme

Introduction. Acid sphingomyelinase deficiency (ASMD, also known as Niemann-Pick Type A and Type B disease) is a rare, inherited metabolic disorder. Liver-related issues, including cirrhosis and variceal haemorrhage, are a leading cause of early mortality in individuals with chronic forms of ASMD. Due to the rarity of this lysosomal storage disorder, there can be a lack of awareness that adults with chronic ASMD disease are at significant risk of cirrhosis, portal hypertension, and variceal bleeding. This case highlights an unusual presentation of recurrent variceal bleeding in an adult with cirrhosis and portal hypertension due to chronic visceral ASMD. *Case Presentation.* A patient with severe splenomegaly was diagnosed with ASMD at age of 25. At age 64 they had multiple hospital admissions for hematochezia (originally diagnosed as ischemic colitis) accompanied by hypotension (blood pressure 91/45 mmHg), anemia (hemoglobin 8.5g/dL, ref 12-16; INR 1.4, ref $\leq$1.2), and mild renal insufficiency (creatinine 1.33mg/dL, ref 0.51-0.95). Colonoscopy did not reveal a source of bleeding. Computerized tomography scanning imaging showed diffuse venous collaterals and ascites. Arteriographies during subsequent episodes of bleeding were negative for active arterial intestinal bleeding. Recurrent gastrointestinal bleeding was found to originate from a varicose vein cluster connected to the right iliac vein and the superior mesenteric vein, located in the submucosa of a small intestinal loop. Multiple varices were secondary to portal hypertension in the context of cirrhosis. The patient died from recurrent variceal bleeding that exacerbated liver failure worsened by pneumonia and hypovolemic and septic shock. *Conclusions.* The variceal bleeding in this patient was atypical in that it originated from venous collaterals bleeding into the small intestine rather than the more typical gastroesophageal varices observed in ASMD. With long standing liver dysfunction and gradual development of portal hypertension, intestinal varices rather than occult intestinal bleeding due to ischemia should be considered in ASMD patients presenting with either hematochezia or hematemesis.

1. Background

Acid sphingomyelinase deficiency (ASMD, also known as Niemann-Pick Type A and Type B disease) is a rare, inherited metabolic disorder resulting in sphingolipid accumulation in nervous and visceral tissues and progressive multisystem disease [1]. Biallelic mutations in *SMPD1*, the gene encoding acid sphingomyelinase (ASM; EC3.1.4.12), give rise to a spectrum of disease phenotypes characterized by differences in the rate of disease progression and the extent of neurological and other organ system involvements. Infantile-onset neurovisceral ASMD is uniformly fatal (OMIM#25707), chronic visceral ASMD (OMIM#607616) has early childhood-adulthood onset with progressive visceral disease without neurodegeneration, and an intermediate phenotype has visceral disease and slowly progressing neurological symptoms [2]. Nonneurological manifestations include hepatosplenomegaly, liver dysfunction, dyslipidemia, cardiac valve insufficiency, interstitial lung disease, osteopenia/osteoporosis, and hematologic abnormalities [2]. There are no approved treatments for

ASMD, and chronic ASMD management aims to prevent long-term complications related to liver and lung disease. Enzyme replacement therapy for chronic forms of ASMD is in clinical development [3].

Liver-related issues including cirrhosis and variceal haemorrhage are a leading cause of early mortality in individuals with chronic forms of ASMD [4–6]. Variable degrees of liver fibrosis were found in 17 adults undergoing liver biopsy during screening for enrolment in a phase 1 ASMD clinical trial, with cirrhosis present in two individuals that had no clinical symptoms of liver failure [7]. Successful liver transplantation has been performed in adults with chronic ASMD that had cirrhosis or liver failure [6, 8–10]. Since the liver is so prominently affected in ASMD, hepatologists or gastroenterologists are typically consulted and involved in management of patients with chronic ASMD forms. The following case report describes an adult with chronic visceral ASMD and an unusual presentation of gastroenterology symptoms resulting from liver disease.

2. Case Presentation

An adult with severe splenomegaly was diagnosed with ASMD at age of 25 while being hospitalized to undergo splenectomy for what was thought to be autoimmune thrombocytopenia. Other ASMD symptoms included hepatomegaly, thrombocytopenia, mixed dyslipidemia, interstitial lung disease (Figure 1(a)), and osteoporosis. The individual was admitted to hospital at age of 53 for *Streptococcus pneumoniae* septic shock with multiorgan failure, hepatic encephalopathy, and disseminated intravascular coagulation and received ventilation for acute respiratory distress syndrome and temporary hemodialysis for acute renal insufficiency.

At age of 64 they were admitted to hospital for hematochezia with a tentative diagnosis of ischemic colitis and admitted again one year later for hematochezia accompanied by hypotension (blood pressure 91/45 mmHg), anemia (hemoglobin 8.5g/dL, ref 12-16; INR 1.4, ref ≤1.2), and mild renal insufficiency (creatinine 1.33mg/dL, ref 0.51-0.95). Gastroscopy revealed one esophageal varix with a red spot in the absence of acute bleeding stigmata. Colonoscopy did not reveal a source of bleeding. Computerized tomography scanning imaging showed diffuse venous collaterals and ascites (Figure 1(b)). Serum-ascites albumin gradient was high (>1.1g/dL). Arteriographies during subsequent episodes of bleeding were negative for active arterial intestinal bleeding. Recurrent gastrointestinal bleeding was found to originate from a varicose vein cluster (Figure 1(c)) connected to the right iliac vein and the superior mesenteric vein, located in the submucosa of a small intestinal loop. Despite laparoscopic suturing of venous collaterals, another episode of bleeding occurred 1 month later leading to admission to the intensive care unit with hypovolemic shock, overwhelming pneumonia, deteriorating liver function/hepatic encephalopathy, anemia (hemoglobin 4.8g/dL; INR 3), lactic acidosis (lactate 9.6mmol/L, ref 0.5-2.2), and high bilirubin (7.54mg/dl, ref≤1).

Cirrhosis was suspected from the clinical course and was supported by direct visualization of the liver during laparoscopy. Liver biopsy indeed showed micronodular cirrhosis with elements of nonalcoholic steatohepatitis and many hepatocytes were filled with vacuoles having transparent cytoplasm (Figure 2(a)). Hepatic venous pressure gradient was 15mmHg, consistent with portal hypertension. Deterioration of hemodynamics and liver function resulted in death. On autopsy, lung pathology showed diffuse infiltration of foamy histiocytes in alveolar spaces and interstitium without inflammatory infiltrate (Figure 2(b)).

3. Discussion

This case highlights an unusual presentation of recurrent variceal bleeding in an adult with cirrhosis and portal hypertension due to chronic visceral ASMD. Individuals with chronic ASMD are at risk of liver-related morbidity and mortality as identified in natural history studies [6], patients undergoing liver biopsy during screening for enrolment in clinical trials [7], and in case reports [5, 10–14]. In a study of 103 adults with chronic visceral ASMD, 9 (9%) had cirrhosis or liver failure requiring liver transplantation [6]. Liver-related issues, including cirrhosis and variceal haemorrhage, are leading causes of early mortality in individuals with chronic forms of ASMD [4].

The patient in the present case died from recurrent variceal bleeding that exacerbated liver failure worsened by pneumonia and hypovolemic and septic shock. Multiple varices were secondary to portal hypertension in the context of cirrhosis. The variceal bleeding was atypical in that it originated from venous collaterals bleeding into the small intestine rather than the more typical hematemesis observed in ASMD. With long standing liver dysfunction and gradual development of portal hypertension, intestinal varices rather than occult intestinal bleeding due to ischemia should be considered in ASMD patients presenting with either hematochezia or hematemesis. Individuals with chronic ASMD, especially asplenic patients, should be monitored for varices at all areas of risk including the most common locations such as the gastroesophageal junction and rectum, as well as less common locations including paraumbilical, splenorenal, gastrorenal, gall bladder, and, as in this case, intestinal. Identification of venous collaterals by ultrasound or CT/MRI imaging, screening for esophageal varices according to standard practices for patients with cirrhosis [15] (e.g., endoscopic screening for varices at the time of diagnosis with follow-up every 2-3 years if negative), and nonselective beta blocker therapy to lower portal pressure are recommended. Clinical monitoring and hepatic assessments for chronic visceral ASMD are described in Wasserstein et al. [16].

Due to low awareness of ASMD, the initial surgical liver biopsy assessment of vacuoles for this patient was nonalcoholic steatohepatitis, since vacuoles were interpreted as (microvesicular) steatosis, rather than sphingolipid storage due to ASMD. Similar misclassification has occurred in cholesterol ester storage disease, where lack of awareness among pathologists has resulted in misdiagnoses of nonalcoholic fatty liver disease/steatohepatitis or cryptogenic cirrhosis [17].

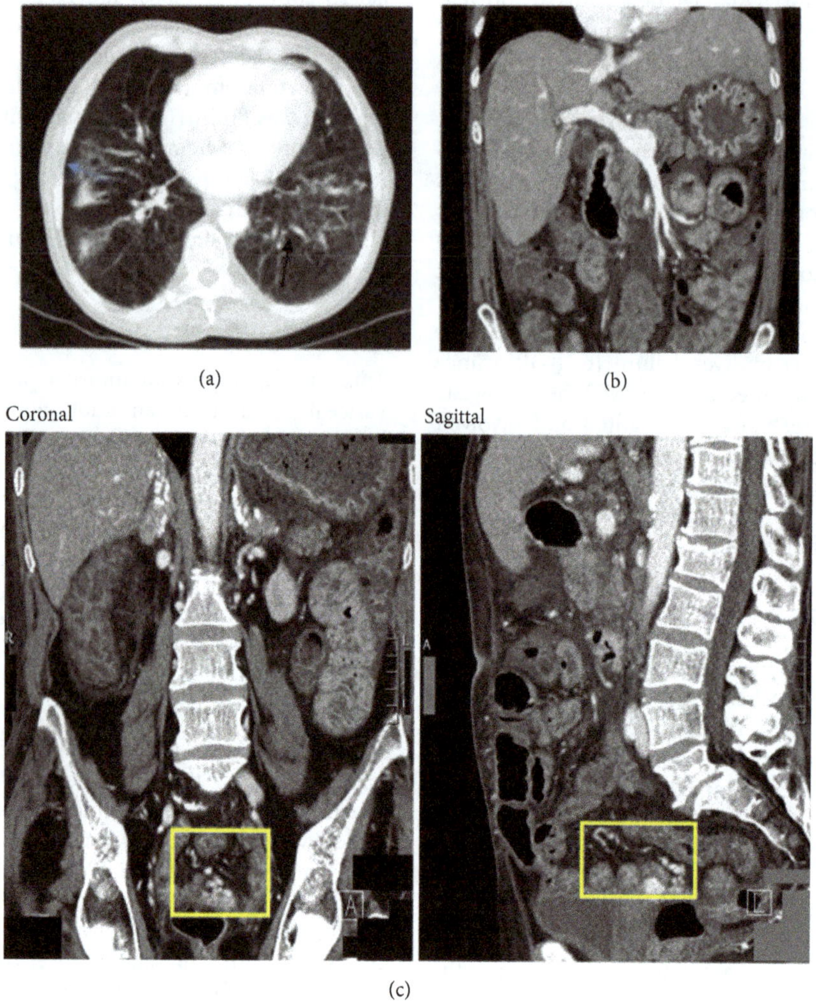

FIGURE 1: *CT of chest (a), abdomen (b), and abdomen/pelvis (c).* (a) Chest CT showing centrilobular emphysema and signs of interstitial lung disease. There are bilateral basal inter- and intralobular septal enhancement (blue arrow) consistent with sphingomyelin deposition seen in ASMD patients. Multiple bronchiectasis (black arrow) is also present. (b) Venous phase of an abdominal contrast CT, showing an enlarged portal vein (arrow) and a moderate amount of ascites fluid in the abdominal cavity. The liver is nodular, enlarged, and steatotic. The patient is asplenic. (c) Coronal and sagittal CT images of abdomen and pelvis show the cluster of varicose veins that are contrast-enhanced (outlined by yellow boxes), situated just above the vaginal lumen, and show extravasation of contrast into the small intestinal lumen.

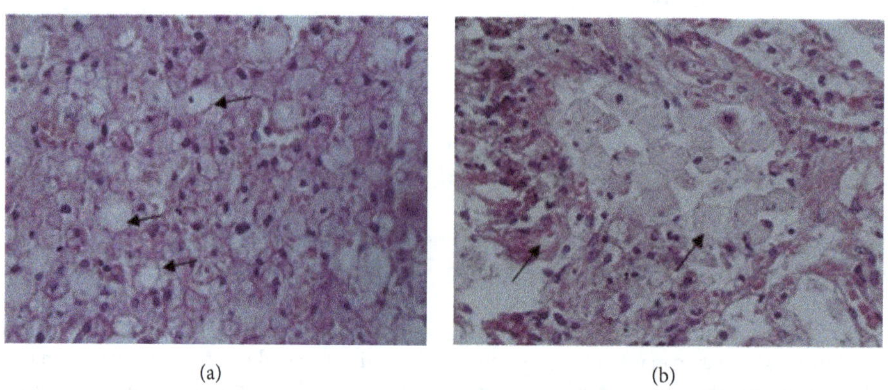

FIGURE 2: *Liver (a) and lung (b) biopsies showing presence of sphingolipid storage due to ASMD.* (a) Hepatocytes filled with vacuoles having transparent cytoplasm (arrows, hematoxylin and eosin staining, 40X). (b) Lung section showing diffuse infiltration of foamy histiocytes in alveolar spaces, as well as the interstitium, without inflammatory infiltrate (arrows, hematoxylin and eosin staining, 40X).

4. Conclusion

Due to the rarity of this lysosomal storage disorder, there can be a lack of awareness among gastroenterologists and hepatologists that adults with chronic ASMD disease are at significant risk of cirrhosis, portal hypertension, and variceal bleeding. This case highlights the fact that adults with ASMD and severe liver dysfunction may develop variceal bleeding at multiple sites in the intestine and viscera rather than more commonly occurring gastroesophageal varices. With long standing liver dysfunction and gradual development of portal hypertension, intestinal varices rather than occult intestinal bleeding due to ischemia should be considered in ASMD patients presenting with either hematochezia or hematemesis.

Abbreviations

ASM: Acid sphingomyelinase
ASMD: Acid sphingomyelinase deficiency
INR: International normalized ratio
SMPD1: Sphingomyelin phosphodiesterase 1 gene.

Authors' Contributions

David Cassiman, Louis Libbrecht, Wouter Meersseman, and Alexander Wilmer provided and analysed patient data. All authors participated in manuscript development and writing and approved the final manuscript.

Acknowledgments

The authors respectfully acknowledge the individual whose case was presented in this manuscript and thank Patrice C. Ferriola, PhD, for assistance in preparation of the manuscript. Funding was provided by Sanofi Genzyme. Patrice C. Ferriola, PhD (KZE PharmAssociates, LLC), provided assistance in preparation of the manuscript and was funded by Sanofi Genzyme.

References

[1] E. H. Schuchman and R. J. Desnick, "Types A and B Niemann-Pick disease," *Molecular Genetics and Metabolism*, vol. 120, no. 1-2, pp. 27–33, 2017.

[2] M. M. McGovern, R. Avetisyan, B.-J. Sanson, and O. Lidove, "Disease manifestations and burden of illness in patients with acid sphingomyelinase deficiency (ASMD)," *Orphanet Journal of Rare Diseases*, vol. 12, no. 1, p. 41, 2017.

[3] M. P. Wasserstein, G. A. Diaz, R. H. Lachmann et al., "Olipudase alfa for treatment of acid sphingomyelinase deficiency (ASMD): safety and efficacy in adults treated for 30 months," *Journal of Inherited Metabolic Disease*, vol. 41, no. 5, pp. 829–838, 2018.

[4] D. Cassiman, S. Packman, B. Bembi et al., "Cause of death in patients with chronic visceral and chronic neurovisceral acid sphingomyelinase deficiency (Niemann-Pick disease type B and B variant): literature review and report of new cases," *Molecular Genetics and Metabolism*, vol. 118, pp. 206–213, 2016.

[5] O. Lidove, F. Sedel, F. Charlotte, R. Froissart, and M. T. Vanier, "Cirrhosis and liver failure: expanding phenotype of acid sphingomyelinase-deficient Niemann-Pick disease in adulthood," *Journal of Inherited Metabolic Disease*, vol. 15, pp. 117–121, 2015.

[6] M. M. McGovern, N. Lippa, E. Bagiella, E. H. Schuchman, R. J. Desnick, and M. P. Wasserstein, "Morbidity and mortality in type B Niemann-Pick disease," *Genetics in Medicine*, vol. 15, no. 8, pp. 618–623, 2013.

[7] B. L. Thurberg, M. P. Wasserstein, T. Schiano et al., "Liver and Skin Histopathology in Adults With Acid Sphingomyelinase Deficiency (Niemann-Pick Disease Type B)," *The American Journal of Surgical Pathology*, vol. 36, no. 8, pp. 1234–1246, 2012.

[8] G. R. Coelho, A. M. Praciano, J. P. C. Rodrigues et al., "Liver transplantation in patients with Niemann-Pick disease - single-center experience," *Transplantation Proceedings*, vol. 47, no. 10, pp. 2929–2931, 2015.

[9] M. S. Mendes, F. X. Portela, R. C. Reis, J. D. Castro, J. H. Garcia, and M. A. Holanda, "Liver transplantation in a patient with Niemann-Pick disease and pulmonary involvement," *Jornal Brasileiro de Pneumologia*, vol. 38, pp. 269–271, 2012.

[10] E. J. Smanik, A. S. Tavill, G. H. Jacobs, I. A. Schafer, L. Farquhar, F. L. Weber Jr. et al., "Orthotopic liver transplantation in two adults with Niemann-Pick and Gaucher's diseases: implications for the treatment of inherited metabolic disease," *Hepatology*, vol. 17, pp. 42–49, 1993.

[11] P. Labrune, P. Bedossa, P. Huguet, F. Roset, M. T. Vanier, and M. Odievre, "Fatal liver failure in two children with Niemann-Pick disease type B," *Journal of Pediatric Gastroenterology and Nutrition*, vol. 13, no. 1, pp. 104–109, 1991.

[12] C. Putterman, J. Zelingher, and D. Shouval, "Liver failure and the sea-blue histiocyte/adult Niemann-Pick disease, case report and review of the literature," *Journal of Clinical Gastroenterology*, vol. 15, pp. 146–149, 1992.

[13] J. P. Tassoni Jr., K. A. Fawaz, and D. E. Johnston, "Cirrhosis and portal hypertension in a patient with adult Niemann-Pick disease," *Gastroenterology*, vol. 100, no. 2, pp. 567–569, 1991.

[14] H. Zhou, R. P. Linke, H. E. Schaefer, W. Mobius, and U. Pfeifer, "Progressive liver failure in a patient with adult Niemann-Pick disease associated with generalized AL amyloidosis," *Virchows Archiv*, vol. 426, no. 6, pp. 635–639, 1995.

[15] S. S. Jakab and G. Garcia-Tsao, "Screening and surveillance of varices in patients with cirrhosis," *Clinical Gastroenterology and Hepatology*, vol. 17, no. 1, pp. 26–29, 2019.

[16] M. Wasserstein, C. Dionisi-Vici, R. Giugliani et al., "Recommendations for clinical monitoring of patients with acid sphingomyelinase deficiency (ASMD)," *Molecular Genetics and Metabolism*, vol. 126, no. 2, pp. 98–105, 2019.

[17] M. Pant and K. Oshima, "Cholesteryl ester storage disease: an underdiagnosed cause of cirrhosis in adults," *Annals of Diagnostic Pathology*, vol. 31, pp. 66–70, 2017.

50

Massive Lipomatosis of the Small Intestine Causing Intussusception

Michael Pagacz[1] **Irvin Willis,**[2] **and John Alexis**[1,3]

[1]*A.M. Rywlin, MD Department of Pathology, Mount Sinai Medical Center, Miami Beach, FL, USA*
[2]*Department of General Surgery, Mount Sinai Medical Center, Miami Beach, FL, USA*
[3]*Herbert Wertheim College of Medicine, Florida International University, Miami, FL, USA*

Correspondence should be addressed to Michael Pagacz; michael@pagacz.ca

Academic Editor: Yoshihiro Moriwaki

Lipomatosis is a rare condition characterized by diffuse, unencapsulted adipose tissue deposition. Intestinal involvement is rare, and presentation as intussusception is rarer still. We report a 40-year-old man who presented with abdominal pain and fecal urgency. Abdominal CT scan showed a protuberant ileo-cecal valve, with intussusception of the ileum into the cecum. The mucosal surface of the resected bowel was bulbous and protuberant, showing loss of mucosal folds, and there was an $8 \times 5 \times 5$ cm mass prolapsing into the ileo-cecal valve. Microscopically there was abundant adipose tissue in the submucosa with an unremarkable mucosa. The patient recovered uneventfully with only occasional cramping in the left abdomen.

1. Introduction

Intestinal lipomatosis is a disease of unknown etiology which may remain asymptomatic or present with complications such as intussusception. It is exceedingly rare, and the presentation as intussusception is rarer still [1]. We report a case of a symptomatic man with intestinal lipomatosis of the small bowel presenting as intussusception.

2. Case Report

The patient is a 40-year-old man with a history of gastroesophageal reflux disease and a family history of colon cancer. He presented with severe abdominal pain, fecal urgency, and episodes of diarrhea. He had lost 22 lbs over two months. An abdominal CT and colonoscopy showed a severely lipomatous, bulbous, and protuberant ileo-cecal valve, with intussusception of the ileum into the cecum. Exploratory laparotomy revealed marked enlargement of the ileum due to massive fat deposition, and adhesions between the ascending colon and the right lateral lower abdominal wall. A dilated segment of the ileum and cecum was surgically resected, which demonstrated a bulbous, protuberant, abnormally smooth mucosal surface in the ileum, sharply demarcated from normal large intestinal mucosa at the ileo-cecal valve (Figure 1). There was an $8 \times 5 \times 5$ cm mass protruding through the ileo-cecal valve into the cecum (Figure 2). At the proximal end of the resected specimen there was a short (4 cm) transition from normal small intestinal mucosa to the abnormal, smooth, bulbous mucosa. Microscopically, there was extensive infiltration of mature adipose throughout the submucosa (Figure 3).

3. Discussion

This is an unusual case of lipomatosis of the small intestine presenting as an intussusception of a submucosal mass into the ileo-cecal valve. 90% of cases are localized in the intestinal submucosa, occasionally with reaching muscularis propria, and 10% are subserosal [1]. The etiology of lipomatosis is unknown. Theories include embryonic displacement of adipose tissue, postchemotherapeutic fat deposition, and chronic irritation such as chronic inflammatory bowel disease, low-grade infection, and hamartomatous syndromes [2].

Only fifteen documented cases of diffuse intestinal lipomatosis exist and only two documented cases of

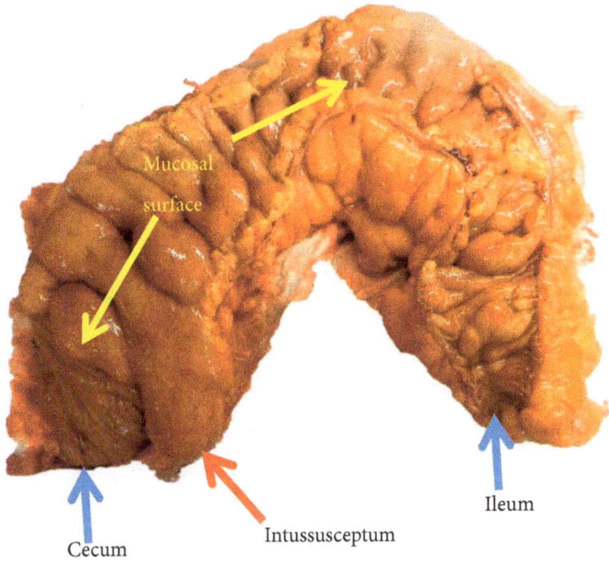

FIGURE 1: Opened bowel with mucosal surface.

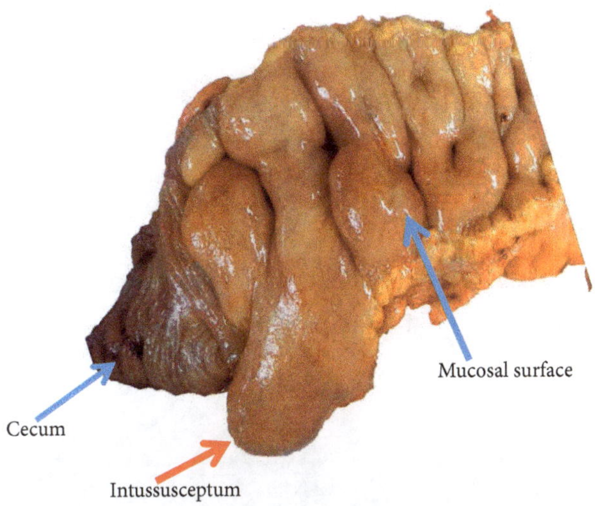

FIGURE 2: Intussusceptum at ileocecal valve.

intussusception caused by diffuse lipomatosis [1]. Most patients in reported cases of intestinal lipomatosis were asymptomatic; however, some presented with subacute intermittent obstruction, colonic perforation, and intussusception, the rarest of complications [3]. Early diagnosis of adult intussusception is difficult because most cases present with nonspecific signs and symptoms and may present in an acute, subacute or chronic manner. The classic triad of intermittent abdominal pain, currant jelly stools, and a palpable tender mass seen in children is rarely present in adults. However, in adults, nausea, vomiting, gastrointestinal bleeding, changes in bowel habits, and abdominal distension are more common [4].

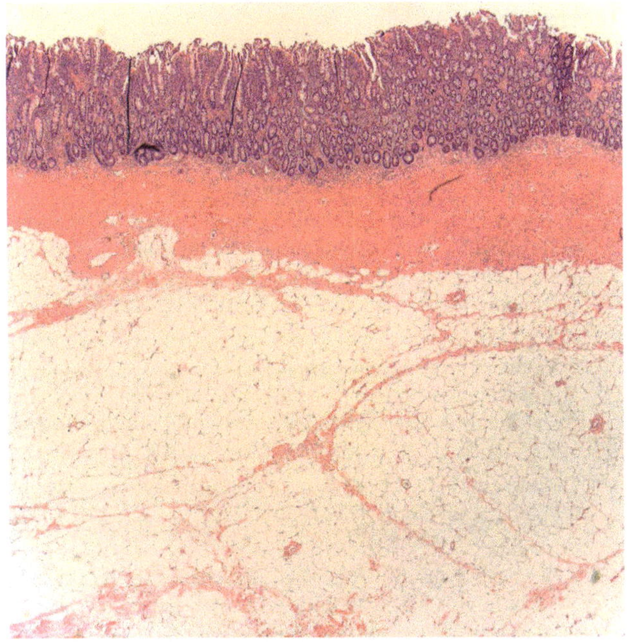

FIGURE 3: Intussuscepted lipomatous mass H&E 4x.

The most useful imaging techniques for evaluating fatty lesions of the intestine are CT scan and ultrasound. Lipomas of the small intestine may appear on CT scan as round, homogeneous, well-circumscribed masses with fat density, while on ultrasonography they usually appear as highly echoic masses. Ultrasonography of intussusception typically shows a multilayered appearance consisting of the alternating hyperechoic and hypoechoic concentric rings that represent alternating layers of mucosa, bowel wall, and mesenteric fat in cross section. The sensitivity and specificity of ultrasonography and CT are similar. Ultrasonography is more useful for the initial diagnosis of intussusception as it is more readily available, enabling it to be used in emergent situations [5].

The prognosis of intussusception is quite variable, depending on the cause. Mortality for adult intussusception is 8.7% in cases with benign lesions, and 52.5% in cases with malignant neoplasms [6]. Invasive management of lipomatosis is not advised unless complications arise such as intussusceptions, obstruction, bleeding, or perforation leading to peritonitis in which case prompt surgical intervention is essential to prevent serious complications such a bowel ischemia and perforation [1, 7].

4. Conclusion

Intussusception in adults is an uncommon condition invariably associated with an underlying cause which needs pathological examination to arrive at a definitive diagnosis. Small bowel lipomatosis is a rare condition that can cause intussusception presenting as obstruction. Prompt diagnosis is crucial as delay in treatment may have serious consequences.

References

[1] K. Kumar, "Rare diagnosis of intestinal lipomatosis complicated by intussusception in an adult: a case report 4. Khan AN, Solomon SS, Childress RD. Composite pheochromocytoma—aganglioneuroma: rare experiment of nature," *Endocrine Practice*, vol. 16, pp. 291–299, 2010.

[2] Y. Bilgic, H. B. Altinsoy, N. Yildirim, O. Alatas, B. H. Kanat, and A. Sahin, "Familial abdominal and intestinal lipomatosis presenting with upper GI bleeding," *Case Reports in Gastrointestinal Medicine*, vol. 2015, Article ID 123723, 4 pages, 2015.

[3] S. Uyulmaz, M. Zünd, U. Caspar, J. Diebold, and K. Slankamenac, "Ileoileal intussusception in unspecific recurrent abdominal pain in adult: A case report," *SAGE Open Medical Case Reports*, vol. 6, Article ID 2050313X1879281, p. 4, 2018.

[4] D. E. Lee and J. Y. Choe, "Ileocolic intussusception caused by a lipoma in an adult," *World Journal of Clinical Cases*, vol. 5, no. 6, pp. 254–257, 2017.

[5] S. R. Jai, F. Bensardi, F. Chehab, D. Khaiz, and A. Bouzidi, "Jejunal lipoma with intermittent intussusception revealed by partial obstructive syndrome," *Saudi Journal of Gastroenterology*, vol. 14, no. 4, pp. 206–207, 2008.

[6] S. Soni, P. Moss, and T. Jaiganesh, "Idiopathic adult intussusception," *International Journal of Emergency Medicine*, vol. 4, no. 8, 2011.

[7] A. Brill and A. Waheed, "Intussusception in adults," *StatPearls* (Internet), StatPearls Publishing, Treasure Island, FL, 2019.

Permissions

All chapters in this book were first published by Hindawi Publishing Corporation; hereby published with permission under the Creative Commons Attribution License or equivalent. Every chapter published in this book has been scrutinized by our experts. Their significance has been extensively debated. The topics covered herein carry significant findings which will fuel the growth of the discipline. They may even be implemented as practical applications or may be referred to as a beginning point for another development.

The contributors of this book come from diverse backgrounds, making this book a truly international effort. This book will bring forth new frontiers with its revolutionizing research information and detailed analysis of the nascent developments around the world.

We would like to thank all the contributing authors for lending their expertise to make the book truly unique. They have played a crucial role in the development of this book. Without their invaluable contributions this book wouldn't have been possible. They have made vital efforts to compile up to date information on the varied aspects of this subject to make this book a valuable addition to the collection of many professionals and students.

This book was conceptualized with the vision of imparting up-to-date information and advanced data in this field. To ensure the same, a matchless editorial board was set up. Every individual on the board went through rigorous rounds of assessment to prove their worth. After which they invested a large part of their time researching and compiling the most relevant data for our readers.

The editorial board has been involved in producing this book since its inception. They have spent rigorous hours researching and exploring the diverse topics which have resulted in the successful publishing of this book. They have passed on their knowledge of decades through this book. To expedite this challenging task, the publisher supported the team at every step. A small team of assistant editors was also appointed to further simplify the editing procedure and attain best results for the readers.

Apart from the editorial board, the designing team has also invested a significant amount of their time in understanding the subject and creating the most relevant covers. They scrutinized every image to scout for the most suitable representation of the subject and create an appropriate cover for the book.

The publishing team has been an ardent support to the editorial, designing and production team. Their endless efforts to recruit the best for this project, has resulted in the accomplishment of this book. They are a veteran in the field of academics and their pool of knowledge is as vast as their experience in printing. Their expertise and guidance has proved useful at every step. Their uncompromising quality standards have made this book an exceptional effort. Their encouragement from time to time has been an inspiration for everyone.

The publisher and the editorial board hope that this book will prove to be a valuable piece of knowledge for researchers, students, practitioners and scholars across the globe.

List of Contributors

Awoke Minwuyelet and Solomon Ayenew
Bichena Primary Hospital, Amhara Region, Ethiopia

Yibeltal Aschale
Department of Medical Laboratory Science, College of Health Science, Debre Markos University, Debre Markos, Ethiopia

Hisham Hurreiz
Al Ain Hospital, Al Ain, UAE

Amira Babikir and Edward Black
Tawam Hospital, Al Ain, UAE

Khaoula Khalil, Fatima Ezzahra Lahlimi and Illias Tazi
Department of Hematology and Bone Marrow Transplantation, Mohammed VI University Hospital, Cadi Ayyad University, Marrakesh 40080, Morocco

Adan Aftab, Nida Saleem, Syed Farhat Abbas, Zafar Ullah and Muhammad Haneef
Shifa International Hospital, H-8/4, Pitras Bukhari Road, Islamabad, Pakistan

Abhishek Polavarapu and Vivek Gumaste
Gastroenterology and Hepatology, Staten Island University Hospital, Northwell Health, Staten Island, New York, USA

Dhineshreddy Gurala, Bindu Mudduluru and Jobin Philipose
Internal Medicine, Staten Island University Hospital, Northwell Health, Staten Island, New York, USA

Pretty Sara Idiculla
Medicine, Sree Gokulam Medical College and Research Foundation, Trivandrum, India

Magda Daoud
Department of Pulmonary and Critical Care, Staten Island University Hospital, Northwell Health, Staten Island, New York, USA

Naureen Narula
Department of Gastroenterology and Hepatology, Richmond University Medical Center, Staten Island, New York, USA

Takeshi Okamoto
Department of Gastroenterology, St. Luke's International Hospital, 9-1 Akashicho, Chuo-ku, Tokyo 104-8560, Japan
Department of Gastroenterology and Hepatology, Department of Internal Medicine, Tokai University School of Medicine, 143 Shimokasuya, Isehara, Kanagawa 259-1143, Japan

Hidekazu Suzuki
Department of Gastroenterology and Hepatology, Department of Internal Medicine, Tokai University School of Medicine, 143 Shimokasuya, Isehara, Kanagawa 259-1143, Japan

Katsuyuki Fukuda
Department of Gastroenterology, St. Luke's International Hospital, 9-1 Akashicho, Chuo-ku, Tokyo 104-8560, Japan

Andrija Karačić, Domagoj Ŝtritof and Branko Bakula
Department of General Surgery, Clinical Hospital Sveti Duh, Zagreb, Croatia

Paula Batur
School of Medicine, University of Zagreb, Zagreb, Croatia

Taro Fukui
Department of Surgery, Saitama Medical Center, Jichi Medical University, Saitama, Japan

Inka Kekez
Department of Radiology, Clinical Hospital Sveti Duh, Zagreb, Croatia

Kermit S. Zhang
Virginia Tech Carilion School of Medicine, Roanoke, VA, USA

Jash Bansal and Vikas Chitnavis
Department of Gastroenterology, Carilion Clinic Memorial Hospital, Roanoke, VA, USA

Anmol Bansal
Department of Radiology, Carilion Clinic Memorial Hospital, Roanoke, VA, USA

Nishant Tripathi, Hirotaka Kato, Tushi Singh, Kishore Karri and Kshitij Thakur
Department of Internal Medicine, University of Kentucky, Lexington, KY, USA

Niki Koirala
Department of Clinical Pharmacy, University of Kentucky, Lexington, KY, USA

Dema Shamoon and Vanessa Sostre
Department of Medicine, St. Joseph's University Medical Center, Paterson, NJ, USA

Varun Patel and Ariy Volfson
Division of Gastroenterology and Hepatology, St. Joseph's University Medical Center, Paterson, NJ, USA

Sahathevan Vithoosan, Ponnudurai Shanjeeban, Joseph Philip Anpalahan, Harindra Karunatilake and Ananda Jayanaga
National Hospital, Colombo, Sri Lanka

Paramarajan Piranavan
Internal Medicine, Saint Vincent Hospital,Worcester, MA 01608, USA

Roie Tzadok
Department of Internal Medicine C, Tel Aviv Sourasky Medical Center, Tel Aviv, Israel

Sharon Levy and Oren Shibolet
Department of Gastroenterology and Hepatology, Tel Aviv Sourasky Medical Center and the Sackler Faculty of Medicine, Tel Aviv University, Tel Aviv, Israel

Jessie Aouizerate
Institute of Pathology, Tel Aviv Sourasky Medical Center, Tel Aviv, Israel

Iqra Haq and Chencheng Xie
Department of Internal Medicine, University of South Dakota Sanford School of Medicine, Sioux Falls, South Dakota, USA

Somashekar G. Krishna
Division of Gastroenterology, Hepatology and Nutrition, The Ohio State University Wexner Medical Center, Columbus, Ohio, USA

Bhaveshkumar Patel and Muslim Atiq
Department of Gastroenterology, University of South Dakota Sanford School of Medicine, Sioux Falls, South Dakota, USA

Thavam Thambi-Pillai
Department of Surgery, University of South Dakota Sanford School of Medicine, Sioux Falls, South Dakota, USA

Karah Odegaard and Kimberlee Buohy
Department of Pathology, University of South Dakota Sanford School of Medicine, Sioux Falls, South Dakota, USA

Hemnishil K. Marella, Jiten P. Kothadia, Nasir Saleem, Bilal Ali, Yousef Abdel-Aziz and Colin W. Howden
Division of Gastroenterology and Hepatology, University of Tennessee Health Science Center, Memphis, TN 38104, USA

Vamsee Mupparaju
Methodist University Hospital, Memphis, TN 38104, USA

Twisha Oza and Abdallah Azouz
Department of Pathology, University of Tennessee Health Science Center, Memphis, TN 38104, USA

Hicham Elmajdoubi, Marouane Baiss, Mohamed El Absi, El Hassan El Faricha El Alami, Mohamed El Ouanani, El Mahjoub Echarrab, Mohamed El Amraoui and Abdelkader Errougani
Surgical Emergency Department, Avicenna Hospital, Mohammed V University, Rabat, Morocco

Yinglin Gao
Internal Medicine, Loma Linda University Medical Center, Loma Linda, CA, USA

Nikhil Gupta and Maisa Abdalla
Gastroenterology Department, Loma Linda University Medical Center, Loma Linda, CA, USA

Olivia Peralta
American University of the Caribbean School of Medicine, Cupecoy, Saint Martin

Christopher Chew
Department of Graduate Medical Education, Northeast Georgia Health System, Gainesville, GA, USA

Matthew Newcomb
Department of Hospital Medicine, Northeast Georgia Health System, Gainesville, GA, USA

Lynna Alnimer and Samira Ahsan
Department of Internal Medicine, Ascension Providence Hospital, Michigan State University/College of Human Medicine, South field, MI, USA

Ali Zakaria, Jalpa Patel and Serge Sorser
Division of Gastroenterology, Ascension Providence Hospital, Michigan State University/College of Human Medicine, South field, MI, USA

Yazan Samhouri
Division of Hematology and Cellular Therapy, Allegheny Health Network Cancer Institute, Pittsburgh, PA, USA

Lyle Goldman
Department of Hematology/Oncology, Ascension Providence Hospital, Michigan State University/ College of Human Medicine, South field, MI, USA

Melanija Ražov Radas
Department of Gastroenterology, Zadar General Hospital, Zadar, Croatia

Aleksandar Knežević
Department of Cardiology, Zadar General Hospital, Zadar, Croatia

Vladimir Trkulja
Department of Pharmacology, Zagreb University School of Medicine, Zagreb, Croatia

Tiago Martins and Kevin Groudan
Baystate Medical Center, Internal Medicine Residency, 759 Chestnut Street, Springfield, MA 01199, USA

Jalaluddin Umar and David Desilets
Baystate Medical Center, Gastroenterology Department, 759 Chestnut Street, Springfield, MA 01199, USA

Hariharan S. Bharadwaj
Baystate Medical Center, Pathology Department, 759 Chestnut Street, Springfield, MA 01199, USA

Ahmad Sharayah, Dileep C. Unnikrishnan and Rishi Raj
Internal Medicine Department, Monmouth Medical Center, Long Branch, NJ 07740, USA

Akhila Arya Perumangote Vasudevan
Internal Medicine Department, Govt Medical Collage, Kozhikode, India

Noor Hajjaj
Faculty of Medicine, University of Jordan, Amman, Jordan

Kenneth Belitsis
Gastrointestinal Department, Monmouth Medical Center, Long Branch, NJ 07740, USA

Zaid Imam, Majd Khasawneh, Hira Iftikhar and Ziad Sayedahmad
Departments of Internal Medicine, William Beaumont Hospital, Royal Oak, MI, USA

Diana Jomaa
Oakland University William Beaumont School of Medicine, Royal Oak, MI, USA

Szczepan Cierniak
Military Institute of Medicine in Warsaw, Department of Pathology, Warsaw, Poland

Maciej Gonciarz and Michał Krogulecki
Military Institute of Medicine in Warsaw, Department of Gastroenterology and Internal Medicine, Warsaw, Poland

Dorota Brodowska-Kania and Grzegorz Kamiński
Military Institute of Medicine in Warsaw, Department of Endocrinology and Radioisotope erapy, Warsaw, Poland

Chukwunonso Chime, Ahmed Baiomi, Kishore Kumar, Harish Patel, Anil Dev and Jasbir Makker
Department of Gastroenterology, Bronx Care Health Systems–Affiliate of Mount Sinai Hospital Systems, Bronx, NY 10457, USA
Department of Medicine, BronxCare Hospital Center, Bronx, NY 10457, USA
Department of Internal Medicine, Bronx Care Health Systems–Affiliate of Mount Sinai Hospital Systems, 1650 Grand Concourse, Bronx, NY 10457, USA

Shurouq H. Alqrinawi and Mohammed Aljawad
Multiorgan Transplant Unit, King Fahd Specialist Hospital, Dammam, Saudi Arabia

Nuralhuda Akbar and Hind AlFaddag
Department of Medicine, Dammam Medical Complex, Dammam, Saudi Arabi

Shahrazad Akbar and Lujayn Akbar
Department of Medicine, King Fahd Hospital of the University, Khobar, Saudi Arabia

Sohail A. Butt
Blood Bank, Dammam Regional Laboratory, Dammam, Saudi Arabia

Neethi Dasu, Brian Blair and C. Jonathan Foster
Department of Gastroenterology, Jefferson Health New Jersey, Cherry Hill, NJ, USA

Colin Smith
Department of Gastroenterology, Jefferson Medical College of "Thomas Jefferson University, Philadelphia, PA, USA

Mira M. Lotfalla, Andrew L. Folpe, Karen J. Fritchie, Patricia T. Greipp, Kevin C. Halling, Taofic Mounajjed, Jorge Torres-Mora and Rondell P. Graham
Department of Laboratory Medicine and Pathology, Mayo Clinic, Rochester, MN, USA

Gretchen G. Galliano
Anatomic Pathology, Ochsner Health System, New Orleans, LA, USA

Priyanka Priyanka
Department of Medicine, WV University Hospital, Morgantown,WV, USA

William Hsueh and John Nasr
Department of Medicine, Division of Gastroenterology, WVU University Hospital, Morgantown, WV, USA

Katongo Mutengo
Department of Internal Medicine, Livingstone Central Hospital, Ministry of Health, Livingstone, Zambia

Francis Mupeta
Infectious Diseases Unit, Department of Internal Medicine, University Teaching Hospital, Lusaka, Zambia

Owen Ngalamika
Dermatology and Venereology Section, University Teaching Hospital, University of Zambia, School of Medicine, Lusaka, Zambia

Masaya Iwamuro
Department of Gastroenterology and Hepatology, Okayama University Graduate School of Medicine, Dentistry, and Pharmaceutical Sciences, Okayama 700-8558, Japan

Takahide Takahashi
Division of Medical Support, Okayama University Hospital, Okayama 700-8558, Japan

Yoko Ota
Department of Pathology & Experimental Medicine, Okayama University Graduate School of Medicine, Dentistry, and Pharmaceutical Sciences, Okayama 700-8558, Japan

Takehiro Tanaka
Department of Pathology, Okayama University Graduate School of Medicine, Dentistry, and Pharmaceutical Sciences, Okayama 700-8558, Japan

Noboru Asada
Department of Hematology and Oncology, Okayama University Hospital, Okayama 700-8558, Japan

Shuya Yano
Department of Gastroenterological Surgery, Okayama University Graduate School of Medicine, Dentistry, and Pharmaceutical Sciences, Okayama 700-8558, Japan

Mayu Uka
Department of Radiology, Okayama University Hospital, Okayama 700-8558, Japan

Rei Nakamura
Department of Nephrology, Rheumatology, Endocrinology and Metabolism, Okayama University Graduate School of Medicine, Dentistry, and Pharmaceutical Sciences, Okayama 700-8558, Japan

Yoshiro Kawahara
Department of Practical Gastrointestinal Endoscopy, Okayama University Hospital, Okayama 700-8558, Japan

Grace E. Kim
Department of Internal Medicine, University of MarylandMedical Center, Baltimore, MD 21201, USA

John D. Morris and Peter E. Darwin
Division of Gastroenterology and Hepatology, University of MarylandMedical Center, Baltimore, MD 21201, USA

P. Thineskaran, K. Abiramy, T. Kumanan, V. Sujanitha, N. Suganthan and G. Selvaratnam
University Medical Unit, Teaching Hospital, Jaffna, Sri Lanka

Elias Estifan and Ashima Kapoor
Department of Internal Medicine, St. Joseph's University Medical Center-New York Medical College, USA

Yana Cavanagh and Matthew Grossman
Department of Gastroenterology, St. Joseph's University Medical Center-New York Medical College, USA

Timothy R. Koch and Elizabeth A. Zubowicz
Center for Advanced Laparoscopic General & Bariatric Surgery, MedStarWashington Hospital Center and Georgetown University School of Medicine,Washington, DC 20010, USA

John B. Gross Jr.
Division of Gastroenterology and Hepatology, Mayo Clinic, 200 First Street S.W., Rochester, MN 55905, USA

Hafsa Abbas
Division of Gastroenterology, BronxCare Hospital Center, Bronx, NY 10457, USA

Masooma Niazi
Department of Pathology, BronxCare Hospital Center, Bronx, NY 10457, USA

Trupti Vakde
Division of Pulmonary and Critical Care, Department of Medicine, BronxCare Hospital Center, Bronx, NY 10457, USA

Sridhar Chilimuri
Department of Medicine, BronxCare Hospital Center, Bronx, NY 10457, USA

Marion Alhenc-Gelas, Romain Cohen and Thierry André
Sorbonne Université, Department of Medical Oncology, AP-HP, Hôpital Saint-Antoine, F-75012 Paris, France

Pascale Cervera
Sorbonne Université, Department of Pathology, AP-HP, Hôpital Saint-Antoine, F-75012 Paris, France

Jean-Christophe Vaillant
Sorbonne Université, Department of Digestive and Hepatobiliary Surgery, AP-HP, Pitié-Salpêtriêre Hospital, F-75013 Paris, France

Mohammad Bagher Jahantab, Vahid Salehi, Saadat Mehrabi, Lotfolah Abedini and Mohammad Javad Yavari Barhaghtalab
General Surgery Department, Shahid Beheshti Hospital, Yasuj University of Medical Sciences, Yasuj, Iran

Daniel Ramirez and Graham Appelbe
Department of Internal Medicine, Ascension Genesys Medical Center, Grand Blanc, MI, USA

Venkatramana Vattipally
Department of Radiology, Ascension Genesys Medical Center, Grand Blanc, MI, USA

Justin Miller
Department of Gastroenterology, Ascension Genesys Medical Center, Grand Blanc, MI, USA

Abdullah Sohail and Ahmad Khan
West Virginia University Charleston Division, Charleston, West Virginia, USA

Hamza Shah
Charleston Area Medical Center, Charleston, West Virginia, USA

Ragheb Rezko
West Virginia University, Morgantown, West Virginia, USA

Karl Andersen and Sarah Burroughs
Advocate Lutheran General Hospital, 1775 Dempster Street, Park Ridge, IL 60068, USA

Assad Munis, Ryan T. Hoff and Alan Shapiro
Department of Internal Medicine, Division of Gastroenterology, Advocate Lutheran General Hospital, 1775 Dempster Street, Park Ridge, IL 60068, USA

Mary Junak, Hunter Jecius and Jennifer Erdrich
Institutional Mailing Address, University of Arizona, Department of Surgery, Tucson, AZ 85724, USA

Ansar Aziz, Tayyab Waheed and Olubunmi Oladunjoye
Reading Hospital Tower Health, West Reading, PA, USA

Adeolu Oladunjoye
Boston Children's Hospital, Boston, MA, USA

Midhat Hanif and Fareena Latif
Independent Researcher, West Reading, PA, USA

Haider A. Naqvi, Muhammad Nadeem Yousaf and Fizah S. Chaudhary
Department of Medicine, Medstar Union Memorial Hospital, Baltimore, MD 21218, USA
Department of Medicine, MedStar Good Samaritan Hospital, Baltimore, MD 21239, USA
Department of Medicine, MedStar Franklin Square Medical Center, Baltimore, MD 21237, USA
Department of Medicine, MedStar Harbor Hospital, Baltimore, MD 21225, USA

Lawrence Mills
Department of Gastroenterology, MedStar Good Samaritan Hospital, Baltimore, MD 21239, USA

Konstantinos Miltiadou, Dimitrios Lygkos, Alexandros Chatzidakis, Evripidis Rizos, Ioannis S. Papanikolaou and Konstantinos Triantafyllou
Hepatogastroenterology Unit, 2nd Department of Internal Medicine-Propaedeutic, Research Institute and Diabetes Center, Medical School, National and Kapodistrian University, Attikon University General Hospital, Athens 124 62, Greece

Zisimangelos Solomos
Doctors of the World, Greek Delegation, Athens 105 53, Greece

Haozhe Sun and Nikhitha Mantri
Department of Internal Medicine, Bronx Care Health Systems–Affiliate of Mount Sinai Hospital Systems, 1650 Grand Concourse, Bronx, NY 10457, USA

Ali N. Hussain
Division of Gastroenterology, Bronx Care Health Systems–Affiliate of Mount Sinai Hospital Systems, 1650 Grand Concourse, Bronx, NY 10457, USA

Naeem Abbas
Department of Gastroenterology, Advantage Care Physician, 260WSunrise Highway Stream Valley, Rosedale, NY 11581, USA

Juan D. Salcedo and Jordan S. Goldstein
Department of Internal Medicine, University of Miami Miller School of Medicine, Miami, FL, USA

Jose M. Quinonez
University of Miami Miller School of Medicine, Miami, FL, USA

Maria Antonietta Mosetti
Division of Hospital Medicine, University of Miami Medical Towers, University of Miami Miller School of Medicine,Miami, FL, USA

Matthew H. Kemm, Cory D. Manly, Thanh D. Hoang, Vinh Q. Mai and Mohamed K. M. Shakir
Division of Endocrinology, Department of Medicine,Walter Reed National Military Medical Center, Bethesda, USA

Ishani Shah
Department of Internal Medicine, Creighton University St. Joseph's Hospital and Medical Center, Phoenix, AZ, USA

Neil Vyas and Kambiz S. Kadkhodayan
Department of Gastroenterology, Creighton University St. Joseph's Hospital and Medical Center, Phoenix, AZ, USA

David Cassiman
Department of Gastroenterology-Hepatology and Metabolic Center, University of Leuven, Belgium

Louis Libbrecht
Laboratory of Hepatology, University of Leuven, Belgium
Department of Pathology, University Hospital Saint-Luc, Brussels, Belgium

Wouter Meersseman
General Internal Medicine-Metabolic Diseases, University Hospital Gasthuisberg, Leuven, Belgium

Alexander Wilmer
Medical Intensive Care, University Hospital Gasthuisberg, Leuven, Belgium

Michael Pagacz
A.M. Rywlin, MD Department of Pathology, Mount Sinai Medical Center, Miami Beach, FL, USA

Irvin Willis
Department of General Surgery, Mount Sinai Medical Center, Miami Beach, FL, USA

John Alexis
Herbert Wertheim College of Medicine, Florida International University, Miami, FL, USA

Index

www.ingramcontent.com/pod-product-compliance
Lightning Source LLC
LaVergne TN
LVHW082203200926
848484LV00008B/2207
* 9 7 9 8 8 8 7 4 0 6 3 8 1 *